INTRODUCTION TO MANAGED CARE

INTRODUCTION TO MANAGED CARE

Health Maintenance Organizations,
Preferred Provider Organizations,
and Competitive Medical Plans

Revised and Expanded Edition
(Originally published as
*Medical Group Practice and
Health Maintenance Organizations*)

ROBERT G. SHOULDICE

INFORMATION RESOURCES PRESS I**R**/**P**®

Published November 1992. Second Impression February 1993.
Third Impression October 1994.
Printed in the United States of America.

Available from
Information Resources Press
1110 North Glebe Road
Suite 550
Arlington, Virginia 22201

Library of Congress Catalog Card Number 91-073438

ISBN 0-87815-062-5

Parts of the present work appeared in a slightly different version in *Medical Group
Practice and Health Maintenance Organizations,* © by Information Resources Press.

To Richard John Hughes

THE AUTHOR

Robert George Shouldice is Professor Emeritus in the Department of Health Services Administration, The George Washington University, from which he retired in the Fall of 1990. During his tenure at The George Washington University, he developed and administered courses in the organization and management of health services institutions, health maintenance organizations, and ambulatory health services administration.

Introduction to Managed Care and its predecessor, *Medical Group Practice and Health Maintenance Organizations*, are based on notes and modifications that Dr. Shouldice prepared for the courses he gave at The George Washington University. In 1979, *Medical Group Practice and Health Maintenance Organizations* was awarded Honorable Mention in the category of "Books for Allied Health Professionals" by the American Medical Writers Association.

Until 1990, Dr. Shouldice contributed a regular column, "Alternative Delivery Systems," to the *Medical Group Management Journal*. He is the author of 18 published reports and articles in his fields of expertise.

He recently completed a consultancy for the government of Indonesia on the social financing of health services in that country. He has presented papers at professional meetings and has served as an expert witness for law firms and as consultant, advisor, and reviewer to more than 100 other agencies, institutions, and organizations.

Dr. Shouldice holds a doctorate in business administration from The George Washington University (GWU) and an MBA in health administration, also from GWU. He is a member of the American College of Health Care Executives (Faculty Associate), the Medical Group Management Association, the American Hospital Association (AHA), and the AHA Society for Ambulatory Care Professionals.

PREFACE

Professor Shouldice spent approximately five years researching and writing this book and is responsible for its entire content. Because of a debilitating illness, however, he asked that we write this preface for him.

In the 1960s, health industry leaders began to recognize the potential of prepaid group practice plans as mechanisms to contain the dramatic rise in health service costs. Studies of existing plans completed in the 1950s and 1960s provided clear evidence that medical group practice and prepaid group practice were effective in controlling costs and the quality of care. The Federal Government, in attempting to restrain the runaway costs of Medicare and Medicaid programs, provided impetus for expanding the number of prepaid health plans.

The term "health maintenance organization" (HMO) was coined during the Nixon administration. Supporting legislation was enacted to develop and expand HMOs, and the concept of the HMO program as a major element of the nation's health programs has been supported by each succeeding administration. The emphasis has been steadily away from traditional institutional inpatient care toward ambulatory and preventive services, which creates a need to study the management of group practice and prepaid group practice in medicine.

In the 1970s, the initiative to control escalating health costs was still mostly experimental. In 1978, only 180 HMOs, many of them demonstration projects, were in operation; in 1990, the number of HMOs had grown to 590 organizations serving 32 million members, or more than 1 in 8 Americans.

The predecessor to this book, *Medical Group Practice and Health Maintenance Organizations*, was the product of a course in the development and management of HMOs, conducted by the graduate program in health care administration at The George Washington University. The course was structured around the numerous studies and articles written about prepaid group practice. The book was shaped to meet the needs of students in the program, managers in the field, and governmental officials. *Introduction to Managed Care*, designed as a textbook for students of health services administration and a handbook for managers of HMOs, preferred provider organizations (PPOs), and competitive medical plans (CMPs), looks at the theory of managed care as well as the nuts-and-bolts of how managed care programs are created, organized, and operated in the 1990s.

Introduction to Managed Care revises and expands on *Medical Group Practice* by looking at prepaid health care not as an experiment but as an integral and growing part of the U.S. medical delivery system. The reader of both the original and this updated text will find more differences than similarities. These differences reflect the dramatically changing methods of providing and financing health services. Beginning with the HMO development in the late 1970s, health care managers have experienced the introduction of PPOs and the federally sponsored CMPs. Also, in the late 1980s, the managed care field began to develop hybrid model HMOs, point-of-service benefits packages, and combinations of closed-panel packages, along with regular indemnity insurance programs. Even though these terms are used interchangeably, they all describe one of the managed care models.

The arrangement of the book allows the reader to put each of the models in perspective. The chapters dealing with the historical development, laws and legislation, and organizational development are written as general reviews, while chapters dealing with marketing, financing, rating and rate making, physician/health plan operations, consumer participation, and providers are emphasized. To enhance the book, many illustrative charts, graphs, and tables are included; in some instances, important concepts are depicted in graphic form only or in tables, since these forms of presentation are deemed to make these points most effectively and clearly. The literature on managed care organizations has proliferated since publication of the first edition and is cited in the references at the end of each chapter.

A project of this magnitude would have been impossible without the financial and collegial support Dr. Shouldice received from The George Washington University. Dr. Shouldice especially wishes to thank Chairman Richard Southby, Professor Kurt Darr, and his teaching and research fellows who were invaluable to him, including Gracie Millender, Julia Hawley, and Norah Singpurwalla, among others. Technical assistance was provided by the Medical Group Management Association, the Group Health Association, and the DHHS Office of Prepaid Health Care. Dr. Shouldice also wishes to acknowledge friends who added to the quality of the text, including Richard John Hughes, Katherine Henneberger Delahunty, and Lee Sommers, who offered support and encouragement.

As noted, the predecessor to *Introduction to Managed Care, Medical Group Practice and Health Maintenance Organizations,* had its genesis in Dr. Shouldice's HMO course at The George Washington University. Although he has maintained an active consulting practice, teaching has been the source of his greatest professional satisfaction and commitment. He enjoys the camaraderie of his students and provides encouragement and often inspiration as well. He is generous in the sharing of knowledge, a sharing that is extended to colleagues as well as to students. Despite his illness, he has striven to produce this latest book as a further contribution to the intellectual and professional community in which he has enjoyed so rich a life.

Ms. Gene P. Allen
Publisher
Information Resources Press

CONTENTS

FIGURES

TABLES

ACRONYMS

AAAHC	Accreditation Association for Ambulatory Health Care, Inc.
AAPCC	adjusted average per capita cost
AAPPO	American Association of Preferred Provider Organizations
AC/AHC	Accreditation Council for Ambulatory Health Care
ACR	adjusted community rate
ADS	alternative delivery system
AGPA	American Group Practice Association
AHA	American Hospital Association
ALOS	average length of stay
AMA	American Medical Association
AMCRA	American Managed (Medical) Care and Review Association
AMH	*Accreditation Manual for Hospitals*
ASO	administrative services only
AVG	average visit group
BC/BS	Blue Cross/Blue Shield
CEO	chief executive officer
CHAMPUS	Civilian Health and Medical Program of the Uniformed Services
CMM	cumulative member months
CMP	competitive medical plan
CMS	Community Medical Services of Seattle
COB	coordination of benefits
COBRA	Consolidated Budget Reconciliation Act
CON	certificate of need
COO	chief operating officer
CPI	consumer price index
CPR	customary, prevailing, and reasonable charges

CPS	California Physicians' Service
DHEW	Department of Health, Education, and Welfare
DHHS	Department of Health and Human Services
DRG	diagnostic-related group (groupings)
EPO	exclusive provider organization
FEHBP	Federal Employees Health Benefits Program
FEP	Federal Employees Plan
FFS	fee-for-service
FMC	Foundation for Medical Care
FTC	Federal Trade Commission
FTE	full-time equivalent
FTEP	full-time equivalent physician
GHA	Group Health Association
GHAA	Group Health Association of America, Inc.
GHC	Group Health Cooperative
GHI	group health insurance
HBO	health benefit organization
HCFA	Health Care Financing Administration
HIAA	Health Insurance Association of America
HIE	Health Insurance Experiment
HIO	health insuring organization
HIP	Health Insurance Plan of Greater New York
HMO	health maintenance organization
HMOS	Health Maintenance Organization Service
HSO	health services organization
IBNR	incurred but not reported
ICDA	*International Classification of Diseases*
IHCC	Integrated Health Care Corporation
IMC	International Medical Centers, Inc.
IP	inpatient
IPA	individual practice association; *also* individual practice arrangement
JCAH	Joint Commission on Accreditation of Hospitals
JCAHO	Joint Commission on Accreditation of Healthcare Organizations
LOS	length of stay
LTC	long-term care
MCO	managed care organization
MECA	Medicare Expanded Choice Act
MES/H	Medical Staff/Hospital Venture Organization
MGMA	Medical Group Management Association
MIG	medically insured group
MIS	management information system

MMD	Marion Merrell Dow, Inc.
NCQA	National Committee for Quality Assurance
OAA	old age assistance
OBRA	Omnibus Budget Reconciliation Act
OEO	Office of Economic Opportunity
OHMO	Office of Health Maintenance Organizations
OP	outpatient
OPHC	Office of Prepaid Health Care
OPM	Office of Personnel Management
OR	operating room
PC	professional component (of services)
PDIS	patient-doctor interaction scale
PERT	Program Evaluation and Review Technique
PGP	prepaid group practice
PHP	private health plans; *also* prepaid health plans
PHPO	private health plan option
PIP	prepaid individual practice
PMPM	per member per month
PMPY	per member per year
PPA	preferred provider arrangement
PPO	preferred provider organization
PRO	professional review organization; *also* peer review organization
PSRO	Professional Standards Review Organization
QA	quality assurance
QA/UR	quality assurance/utilization review
QRO	quality review organization
RBRVS	resource based relative value scale
RFC	request for contract
RFP	request for proposal
RVS	relative value system (study)
S/HMO	Social Health Maintenance Organization
SNF	skilled nursing facility
SOBRA	Sixth Omnibus Budget Reconciliation Act
SOP	standard operating procedures
SSA	Social Security Administration
TC	technical component (of services)
TEFRA	Tax Equity and Fiscal Responsibility Act
TPA	third-party administrator
UCR	usual, customary, and reasonable
UR	utilization review

1

HEALTH MAINTENANCE ORGANIZATIONS AND ALTERNATIVE DELIVERY SYSTEMS

Free enterprise in the health services industry has fostered the development of several alternative delivery structures generically called *managed care organizations* (MCOs) or *alternative delivery systems* (ADSs). Traditionally, physicians and hospitals have provided services for fees that were paid directly by the recipients of care or through the philanthropy of private citizens and organizations. As the structure of American society became more complex, the traditional one-on-one delivery system evolved into today's integrated system of complex, highly technological delivery components with several sophisticated payment structures. A basic discussion of these alternative systems, which include the health maintenance organization (HMO), the preferred provider organization (PPO), and the competitive medical plan (CMP) as health delivery concepts, first requires an understanding of the three most common delivery and financing systems.

Health Delivery and Financing Structures

PRIVATE PAY

In 1984, approximately 16 percent of the civilian population under age 65 (33 million people) was without some form of private health insurance. By the end of 1988, more than 31.5 million Americans—approximately 13.0 percent of the total U.S. population and 14.7 percent of the under age 65 population—were without health care insurance coverage[1] (see Figure 1-1). Although these

---

[1] Health Insurance Association of America. *Source Book of Health Insurance Data 1990.* Washington, D.C., HIAA, 1991, p. 13.

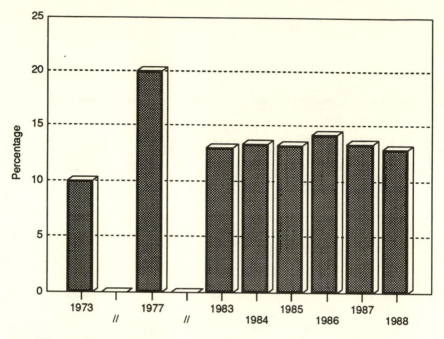

NOTE: 1973, 1977 figures are approx.

SOURCE: Health Insurance Institute, *Source Book of Health Insurance Data 1974–75*, New York, HII, 1975, p. 19; and Health Insurance Association of America, *Source Book of Health Insurance Data 1990*, Washington, D.C., HIAA, 1991, p. 22.

FIGURE 1-1 Percentage of persons in the United States without health insurance coverage: 1973–1988.

self-pay persons may have had some public financing of health services, many continued to be directly responsible for payment of their medical care, as indicated in Figure 1-2. Health services managers are aware that many private-pay patients are unable to pay out-of-pocket expenses for required health services and cannot afford to purchase adequate health insurance coverage. Generally, the self-responsible private-pay patient, because no third party such as government or an insurer is involved in payment to providers, has become the "balancing factor" for most provider organizations; payments from these patients are one of the few sources of revenue that hospitals, for example, can vary as the financial situation warrants without third-party approval or interference. In states that continue rate-review activities under a waiver from federal diagnostic-related group (DRG) payment regulations, even charges to private-pay patients are being monitored and controlled.

In many situations, private pay really means "no payment," and these accounts receivable become bad debt write-offs. Health services organizations

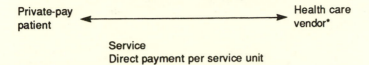

*The term "health care vendor" encompasses all providers of health care—physicians and other health care personal providers, hospitals, clinics, other institutions, and delivery programs.

FIGURE 1-2 Private-pay health services structure.

attempt to cover such losses through higher fees to patients who use other financing methods.

TRADITIONAL THIRD-PARTY FINANCING SYSTEMS

Service Plans

Blue Cross and Blue Shield (BC/BS) plans are considered "service plans." The Great Depression forced the nation's hospitals to depend less on philanthropic revenues and more on patient-payment revenues for their services. Hospitals were faced with declining occupancy rates and losses of revenue. Concurrently, patients were faced with substantial losses of income and mounting debts, including those for medical care. A scheme was needed to protect patients from the economic consequences of hospitalization. Several innovative approaches, including the service plan device, were developed to protect families from high hospitalization costs and to stabilize the financial situation of hospitals.

The Blue Cross movement began with a group of 1,250 school teachers who formed an arrangement with Baylor Hospital to provide them with hospital care on a prepayment basis. The considerations of social responsibility and humanitarianism inherent in the Baylor Hospital experiment also were incorporated into the Blue Cross plans that were initiated as a result of this experiment. It is from the social insurance function of income redistribution and risk assumption by local Blue Cross plans that the present Blue Cross programs have evolved. This service plan concept had a profound effect on the traditional underwriters of insurance—commercial carriers—by introducing insurance for hospital and surgical care. By 1933, the Blue Cross service plan and the group hospitalization prepayment principle had been adopted by the American Hospital Association (AHA).

Autonomous local Blue Cross plans were loosely joined through the national Blue Cross Association located in Chicago, Illinois. Boards of directors represented local hospitals, physicians, and the general public. Such a system permitted quicker, more accurate, and more acceptable responses to local

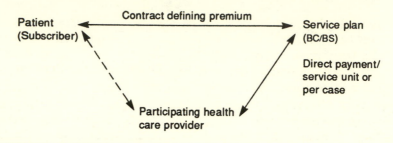

FIGURE 1-3 Blue Cross/Blue Shield plans—financing.

situations than a national body could provide. Most important, the Blue Cross plans stressed hospital benefits in the form of service rather than a cash indemnity (a benefit, usually cash, paid by a private insurer for an insured loss).[2] Blue Cross plans also provided for "full service" and "full coverage" benefits packages in recognition of a perceived responsibility to provide *total* hospital expense coverage to subscribers.

More commonly referred to as "first dollar, first day" coverage, BC member benefits begin with the first dollar of care rendered on the first day of a hospital stay—a relatively expensive but socially valuable insurance arrangement. These characteristics have changed very little over the 60-plus years that Blue Cross plans have been in existence.

As nonprofit hospital service organizations, regional Blue Cross plans affiliate on a contractual basis with local hospitals; in essence, hospitals entering into such an association with Blue Cross agree to accept the Blue Cross reimbursement schedule for hospital services that are provided to Blue Cross member patients (i.e., they become participating hospitals with Blue Cross) and are usually paid directly by Blue Cross. These relationships are illustrated in Figure 1-3.

Four reimbursement formulas are used by Blue Cross;[3] they are based on:

1. The retail charges of the hospital for services provided
2. The cost of the services provided
3. A uniform daily rate to all hospitals
4. A prospective pricing system known as diagnostic-related group (DRG) payment on a per-case basis

---

[2] Sylvia A. Law. *Blue Cross: What Went Wrong?* 2nd Edition. New Haven, Conn., Yale University Press, 1976, pp. 6–25.

[3] Fredric R. Hedinger. *The Social Role of Blue Cross as a Device for Financing the Cost of Hospital Care: An Evaluation.* Ames, Ia., Graduate Program in Hospital and Health Administration, University of Iowa, 1966, p. 74. Health Care Research Series No. 2

Blue Shield plans, like hospital service plans, are nonprofit medical service plans that have developed along the lines of the Blue Cross model. Prior to the Great Depression, the lack of adequate medical resources in the northwest United States encouraged the growth of various industrial contract practices. In Washington State, the lumber industry had been contracting with physicians for the care of its workers since the early 1900s. In response to the growing number of private physician/employer contracts, county medical service bureaus were established "through which all medical contracts were channeled so that free choice would be preserved and the profession might have at least some nominal control over the practices."[4] The ultimate objectives of the medical service bureaus were to meet and, if possible, control the competition of employer-sponsored medical service programs. Thus, the medical service bureaus became the forerunners of the present local medical societies as well as the Blue Shield plans.

In 1934, following the example of the American Hospital Association in adopting the group hospitalization prepayment principle, the American Medical Association's (AMA) House of Delegates adopted a set of principles to provide guidance in the development of medical service (Blue Shield) plans. By 1938, AMA recommended that its local medical societies develop medical service plans, the first of which were the California Physicians' Service and the County Medical Society in Oregon and Washington. It is now recognized that these activities were principally undertaken by AMA to prevent the Blue Cross plans from underwriting physician services.

Blue Shield complements Blue Cross hospital coverage. Enrollment in a Blue Shield plan provides coverage for physician services that are identified in a contract between an individual or his/her employer and Blue Shield. All physicians in the region are usually eligible to participate in the regional Blue Shield plan; physicians who do participate agree to accept payment from Blue Shield for the services they provide to Blue Shield subscribers. As shown in Figure 1-4, reimbursement by Blue Shield follows the provisions of the provider agreement between the physician and Blue Shield and may include reimbursement on a Blue Shield fee schedule, based on service units provided by the physician, or a profile of the individual physician's Blue Shield billing practices and the level of his/her charges for services billed.

In the recent past, several changes have occurred and continue to occur relative to service plans. Independent and separate Blue Cross and Blue Shield plans have joined together to form single corporations so as to pool resources and become more effective in competing with alternative delivery systems.

---

[4] William A. MacColl. *Group Practice and Prepayment of Medical Care*. Washington, D.C., Public Affairs Press, 1966, p. 37.

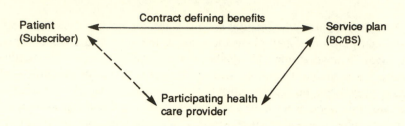

FIGURE 1-4 Blue Cross/Blue Shield plans—health services delivery.

Also, the unwritten agreement that autonomous regional plans will not compete with other regional BC/BS plans and will honor franchised geographic areas has been violated; some plans are actively marketing their health insurance products in neighboring BC/BS service areas. This has resulted in lawsuits in the BC/BS family. Such service-area infringements may be a symptom of the cutthroat competitive environment the field has experienced since 1980.

In the early 1970s, BC/BS plans entered the alternative delivery systems market with their own health maintenance organizations. Their objective was to be more effective in controlling their existing market share. As of December 31, 1989, the "Blues" operated 92 plans, with a total membership of 4.5 million. Of the 590 HMOs operating in the United States, approximately 15 percent are BC/BS plans, accounting for approximately 14 percent of all individuals enrolled in HMOs.[5]

The relationships described in the preceding paragraphs are illustrated in Figures 1-3 and 1-4.

Indemnity Plans

Before the Great Depression, insurance companies were interested in insuring individuals only against loss of income due to inability to work as a result of sickness, accident, or loss of life. With the development of the Blues family in the 1930s, commercial carriers recognized the large market for health insurance and realized that their expertise in risk-pooling and actuarial techniques would be of great advantage in entering this new market. Beginning in 1940, both life and casualty carriers began to write health insurance.

---

[5] Blue Cross Association, Chicago, Ill., personal communication, May 6, 1987; and the Office of Prepaid Health Care, Health Care Financing Administration, U.S. Department of Health and Human Services, Washington, D.C., personal communication, May 6, 1987. In May 1986, there were 3.5 million BC/BS members involved in BC/BS HMOs from a total of 21 million HMO enrollees in the United States.

Unlike BC/BS arrangements, commercial carriers do not establish working agreements with, or profiles of, hospitals and physicians. The individual subscriber or his/her employer enters into a contractual agreement with the insurance company or indemnity carrier. The carrier identifies the underwriting risk of its subscribers and is then able to accurately predict its costs and calculate the premiums it must charge. Monthly or other periodic premium payments based on these costs are then prepaid by the subscriber or his/her employer before the subscriber receives health care services.

Indemnity plans reimburse the insured patient (or beneficiary) with stipulated sums of money to be applied against expenditures for the insured risks. Note that the contractual arrangement is with the insurance company and the patient only (or with his/her employer on behalf of the employee and his/her dependents); therefore, the insurance company pays the patient directly. These payments, as stipulated in the policy, can be reimbursement for the patient's expenditures for health services or for loss of income during illness, or both. Subscribers bear sole responsibility for identifying their need for care, locating the providers of such care, and, in most instances, paying for the care. It is only after care has been received and paid for that the indemnity carrier reimburses the patient. The vendor of care has an indirect relationship with the insurance company regarding provision and payment for care, as indicated by the broken lines in Figures 1-5 and 1-6.

As these figures show, the major difference between Blue Cross plans and commercial insurers is that the former have contractual arrangements with hospitals and, through Blue Shield, with physicians, while commercial carriers have no such relationships. Both delivery systems provide the patient/enrollee with a free choice of vendor, although Blue Cross enrollees are limited to BC participating hospitals if they desire full payment for services, and Blue Shield enrollees are limited to BS participating physicians. These limitations are minimal, however; 91 percent of the short-term nonfederal hospitals are

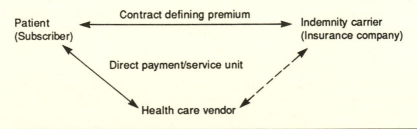

FIGURE 1-5 Commercial indemnity plans—financing.

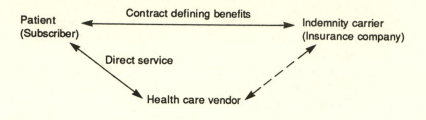

FIGURE 1-6 Commercial indemnity plans—health services delivery.

affiliated with a local Blue Cross plan.[6] Although cash benefits for health services usually are paid to the insured patient by commercial carriers, they also can be made directly to the providers of care through an arrangement called an *assignment of benefits,* or *an authorization to pay benefits.*

Three concepts are basic to Blue Cross plans: service benefits, full coverage benefits packages, and community rating methods.[7] Although community and experience rating will be explained more fully in Chapter 11, it is important to remember that Blue Cross plans, to compete with commercial carriers or because of the logistics of service delivery, will provide, under certain conditions, service and/or cash benefits and partial coverage, and they have adopted experience-rating methods. Thus, the practices of Blue Cross/Blue Shield and commercial insurers have slowly but inevitably converged.

Government-Sponsored Programs

Federal, state, and local governments have assumed a larger role in health services financing through "public insurance" programs. In 1988, of the total $539.9 billion national health expenditures, approximately 42 percent ($227.5 billion) consisted of public funds.[8] Included in this figure are funds for Medicare and Medicaid programs, Public Health Service programs, and county and state welfare assistance programs, among others. Under these programs, service benefits are provided to recipients who have met eligibility requirements; fees are generally paid directly to the provider of care by the governmental agency and are based either on charges for the specific services rendered or on a contractual amount agreed to beforehand. In some instances,

---

[6] American Hospital Association, *Hospital Statistics,* Chicago, Ill., AHA, 1973, p. 300; and Blue Cross Association, Chicago, Ill., personal communication, May 21, 1987.

[7] Hedinger. *The Social Role of Blue Cross,* p. 47.

[8] Health Insurance Association of America. *HIAA Health Trends Chart Book 1990.* Washington, D.C., HIAA, 1990, p. 3.

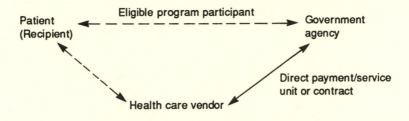

FIGURE 1-7 Government-sponsored programs—financing.

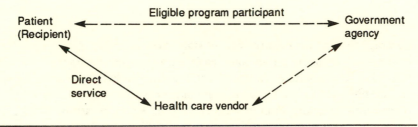

FIGURE 1-8 Government-sponsored programs—health services delivery.

the recipient is required to pay a nominal charge (copayment or deductible) for the services rendered. Figures 1-7 and 1-8 illustrate the patient, health services vendor, and paying agency relationships under government-sponsored programs.

Worker's Compensation Programs

All state legislatures have enacted worker's compensation or statutory disability benefit laws that provide for health insurance coverage of employees who are injured or become ill while "on the job" during the course of employment. The employee is covered from the first moment on the job and at all times during employment. There are no waiting periods or limitations because of full- or part-time employment; coverage is instantaneous and benefits are automatic. Benefits are established by state laws; consequently, there is little red tape for the employee in being compensated for loss. Benefits include all reasonable medical care, rehabilitation services necessary to return the injured employee to work, and partial replacement of lost wages.

In some states, a monopolistic state fund has been created from which payments are made; in other states, private health insurers are permitted to write

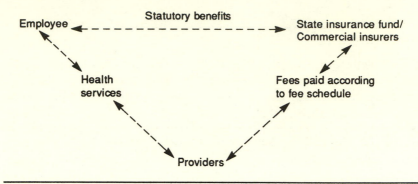

FIGURE 1-9 Worker's compensation financing and delivery.

coverage to meet the requirements of state laws. In several states, commercial insurers can compete on an equal basis with the state insurance fund. These relationships are outlined in Figure 1-9. Because worker's compensation benefits are provided to employees who are hurt or become ill while on the job, all other forms of health insurance coverage (i.e., Blue Cross/Blue Shield, HMO, indemnity coverage) might be classified as "off the job" and in effect when individuals are not "at work." Coverage by worker's compensation involves the issue of whether the injury occurred *on the job in the course of employment*, a key phrase in qualifying for compensation. If this test cannot be met, other insurance coverages would apply.

Funds for worker's compensation coverage come from premiums paid by employers and from state and local taxes. In general, premium rates are adjusted annually by statute, although interim changes also may be made (for example, if state regulatory agencies change fee schedules for physicians treating injured employees). Employers can contain or reduce their premiums by controlling accidents and the costs of accidents through positive programs to reduce employee injuries, creating a safe work environment, providing educational programs, conducting safety inspections, and counseling employees on safe work practices. Experience rating is applied automatically in some states to create individual employer premiums. In 1988, state and local governments spent $9.668 billion and the Federal Government spent $300 million for hospital and medical expenditures under worker's compensation programs.[9]

---

[9] Health Insurance Association of America. *Source Book of Health Insurance Data 1990*, p. 43.

ALTERNATIVE DELIVERY SYSTEMS/MANAGED CARE ORGANIZATIONS

The final method of delivery and financing of health services in the United States is through a class of innovative approaches, including HMOs, PPOs, and CMPs. These organizations are described as "managed care organizations (MCOs)" because of their emphasis on creating structures that enhance *control and management* of the financing and delivery of health services. Two of these—HMOs and CMPs—establish the greatest control of providers by placing them "at risk" for over-utilization of services, thus requiring physicians to limit utilization by changing their practice patterns. All of the nontraditional systems provide incentives for consumers to alter their customary patterns of selecting and using health services. In the following sections, health maintenance organizations are addressed, while PPOs and CMPs are reviewed in Chapters 3 and 5, respectively.

Direct-Service Plans

More commonly called health maintenance organizations, direct-service organizations have, in the past, also been referred to by various other titles: prepaid group practice plans, prepaid individual practice plans, prepaid health plans, independent health insurance plans, and health insurance plans other than Blue Cross/Blue Shield or insurance companies.[10] To simplify terminology, health maintenance organization or HMO will be used to identify these direct-service plans.

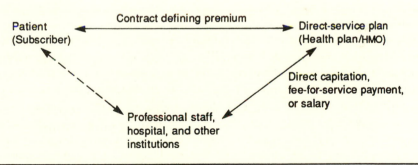

FIGURE 1-10   Health maintenance organization—financing.

---

[10] Louis Reed and Maureen Dwyer. *Directory of Health Insurance Plans Other than Blue Cross or Blue Shield Plans or Insurance Companies, 1970 Survey.* Washington, D.C., Office of Research and Statistics, Social Security Administration, U.S. Department of Health, Education, and Welfare, 1971.

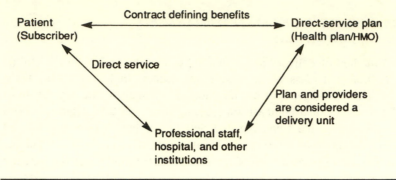

FIGURE 1-11   Health maintenance organization—health services delivery.

Compared to the "Blues" and commercial carriers, HMOs are a relatively small group of health insurers/providers. As of July 1, 1989, 32.5 million people, or approximately 13.2 percent of the U.S. population, were enrolled in 590 HMOs.[11] These health plans combine the functions of the insurance carrier and the providers of hospital services, including physician care, in a single organization. Consequently, HMOs compete directly with BC/BS plans and commercial insurers, as well as with major providers (solo physicians, medical group practices, hospitals, and urgent care centers, among others). Competitive activity before the 1970s was limited to localized geographic areas, primarily the Far West and Northwest; Detroit, Michigan; Cleveland, Ohio; the District of Columbia; and New York City. During the 1970s and 1980s, however, HMOs spread to virtually every major metropolitan community and even to many rural areas of the United States.

As illustrated in Figure 1-10, subscribers (members) pay health insurance premiums to the HMO (health plan). The HMO establishes close relationships with both inpatient and outpatient providers of care—usually via contractual agreements. When care is required, the HMO directly furnishes services through its professional staff and affiliated organizations, as shown in Figure 1-11. Since all costs have been prepaid through a premium, the HMO does not charge subscribers for specific services rendered. Hospitals and physicians may have contractual relationships with the health plan and are usually paid by the HMO, either on a fee-for-service basis, a capitation basis, or even a salary basis. *Capitation* is the negotiated (prospective payment) fee charged by the actual health services vendor for accepting the responsibility of providing services *per*

---

[11] Lynn Gruber, Maureen Shadle, and Kirk Pion. *The InterStudy Edge.* Excelsior, Minn., InterStudy, Vol. 4, 1989, pp. 1–2, 11–12, 18.

person for a specified time period, for example, $30 per member per month (PMPM).

This close association between the health services providers and the health plan exemplifies one of the fundamental characteristics of HMOs—for the member/patient, the HMO is not merely an insurer, it is also *the provider* of health services; the HMO must guarantee the availability of the services described in the subscriber contract. Unlike the BC/BS or private insurance carrier arrangements, it is the responsibility of the HMO to furnish the providers of health services and to pay them for providing such services.

The HMO Concept, Characteristics, and Philosophy

The HMO concept combines a financing mechanism and a delivery system under the control and direction of a single management entity—the health plan. An HMO is defined as any organization, either for-profit or nonprofit, that accepts responsibility for providing and delivering a predetermined set of comprehensive health maintenance and treatment services to a voluntarily enrolled population for a prenegotiated and fixed periodic premium payment. HMOs consist of three components: the health plan (which provides organization and management); the providers (physicians, hospitals, and others); and the consumers (subscribers, members, or enrollees).

The HMO Act of 1973, Public Law 93-222 and its amendments, provides a specific definition of HMOs that meets the federal requirements of the law. These regulations are discussed in Chapter 2. They provide the basis under which an HMO that meets all of the federal requirements under the HMO Act and its amendments can become "qualified." Not all HMOs are federally qualified; as of July 1, 1989, 307 or 52 percent of all HMOs had federal qualification.[12]

To understand HMOs, one needs to know the philosophy and goals of such organizations. HMOs are established to:

1. Promote alternatives to the existing fee-for-service system and provide a choice of health delivery *and* insurance systems
2. Attempt some reforms and changes in the existing health services system, so as to effect greater organizational efficiencies and more effectively control the quality of care

---

[12] Ibid., p. 17.

3. Promote cost control and containment by creating financial incentives for both providers and enrollees

4. Promote quality services through a free market system, allowing people to choose among competing health plans, and the HMO to use the "managing" primary care physician to control the amount and quality of patient services

5. Create a vertically integrated system of care with constant accessibility and a single entry point

6. Control costs and, thus, premiums through risk sharing with providers and the use of financial incentives to manage patient care

HMOs are also defined by understanding their most common characteristics.

1. *An organized system*—financing combined with delivery of services, including primary, specialty, ambulatory, and inpatient services

2. *Comprehensive benefits*—including inpatient, outpatient, extended care, home health, and mental health services, as well as drug coverage

3. *Voluntary enrollment*—members are given dual or multiple choice(s) of health plans, including traditional service and indemnity plans

4. *Defined geographic service area*—enrollment and service delivery, limited geographically to assure adequate availability and accessibility of health services

5. *Risk assumption*—by the HMO *and* providers that creates incentives to control costs; this is accomplished through *capitation* payments to providers of care, through *sharing* in risk pools (positive financial incentives), and/or withholds (negative financial incentives) from fee-for-service payments to providers

6. *Prepayment*—of premiums that are based on actuarial data and usually created by a modified community-rated method and paid by employers or other organizations

7. *Medical group practice*—physicians practicing in autonomous and self-governing medical groups, who are paid through a capitation arrangement; or physicians practicing in group-like arrangements as salaried employees of the HMO or under contract to the HMO using an individual practice association (IPA)

8. *Cost containment*—incentives to emphasize changes in physician practice patterns that lead to reduced utilization, especially of hospital use

9. *Enhanced management*—of quality, costs, and patient services through the use of managing physicians (gatekeepers), a single entry point into the health services system, and an organizational structure with clearly identifiable focal points of responsibility for all managerial, administrative, and service functions

Although these characteristics are evident in individual HMOs, there is great flexibility in sponsorship, method of paying providers, delivery of services, benefits, and profit status. The strength of the HMO concept is its ability to mold the health plan's form and style to local conditions while maintaining the basic features common to all HMOs.

HMO, therefore, is an umbrella term that includes two general types of prepaid health plans, according to a classification by type of physician participation; these are prepaid group practice plans and prepaid individual practice plans. They are described in the sections that immediately follow. The Federal Government also classifies qualified HMOs according to physician participation but uses three categories: group, staff, and IPA models. Others add a fourth category to the federal grouping—"network" models. The federal models are described in Chapter 4.

A *prepaid group practice* (PGP) plan is developed around a medical group practice of physicians and dentists, usually in a multispecialty arrangement and identified as a "group" or "staff" model HMO. As defined by the American Medical Association, medical group practice describes the provision of medical services by a number of physicians working in systematic association, with the joint use of equipment and technical personnel and a centralized administration and financial organization. The PGP plan may be sponsored by the group practice; the physicians develop the insuring mechanism and make it available to their patients and others either on an individual or a group basis. Premium payments are pooled, and physician salaries are drawn from this revenue. The PGP also may be sponsored by nonphysician groups; the Health Insurance Plan (HIP) of Greater New York is an example of a prepaid group practice developed by a city. HIP, as the responsible organization, contracts with physician groups throughout metropolitan New York City to provide care to HIP members. Payment to physicians is on a capitation basis.

Prepaid individual practice (PIP) plans, in contrast, use the services of individual, solo practitioners in their private office settings; they are identified as IPA model HMOs in Chapter 4. These individual practice approaches are a compromise between the traditional fee-for-service solo practitioner system and the prepaid group or solo practitioner system. Historically, PIPs were established through local and state medical societies, by small groups of local physicians, or by groups of community residents.

The first type, called Foundations for Medical Care (FMCs) or IPAs, are developed by local and state medical societies. The FMCs or IPAs are associations of physicians that organize and develop a management and fiscal structure and determine a fee schedule for individual physicians who join the association. The new organization, usually a separate corporation under physician control, may then contract with a health plan to provide services to members, or may actually become the managing organization (health plan) that establishes

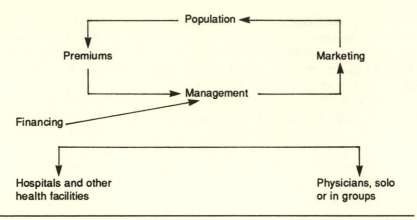

FIGURE 1-12 HMO schema.

benefits and premium structures, markets the health plan, completes peer reviews, and makes payment of claims. All local physicians may be eligible for participation as providers in the health plan; they are paid by the health plan, not the patient (member), on a discounted fee-for-service basis, unlike other HMO types, which compensate their providers via a capitation or salary arrangement.

HMOs are four-way arrangements between the enrolled population; a medical group or IPA—solo practitioners, hospital(s), and other health facilities; a management organization; and a financing mechanism.[13] These HMO components are arranged as shown in Figure 1-12. An interested group of physicians and laymen joins together with a common intent—HMO development. The group develops the prepaid plan, first identifying and obtaining financing. Gradually, over a period of from one to five years, the management group formulates a benefits package and corresponding premium structure and identifies target populations to whom the plan will be marketed. The benefits package is then marketed to that audience. Premiums collected from enrollees are used by the HMO to defray the cost of care provided. This cyclical process continues as the plan is marketed, as new members are enrolled, and as member services are financed. Health services are guaranteed by the plan through its contractual relationships with the plan's physicians and other health services vendors. As the plan grows with the addition of new enrollees, it generates new resources to provide more services, reduce the cost of the existing benefits package, and create a profit/surplus from operation.

---

[13] Beverlee A. Myers. *Health Maintenance Organizations: Objectives and Issues.* Washington, D.C., U.S. Government Printing Office, 1972. DHEW Publ. No. (SHM) 73-13002

Prepayment: Fee-for-Service Versus Capitation

The traditional method of providing ambulatory health services is a one-on-one relationship between private solo physicians and their patients. Charges for services are paid by the patients or their insurance programs on a fee-for-service (unit-of-service) basis. The more units of service that are provided, the higher the total fee collected by the physician. When BC/BS and commercial insurers enter into a relationship, the patient prepays for his/her health services, which may or may not be required at a later date. The responsibility for arranging and obtaining services remains with the subscriber, but payment flows from the insurer on a per-unit-of-service basis.

If BC/BS plans and private insurance carriers are prepaid by periodic premiums, how do these delivery structures differ from HMOs, whose subscribers also prepay on a periodic basis? As Figure 1-13 shows, there is little difference between the systems at this level. Subscribers pay premiums to their insurance plans: individuals pay their own premiums, and persons included in group contracts have their premiums totally (noncontributory) or partially (contributory) paid on a capitation basis. The difference between the two systems is in the interaction of the specific health plan and the providers of care. Again, the HMO stresses the total-system, direct-service approach. Within this structure,

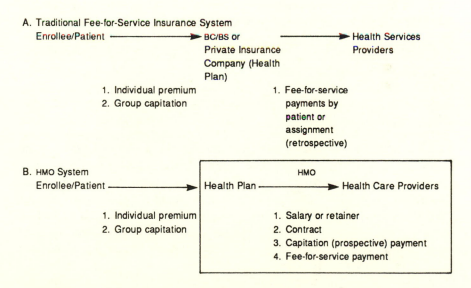

FIGURE 1-13 Premium movement to providers.

the providers can be paid on a salary or retainer, per capita, per case, or fee-for-service basis. Although any of these payment approaches may be used, the HMO provider is always placed at risk and given financial and nonfinancial incentives to hopefully choose the most appropriate level and amount of care.

Without commenting on the value of either system to society, the major difference between the traditional fee-for-service system and the HMO system centers on the provider's incentives in the fee-for-service system: the more units of service rendered, the higher the provider's revenue. Conversely, under the HMO system, the fewer units of service provided, the greater the savings to the plan. These savings may be shared with the providers as incentive payments and bonuses, may be used to provide additional benefits to members, may be used to reduce premiums, or may be realized as surplus or profit from the system, like the traditional fee-for-service system. Under the HMO system, incentive payments to physicians are used as an inducement for them to change their practice patterns and generally function more efficiently, to reduce overuse where possible, and to help control costs.

Cost containment within the concepts of good patient care is one of the major goals of HMOs. Thus, HMOs change the methods by which physicians are paid. These methods include capitation; discounted fee-for-service payments tied to withholds, to be returned if utilization is at an appropriate level; and bonuses tied to levels of use. They are used by HMOs to control their operating costs. Figure 1-13 identifies the major differences between the two systems and, more importantly, emphasizes the parallelism between them. This similarity is further emphasized when one considers the fee-for-service IPA approach and the fact that both systems use common components of the industry. Thus, the HMO is more an alternative delivery *concept* than an alternative delivery *system*—a different way of thinking about and arranging the current health delivery components.

Summary

A discussion of alternative delivery systems requires an understanding of the health delivery structures being used today. A *private pay* or *self-responsible system* is used by approximately 13 percent of the total civilian population. Under this system, the patients directly pay health services providers for direct service. A second and more common health delivery/financing structure consists of health insurance programs that are used to underwrite the cost of health services. These include the service plans, indemnity plans, and government-sponsored programs.

Service plans, which include Blue Cross and Blue Shield, are the traditional hospital and medical or physician insurance plans. Benefits usually are provided in the form of health services to members, with fees paid directly to the participating provider of care. Subscribers to these plans are free to identify and choose among participating providers. Indemnity plans are provided by commercial insurance companies or private carriers who, following the lead of BC/BS, insure the costs of both physician and hospital care. Members are free to select their providers of care and are reimbursed for the cost; under certain conditions, patients may assign their cash payment to the provider.

Government-sponsored programs are financed and operated by federal, state, and local governments. These include Medicare, Medicaid, the Federal Employees Health Benefits Program, CHAMPUS, county and state welfare programs, and worker's compensation programs. Eligible program participants receive service benefits, and their fees generally are paid directly to the providers of care by the government.

Over the last two decades, BC/BS organizations, as well as Medicare (through competitive medical plans) and Medicaid programs, have become involved with a third method of health services delivery and financing known as alternative delivery systems or "managed care organizations." The major organizations that are included in this system are known as *direct service plans* or health maintenance organizations, competitive medical plans, and preferred provider organizations. HMOs and CMPs assume risks for members' medical services and attempt to pass some level of risk to providers, while PPOs generally do not assume risk. HMOs comprise a relatively small group of health insurers/providers—approximately 13.2 percent of the U.S. population was enrolled in HMOs as of July 1, 1989. These plans are characterized by the unique development of a single organization to provide inpatient, outpatient, and other health services. Thus, the HMO concept is both a financing mechanism and a health care delivery system under the control of a single management group. The HMO may be defined as either a for-profit or not-for-profit organization that accepts responsibility for providing and delivering a prenegotiated set of comprehensive health services to a voluntarily enrolled group for a periodic premium.

HMO is an umbrella term that identifies several models, including prepaid group practice (PGP) plans, prepaid individual practice (PIP) plans, individual practice associations (IPAs), and Foundations for Medical Care (FMCs). The major differences between group practice and individual practice plans are in the areas of sponsorship, physician practice patterns, and provider reimbursement methods. PGPs are generally sponsored by private physician groups and other nonphysician organizations, whereas PIPs and IPAs usually are sponsored by local medical societies or individual physicians who have banded together to assure their economic welfare. Physicians practice as a group in PGPs versus as individuals in PIPs, IPAs, and FMCs. Finally, capitation is used as the payment mechanism for PGP physicians, while the traditional discounted fee-for-service approach with a withhold is used in PIPs. Thus, identifying an HMO is somewhat complicated, because of the variety of models that are available; in fact, the Federal Government has its own identification method that uses group model, staff model, and IPA models to describe HMOs. This flexibility in sponsorship, delivery, and payment, however, is one of the characteristics that makes the HMO concept attractive and a strong competitor for the traditional systems.

The objective of HMOs is to organize the health delivery components so the plan can market its product—the benefits package—and provide direct, comprehensive health services to its enrollees. Moreover, in the process of providing quality health services, the goal of the HMO is to reduce and/or contain the costs of furnishing health care by providing incentives to the providers to use appropriate levels and types of health services, including health maintenance and prevention. One mechanism used by the prepaid group practice HMO model to help control costs and to provide efficiency incentives is capitation—the price per person charged by the health provider for services rendered during a specified time period, usually a month.

Both fee-for-service plans and the HMO system use prepayment in the form of health insurance. The HMO system is unique, however, in its use of capitation payments for both physicians and hospitals, as well as traditional fee-for-service payments, with a withhold that places providers at risk. The use of identical components, such as medical group practice and prepaid health insurance, emphasizes the parallelism between the two systems. The HMO does not create a new delivery component but provides an alternative method of arranging the current ones. These alternative patterns are now frequently being used by the Blues and Medicare and Medicaid, a practice which suggests that the two systems—traditional fee-for-service and capitated approaches—are merging into a new, integrated health delivery and financing system in the United States.

References

Brown, Lawrence D. "Introduction to a Decade of Transition." In: *Health Policy in Transition: A Decade of Health Politics, Policy and Law*. Edited by Lawrence D. Brown. Durham, N.C., Duke University Press, 1987.

Dearing, Walter P. *Developments and Accomplishments of Comprehensive Group Practice Prepayment Programs*. Washington, D.C., Group Health Association of America, Inc., 1963, pp. 1–10.

Enthovan, Alain C. *Health Plan: The Only Practical Solution to the Soaring Cost of Medical Care*. Reading, Mass., Addison-Wesley, 1980.

Feldman, Roger. "Health Insurance in the United States: Is Market Failure Avoidable?" *Journal of Risk and Insurance, 54*(2):298, 1987.

Frech, H. E., III, and Paul B. Ginsburg. "Competition Among Health Insurers Revisited." *Journal of Health Politics, Policy and Law, 13*(2):279, Summer 1988.

Goldberg, Lawrence G., and Warren Greenberg. "The Competitive Response of Blue Cross to the Health Maintenance Organization." *Economic Inquiry, 18*(1):55–68, January 1980.

Greenberg, Warren, ed. *Competition in the Health Sector: Past, Present and Future.* Gaithersburg, Md., Aspen Publishers, Inc., 1978.

Hedinger, Fredric R. *The Social Role of Blue Cross as a Device for Financing the Cost of Hospital Care: An Evaluation.* Ames, Ia., Graduate Program in Hospital and Health Administration, University of Iowa, 1966, pp. 1–13, 17–18, 34–49, 73–76, 82–84. Health Care Research Series No. 2

Law, Sylvia A. *Blue Cross: What Went Wrong?* 2nd Edition. New Haven, Conn., Yale University Press, 1976.

Melhado, Evan M.; Walter Feinberg; and Harold M. Swartz; eds. *Money, Power and Health Care.* Ann Arbor, Mich., Health Administration Press, 1988.

Myers, Beverlee A. *Health Maintenance Organizations: Objectives and Issues.* Washington, D.C., U.S. Government Printing Office, 1972. DHEW Publ. No. (SHM) 73-13002

Nixon, President Richard M. *Health Message from the President of the United States: Relative to Building a National Health Strategy* (February 18, 1971). 92nd Congress, 1st Session. Washington, D.C., U.S. Government Printing Office, 1971, p. 4.

Reed, Louis, and Maureen Dwyer. *Directory of Health Insurance Plans Other than Blue Cross or Blue Shield Plans or Insurance Companies, 1970 Survey.* Washington D.C., Office of Research and Statistics, Social Security Administration. U.S. Department of Health, Education, and Welfare, 1971.

Saward, Ernest W. *The Relevance of Prepaid Group Practice to the Effective Delivery of Health Services.* Washington, D.C., Health Services and Mental Health Administration, U.S. Department of Health, Education, and Welfare, 1969.

University of Chicago, Graduate Program in Hospital Administration, Center for Health Administration Studies, Graduate School of Business. *Health Maintenance Organization: A Reconfiguration of the Health Services System. Proceedings of the Thirteenth Annual Symposium on Hospital Affairs.* Chicago, Ill., 1971, pp. 2–10.

U.S. Department of Health, Education, and Welfare. *Health Maintenance Organizations: The Statements of President Richard M. Nixon and Secretary Elliot L. Richardson of the U.S. Department of Health, Education, and Welfare.* Rockville, Md., DHEW, 1971.

_____. *Towards a Comprehensive Health Policy for the 1970s: A White Paper.* Washington, D.C., U.S. Government Printing Office, 1971, pp. 31–37.

_____, Health Services and Mental Health Administration. *Health Maintenance Organization. The Concept and Structure.* Rockville, Md., DHEW, 1971.

2

HISTORY, PHILOSOPHY, AND LEGISLATIVE ACTIVITIES

The concepts on which today's HMOs are structured have been a part of the medical services delivery system for many years. In this country, early efforts to provide prepaid group practice medical care were undertaken by the Federal Government on behalf of military personnel and merchant seamen. HMO-like organizations for the civilian population began to evolve at the beginning of the twentieth century, with the industrialization of the western United States. Railroads and associated railroad workers' unions realized that it was necessary to provide medical care for their crews as the workers moved farther away from established medical service. Medical care arrangements also were developed in the "company towns" by the mining, lumber, and manufacturing industries. Historical evidence shows that prepaid group practice plans were established for workers to fill the void when adequate solo fee-for-service medical services were not available.

Medical Group Practice Development

Along with the development of medical service delivery organizations, another major HMO element appeared—medical group practices sponsored by physicians. The first was the Mayo Clinic, founded in Rochester, Minnesota in 1887 by Dr. W. W. Mayo and his two sons, W. J. and C. H. Mayo. But probably the first *prepaid* group practice plan was organized by the Western Clinic in Tacoma, Washington around 1910; its members were employees of the lumber mills. The Tacoma area was also the initial site for a chain of 20 prepaid industrial clinics, the first of which was established in 1911. Two of these clinics ultimately became present-day HMOs—the Group Health Cooperative of Puget Sound and the King County Blue Shield alternative delivery system.

Two other medical group practices are significant in HMO development. The Ross-Loos Medical Clinic in Los Angeles, California initiated prepaid medical services in 1929, its first year of operation; today Ross-Loos is the CIGNA Healthplans of California, with more than 536,000 members at the end of 1989. Also in 1929, the Palo Alto Medical Group in Palo Alto, California was formally organized, but did not offer prepaid services until it signed a contract with Stanford University to insure its student body in 1947. The year 1929 was also important in the development of cooperative prepaid plans. During that year, Dr. Michael A. Shadid helped organize a health cooperative in Elk City, Oklahoma. He also played a role in the development of several other prepaid plans in the West and Midwest.

Prepayment as a Social Movement

During the mid-1920s, the prosperity of the nation was reflected by a change in national emphasis from wartime programs to social programs and domestic health issues. Health care costs needed to be controlled, and, according to the 1933 report of the Committee on the Costs of Medical Care, part of the answer was greater use of medical group practices, especially prepaid group practices. By the time the report was released, the economic boom had given way to the Great Depression. As William A. MacColl, M.D. observed, the American public had been seriously challenged to look at the whole social structure under which it lived and to reexamine many of the traditional values and habits threatened with change.[1] The Depression created instability and insecurity, yet it also engendered an atmosphere where change could take place. Prepaid programs offered stability, at least for medical services.

Another outcome of the instability of the 1930s was the development of cooperative arrangements. Group action during the Depression led to the creation of buying clubs (similar to the English and European cooperatives), as well as several prepaid health cooperatives. Passage in 1935 of the Wagner Act, which guaranteed workers the right to organize and bargain collectively, hastened the expansion of labor unions. Health care became a negotiable item at the bargaining table, and the obligation of employers to pay at least a part of their employees' health care costs fostered great interest in the development and control of new health care programs. Providers joined the effort to control health services delivery and financing by establishing Blue Cross and Blue Shield plans, and indemnity insurers expanded their products to include health services insurance coverages. All of these developments can be traced to the

---

[1] William A. MacColl. *Group Practice and Prepayment of Medical Care.* Washington, D.C., Public Affairs Press, 1966, p. 14.

TABLE 2-1　Selected HMO-like Organizations from 1900 to 1975

Plan	Date of Establishment	Sponsor
Western Clinic, Tacoma, Washington	1906, 1910*	Medical partnership
Bridge Clinics in Oregon and Washington†	1911	Individual practitioner
Palo Alto Medical Clinic, Palo Alto, California	1929, 1947*	Medical partnership
Ross-Loos Clinic, Los Angeles	1929	Medical partnership
Community Hospital Association, Elk City, Oklahoma	1929	Cooperative
Group Health Cooperative of Puget Sound (1947), Seattle, Washington (formerly Medical Securities Clinic)	1935	Cooperative (originally a medical partnership)
Group Health Association, Washington, D.C.	1937	Cooperative
Physicians Association of Clackamus County, Gladstone, Oregon	1938	Medical partnership
Kaiser Foundation Health Plan, Oakland, California and Portland, Oregon	1942	Industry
Community Health Center, Two Harbors, Minnesota	1944	Union cooperative
Labor Health Institute, St. Louis, Missouri	1945	Teamsters Union
"Miners' clinics"—nine group practice plans in Pennsylvania, Ohio, and West Virginia	1946	United Mine Workers Union
Health Insurance Plan of Greater New York, New York City	1947	City, physicians, and community
Foundation for Medical Care of San Joaquin County, Stockton, California	1954	Medical society
Community Health Association of Detroit, Michigan	1956	United Auto Workers Union
Group Health Plan of St. Paul, Minnesota	1957	Indemnity insurance company
Community Medical Services, Seattle, Washington†	1960	Sole proprietorship/ medical partnership
Columbia Plan, Columbia, Maryland	1969	Connecticut General Life Insurance Company, The Johns Hopkins University and Hospital, and tne Rouse Company
Harvard Community Health Plan, Boston, Massachusetts	1969	University
Kaiser Foundation Health Plan, Denver, Colorado	1969	Industry, community
Greater Marshfield Community Health Plan, Marshfield, Wisconsin	1971	Physician
Geisinger Health Plan, Danville, Pennsylvania	1972	Hospital
New Mexico Health Care Corporation, Albuquerque	1973	Hospital
Group Health of Arizona, Tucson	1974	Carrier
U.S. Community Health Services, Canoga Park, California	1974	Physician
North Communities Health Plan, Inc., Evanston, Illinois	1975	Consumer

*The second date indicates when the prepayment plan was first offered. The Western Clinic decided to end its capitated contracts in 1976 but reestablished them on a limited basis in mid-1980.

†The Bridge Clinic, established in 1911, was purchased by Dr. John Pieroth in 1946 and sold to Dr. Irwin S. Neiman in 1952. In 1960, Dr. Neiman incorporated the clinic as the Community Medical Services of Seattle (CMS). CMS was purchased in 1972 by Doctors Hospital of Seattle.

competitive activities between early prepaid health plans and the traditional medical industry. Confrontations between these prepaid plans and organized medicine culminated in long court battles over restraint of trade under the terms of the Sherman Antitrust Act. Courts ruled in favor of the prepaid plans in every case.

The group action behind prepaid programs was directed toward stabilizing society, increasing the value obtained from limited incomes, and obtaining products and services as good as or better than those that members could obtain individually. The originators of these new plans wanted a voice in their development on an equal basis with providers, and they wanted assurance of quality, fiscal responsibility, availability, and, most important, security from financial loss. This system, however, could be effective only if fee-for-service payments to physicians were eliminated and the physicians shared in the financial risks of the plan through capitations or salaries with bonus potential. Physicians were to concentrate on professional activities that would enhance the quality of medical care. Finally, the goal of the prepaid programs was to develop parallel interests of patients and physicians, manifested in a program designed to promote good care, preventive and treatment services, and stability in financing.

The Pre-HMO Period

The period between the development of group practices and health plans (prior to 1930) and the evolution of federally supported plans (1970) was one of moderate expansion in prepaid health plans. Table 2-1 provides a list of many of the early plans.[2] Known as HMO prototypes, these early plans greatly influenced the concepts included in P.L. 93-222.

1950 to 1975

Innovative approaches to prepaid medical care continued to appear between 1950 and 1975. The role of labor in these efforts was significant, as collectively bargained health and welfare funds began to spread. During this period, disposable personal income increased to all-time highs, with a resultant ability to pay for and use private insurance. Tables 2-2 and 2-3 illustrate the dramatic

---

[2] The history of many of the plans is given in MacColl, *Group Practice and Prepayment of Medical Care*, pp. 24–54; Jerome L. Schwartz, "Early History of Prepaid Medical Care Plans," *Bulletin of the History of Medicine*, 39(5):450–475, September–October 1965; and Leon Gintzig and Robert G. Shouldice, "Prepaid Group Practice—A Comparative Study," Washington, D.C., The George Washington University, 1971. Part I, Vols. 1–3.

TABLE 2-2　Number of Persons with Private Health Insurance Protection by Type of Coverage in the United States (in thousands)

Year Ended	Hospital Expenses	Surgical Expenses	Regular Medical Expenses (Physician's Expenses)
1950	76,639	54,156	21,589
1955	101,400	85,681	53,038
1960	122,500	111,525	83,172
1965	138,671	130,530	109,560
1970	158,847	151,440	138,658
1973	168,455	162,644	151,680
1974	171,140	166,434	158,170
1975	178,180	169,002	168,334
1976	176,858	167,701	163,342
1977	179,853	168,002	161,289
1978	185,690	174,724	166,840
1979	185,743	177,146	167,163
1980	187,375	178,223	169,529
1981	186,193	176,898	164,084
1982	188,337	180,298	171,642
1983	186,644	179,057	173,100
1984	184,403	*	*
1985	180,089	*	*
1986	180,060	*	*
1987	181,125	*	*
1988	188,000 (est.)	*	*

*Reporting requirements were changed in 1984; thus, these data are not available.

SOURCE: Health Insurance Association of America, *Source Book of Health Insurance Data 1984–1985*, New York, HIAA, 1985, p. 10; and _____, *Source Book of Health Insurance Data 1986–1987*, Washington, D.C., HIAA, 1987, p. 10. The Public Relations Division of the Health Insurance Association of America, Washington, D.C., provided 1986 data on June 15, 1988, and 1987–1988 data on May 11, 1990.

TABLE 2-3　Number of Persons with Private Health Insurance in the United States, 1984–1988 (in thousands)

	1984	1985	1986	1987	1988
Total population	233,445	235,520	238,197	239,209	243,100
Persons covered	202,107	204,235	204,419	205,531	211,600
Private health insurance	177,418	180,089	180,060	181,125	188,400
Employer-related	144,321	147,086	145,784	146,658	153,300
Persons without coverage	31,338	31,285	33,778	33,678	31,500

SOURCE: Health Insurance Association of America. *Source Book of Health Insurance Data 1990*. Washington, D.C., HIAA, 1991, p. 7.

increase in the number of persons with private health coverage. New types of health plans emerged, some sponsored by traditional cooperatives and physician partnerships. Indemnity insurance companies, universities, private companies, cities, and Blue Cross/Blue Shield plans sponsored several HMO-like organizations.

The HMO movement grew at an accelerated rate during this 25-year period. Operational HMOs increased from approximately 20 in 1950 to 33 in 1970 and to 166 in 1975. Dr. Shadid's plan in Elk City and at least four other physician-sponsored group practice plans, however, were some of the casualties.[3]

Federal Government Interest

Costs of health care increased dramatically between 1950 and 1975. In 1950, the average hospital cost per patient day was $15.62, and the total cost of an average hospital stay was $126.52. By 1975, these costs had escalated to $151.20 and $1,164.20, respectively. Similarly, in 1950, individuals spent 4.6 percent of their disposable personal income for health care, including health insurance. By 1975, this percentage had increased to 8.3 percent (and to approximately 12 percent in 1990). According to the Consumer Price Index (CPI), from 1962 to 1975, medical costs rose 59 percent—more rapidly than any major category of personal expenses. Thus, both private groups and public agencies looked for mechanisms that would reduce and contain costs.

Several national studies, in particular the 1967 *Report to the President,* recommended group practice, and especially prepaid group practice, as possible solutions to the cost-of-care crisis. The gestation period for the federal program was relatively short: by March 9, 1970, a position paper was completed by Paul M. Ellwood, Jr., M.D. and his associates at the American Rehabilitation Foundation (later to be called InterStudy) in which he coined the phrase "health maintenance organization."[4] As described in this paper, the HMO concept was to become a major issue of the Nixon administration's health program.

First announced before an executive session of the House Ways and Means Committee on March 23, 1970, and through a press release on March 25, 1970, Alternative C, as the proposal was called, would authorize the Social Security Administration to contract with HMOs to guarantee comprehensive

---

[3] Jerome L. Schwartz. *Medical Plans and Health Care.* Springfield, Ill., Charles C Thomas, Publisher, 1968, p. 23.

[4] Paul M. Ellwood, Jr. "The Health Maintenance Strategy." Minneapolis, Minn., InterStudy, 1970.

health service for the elderly at a fixed rate. The Nixon administration's bill, designed to help establish HMOs, was introduced in March 1971.

1970 to the Present

Per capita disposable personal income continued to rise during the 1970s and 1980s, but so did the cost of medical services. The cost of a patient day in hospital reached $586.33 in 1988, and an average stay was $4,206.73, a 127 percent increase between 1980 and 1988. Employers, unions, federal and state governments, health insurers, and others aggressively worked to develop alternatives to the traditional health insurance programs, which they felt were providing the wrong incentives to physicians and hospitals and, thus, pushing the costs of care higher. Employers, who bore the costs of their employees' health benefits and paid substantial Social Security taxes to support Medicare and Medicaid, were pressing for dramatic changes. The first of these changes was the passage of Title XIII of the Public Health Service Act, better known as the HMO Act of 1973.

Before 1970, fewer than 50 HMO-like organizations were in existence, with an enrollment of less than 2 percent of the health insurance market. After passage of the act, development accelerated, as shown in Table 2-4 and Figures 2-1, 2-2, and 2-3. After reaching a high of 653 in 1988, the number of HMOs has since declined as a result of mergers, consolidations, and terminations. Although HMOs experienced annual membership growth in excess of 20 percent during the early 1980s, the growth rate began to decline in 1987, and enrollment increased only 5 percent from 1988 to 1989. This decline may be attributed to various factors, including: (1) substantial increases in HMO premiums, (2) plan termination of some unprofitable accounts, and (3) decisions of some HMO members to transfer to hybrid HMO products. An additional factor may have been purchaser concerns about the financial stability of the HMO industry, given the Maxicare bankruptcy and the industry's poor

TABLE 2-4 Number of and Enrollment in Health Maintenance Organizations: 1970 to mid-1989

Year	1970	1976	1978	1980	1982	1984	1985	1986	1987	1988	1989
Number of Plans	33	176	203	236	265	337	480	626	653	607	590
Enrollment (millions)	4,000	6,016	7,471	9,100	10,831	16,743	21,000	25,777	30,300	31,940	32,500

SOURCE: Group Health Association of America, Washington, D.C. News Releases; InterStudy, *National HMO Census 1989*, Excelsior, Minn., 1990; and Lynn Gruber, Maureen Shadle, and Kirk Pion, *The InterStudy Edge*, Excelsior, Minn., InterStudy, Vol. 4, 1989, p. 1.

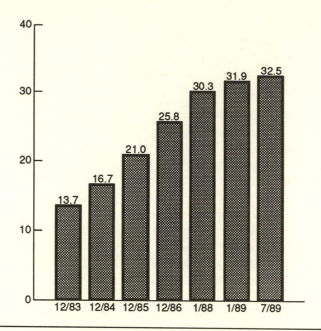

FIGURE 2-1   Growth in HMO enrollment.

financial returns of the prior two years. InterStudy predicts modest enrollment gains will continue as HMOs restructure to improve their profit margins and find new ways to attract new clients. By mid-1989, there were 590 HMOs with a combined enrollment of 32.5 million members, or approximately 13 percent of the U.S. population and 16 percent of all individuals with health insurance coverage.

The HMO industry is currently experiencing a maturing process, with a slowing of membership growth, the consolidation of plans, and the development of HMO products that more closely match purchasers' desires. These include hybrid and open-ended HMOs and triple-option health plans, under which employers are allowed to offer their employees the option of enrolling in an HMO, PPO, or an indemnity insurance program all offered by the same HMO organization.

The following is a profile of the current HMO industry.

- Approximately 60 percent of all HMOs provide physician services through an individual practice arrangement (IPA model HMOs are described in Chapter 4).

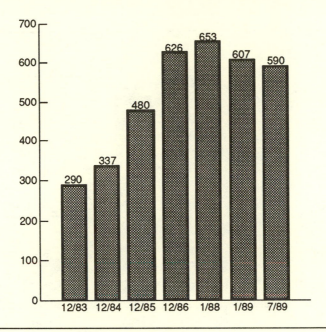

FIGURE 2-2   Growth in number of HMOs.

- As the industry matures, the traditional nonprofit tax status of HMOs is giving way to for-profit arrangements.
- Of 553 HMOs studied, representing 91 percent of the industry's enrollment, the combined net income totaled $182 million in 1989, compared with a loss of $887 million in 1988 for the same HMOs; 55 percent of these plans were profitable in 1989, compared to 32 percent in 1988.
- Based on estimates, the HMO industry lost $1.39 billion before taxes on revenues of $33.3 billion in 1988. This rate of return on revenues (−4.2 percent) is the same as for 1987 in aggregate, when only 38 percent of the industry reported a gross profit.
- In 1989, most plans covered primary care visits, hospitalization, outpatient mental health, home health, and skilled nursing care, among other benefits. Approximately 95 percent of the plans covered pharmacy benefits, and 93 percent covered inpatient mental health services.
- Most HMOs provide hospital care without limits and copays, and the majority of health plans provide primary care without limits or copays (or a nominal copay).

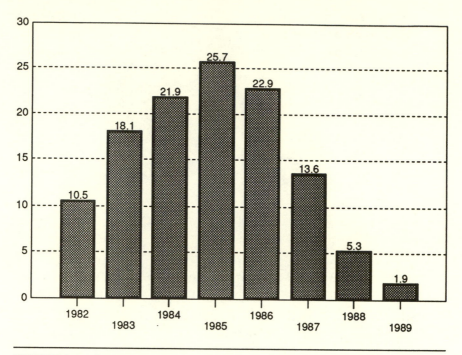

FIGURE 2-3 Annual percentage growth in HMO enrollment, 1982–1989.

- The average monthly premium charged by HMOs in 1989 was approximately $230 for family contracts and $86 for individuals.
- In 1989, the mean monthly premium in the HMO's largest account increased 17.4 percent for single contracts and 18.5 percent for family contracts. Although premium increases for HMOs were higher than in previous years and exceeded the growth in the medical care component of the Consumer Price Index for this period, they were below the reported increases in indemnity premiums (12 to 25 percent in 1988). Premiums in 1989 rose 16 percent, slightly less than the 16.9 percent increase in 1988. Premium increases also occurred in 1987, with a 12 percent increase, compared to 8 percent in 1986 and 3 percent in 1985.
- A 12-year Rand Corporation study suggests that HMO members experience up to 40 percent fewer hospital admissions and save up to 28 percent on health care costs, compared to individuals in the traditional fee-for-service system. Rand also concluded that regardless of the en-

rollee's income level, lower hospitalization rates were not reflected in lower levels of health status.[5]

- In 1987, for people under age 65, HMOs reported 394 hospital days per 1,000 enrollees, compared to the national average of 809; for those over age 65, HMOs reported 1,945 days per 1,000 enrollees, compared to 3,030 days in the traditional fee-for-service system.

- In 1986, HMOs reported that all members made 3.7 physician visits while over age 65 members used 8.3 physician visits. In comparison, the National Center for Health Statistics reported that all U.S. citizens used 3.1 physician visits per person per year and over age 65 citizens used 5.1 visits per person per year.

- In late 1988, nearly 1.82 million Medicare beneficiaries received their health services through HMOs that had Medicare risk contracts or were competitive medical plans (see Chapter 5 for a discussion of CMPs).

- As of June 30, 1989, there were 1.1 million Medicaid beneficiaries in 183 plans, of which 127 were federally or state qualified HMOs.

- Generally, most studies of patient satisfaction indicate that HMO members are as satisfied with health plan services, coverage, and costs as fee-for-service patients; however, people assigned to the HMO setting were less satisfied overall relative to the fee-for-service patients.[6]

- Profitability of HMOs is directly related to their enrollment level, with larger plans achieving economies of scale, especially in lower per-member administrative costs.

Legislative Activity

The Federal Government became actively involved in the HMO concept because the health services industry had problems in meeting three objectives—providing access to care, stabilizing the financing and cost for both purchasers and providers, and assuring a high level of quality. Legislation to help distribute health services more equitably included the Hill-Burton program (P.L. 79-724, the Hospital Survey and Construction Act), the Comprehensive Health Planning and Public Health Services Amendments Act (P.L. 89-749), and

---

[5] Robert G. Shouldice. "Questioning the Quality of Health Services." *Medical Group Management Journal, 35*(2):8–9, 11, March/April 1988.

[6] Allyson Ross Davis; John E. Ware, Jr.; Robert H. Brook; Jane R. Peterson; and Joseph P. Newhouse, "Consumer Acceptance of Prepaid and Fee-for-Service Medical Care: Results from a Randomized Controlled Trial," *Health Services Research, 21*(3):429–452, August 1986; *see also* Robert G. Shouldice and Norah Singpurwalla, "Consumer Satisfaction and Quality of Health Services (Part 2)," *Medical Group Management Journal, 35*(3):8–9, 11, May/June 1988.

the National Health Planning and Resources Development Act (P.L. 93-641), among others. Regarding the second issue—stabilizing the increasing cost of care—regulations were implemented to reduce the demand for care, such as limiting coverage under Medicare; increasing the supply of physicians; increasing the productivity of providers; and changing the method of payment to hospitals, long-term care organizations, physicians, and others. As to the third issue, early attempts to assure quality of care included the passage of P.L. 92-603, which created the Professional Standards Review Organizations (PSROs), P.L. 93-222 (the HMO Act), the Medicare Quality Protection Act of 1986, and others.

In Dr. Ellwood's 1970 position paper, he and his associates presented an outline of the HMO concept:

. . . the health maintenance strategy envisions a series of government and private actions designed to promote a highly diversified, pluralistic, and competitive health industry in which:

— Many different types of health maintenance organizations would provide comprehensive services needed to keep people healthy, offering consumers—both public and private—a choice between such service and traditional forms of care.

— Services would be purchased annually from such organizations through health maintenance contracts (capitation), at rates agreed upon before illness has occurred, with the provider sharing the economic risk of ill health.[7]

Dr. Ellwood and his associates set forth the following steps that should be taken by the Federal Government over a 5- to 10-year period to implement the strategy:

1. Adopt the health maintenance strategy and require both private enterprise and public agencies to join the health industry in implementing the national objective of health maintenance.

2. Provide incentives for the creation of health maintenance organizations.

3. Foster the elimination of any legal barriers that may block the creation of such organizations.

4. Begin purchasing the services offered under Medicare, Medicaid, and other federal reimbursement programs by means of health maintenance contracts rather than by using the present methods of paying for individual medical services.

---

[7] Ellwood. "The Health Maintenance Strategy," pp. 1–2.

5. Build into these contracts a sufficient return to support necessary investments in manpower, facilities, and health services research by contracting with health maintenance organizations.

6. Review the Federal Government's activities in the health field to determine how they currently contribute to, or frustrate, the health maintenance strategy and initiate necessary modifications to support it.[8]

Initially, the HMO concept was proposed by the Nixon administration as a way to contain the costs of the Medicare and Medicaid programs. But, because of their cost-saving potential and the increasing interest and acceptance of the concept, HMOs became the central issue of President Nixon's health program. So strong was the sentiment for HMO development that an HMO office was established within DHEW's Office of the Administrator, Health Services and Mental Health Administration, in May 1971. The HMO office was then followed by the Health Maintenance Organization Service (HMOS), established October 19, 1971, and the current Office of Prepaid Health Care in the Health Care Financing Administration, DHHS. Major HMO functions on the federal level included technical assistance to developing HMOs, backup support for HMO legislation, award and management of planning and development grants, assistance in the development of Title XIX contracts, and evaluation of grants. HMOs operated on reprogrammed funds from October 1971 until the passage of the HMO law in December 1973.[9] DHEW support for HMO grants and contracts for fiscal years 1971, 1972, and 1973 totaled nearly $26 million—$16.9 million for the direct support of 155 HMO projects.[10]

The administration's strategy of 1971 and 1972 was constructed around a program of financial and technical assistance in the planning, development, and expansion of existing and new HMOs. A second aspect of the strategy called for the Federal Government to pay all or part of the premium for specific beneficiary groups, such as Native Americans, Medicare recipients, and the poor. The administration also favored action that would override restrictive state laws that precluded HMO development. Finally, the Federal Government

---

[8] Ibid., p. 2.

[9] The three basic authorities under which HMOs operated include Section 304 of the Public Health Service Act, authorizing grant and contract experimentation with alternative health service delivery forms; Section 314(e) of the Comprehensive Health Planning and Services Act, authorizing health service project grants; and Section 9101(c) of the Regional Medical Programs law.

[10] U.S. Department of Health, Education, and Welfare, Health Services Administration. *Health Maintenance Organization Service: Program Status as of December 1972.* Rockville, Md., DHEW 1973, pp. 9–43.

was to develop guidelines to assist in a rigorous review of HMO operations to ensure that the quality of care met professional standards.

Priority considerations were given to development of HMOs in underserved areas; however, care was taken to avoid the implication that this was to be a demonstration on a particular segment of society. HMOs were not to be forced on anyone. Rather, they were viewed as an innovation in health care delivery that should be made available to everyone on a free-choice basis.

A time-limited demonstration approach was selected as the 1973 HMO strategy; no long-term commitment to a federal subsidy for activities was envisioned.[11] According to DHEW officials, HMOs had been chosen for federal demonstration investment for several reasons: they had proved effective in certain parts of the country; they might improve the effectiveness and efficiency of health services and might contain, if not reduce, the expenditures that government, individuals, and employers pay for health care; they might encourage and attract the participation of federal programs such as Medicare, Medicaid, the Federal Employees Health Benefits Program (FEHBP), and the Civilian Health and Medical Program of the Uniformed Services (CHAMPUS); and they had potential for introducing more competition into the health care field.

The Health Maintenance Act of 1973 and Its Amendments

The present HMO law, P.L. 93-222 (Title XIII of the Public Health Service Act), was signed by President Nixon on December 29, 1973. It amends "the Public Health Service Act to provide assistance and encouragement for the establishment and expansion of health maintenance organizations, health care resources, and the establishment of a Quality Health Care Commission, and for other purposes. . . ."[12] The measure committed the Federal Government to a time-limited demonstration effort and support of HMO development. It authorized the expenditure of $375 million over a five-year period from FY 1974 through FY 1978; several amendments provided additional funding through FY 1981. Development assistance was provided to a limited number of demonstration projects, with the intention that they become self-sufficient within fixed periods. The law's major purpose was to stimulate the interest of consumers and providers in the HMO concept and to help make health care

---

[11] Statement of Frank C. Carlucci Before the Subcommittee on Public Health and Environment, Committee on Interstate and Foreign Commerce, March 6, 1973, pp. 3–4.

[12] U.S. Congress, House of Representatives. *Health Maintenance Organization Act of 1973; Conference Report.* 93rd Congress, 1st session. December 3, 1973, p. 1.

delivery available through HMOs—and to allow people to select for themselves either a prepaid system for obtaining health services or the more traditional approach.[13] Amendments that made the law more workable and that refunded the activities of the federal HMO office were enacted in 1976, 1978, 1980, 1981, 1986, and 1988.

Federal assistance under the HMO legislation was granted to public or private entities only if the HMO met the definitional and organizational requirements of the act. These included the following:

- HMOs are defined as entities that provide basic health services to their enrollees. Prepaid enrollment fees for the basic and supplemental health services must be fixed uniformly under a community-rating system without regard to the medical history of any individual or family.

- Basic health services to be provided enrollees include physician services, inpatient and outpatient hospital services, medically necessary emergency health services, up to 20 visits for short-term outpatient evaluative and crisis-intervention mental health services, medical treatment and referral services for the abuse of or addiction to alcohol and drugs, diagnostic laboratory and diagnostic and therapeutic radiology services, home health services, and preventive health services.

- The HMO may provide supplemental health services, and a nominal copayment may be charged the enrollee at the time of service.

- Basic and supplemental services must be provided by the HMO staff or professional under contract or by any combination of staff, medical group practice, or individual practice association. Unusual or infrequently used services may be provided by physicians outside the plan.

- Services must be available and accessible 24 hours a day, seven days a week. Moreover, a member must be reimbursed for expenses incurred outside the HMO area if it was medically necessary that services be rendered before the member could return to his or her HMO.

- A medical group must be organized as a partnership, professional corporation, association, or other arrangement and must spend the majority of its practice activities with HMO members. Medical group practices pool income from their practice and share net income based on a prearranged income-sharing formula; share medical records, major equipment, and staff; and encourage continuing education of their members.

---

[13] *Statement by the President.* Press Release. San Clemente, Calif., Office of the White House Press Secretary, December 29, 1973, p. 1.

- Individual practice associations (IPAs) are defined as a partnership, corporation, association, or other legal entity that has entered into service arrangements with physicians. Sharing activities are similar to group practices, except that income is not pooled but paid directly to the individual physician.
- The HMO must have a fiscally sound operation, with adequate provisions against risk of insolvency. It must be capable of assuming full financial risk, on a prospective basis, for the delivery of health services to members.
- The HMO must have annual open enrollment periods and must enroll persons who are broadly representative of the various age, social, and income groups in its service area. It cannot refuse to enroll or reenroll members because of health status or need for health services.
- Health education must be provided to the HMO's members, covering the use of health services as well as methods of personal health maintenance, such as proper diet, exercise, the use of medications, and so on.
- The HMO must have an ongoing quality assurance program and must emphasize health outcomes.
- A data reporting system must be used to collect information on the cost of operations; utilization patterns; and the availability, accessibility, and acceptability of the HMO's services.

The act authorized grants and contracts to public and private not-for-profit organizations to assist the feasibility, planning, development, and initial operation of HMOs. Loans also were available to for-profit organizations for the same purposes.

The first HMO development grants were awarded in FY 1975, the last in FY 1981. During that period, a total of $145,186,454 in grants was awarded to 309 separate organizations—$18.1 million in feasibility grants, $28.9 million in planning grants, and $98.1 million in initial development grants. The results of these grants were as follows:[14]

- Of the 309 organizations receiving grants, 117 (37.9 percent) became operational and received federal qualification. These 117 organizations received $111,108,284 (76.8 percent) of the grant funds awarded; 96 are still operating, are still federally qualified, and have a total enrollment of

---

[14] U.S. Department of Health and Human Services, Health Resources and Services Administration, Bureau of Health Maintenance Organizations, Office of Health Maintenance Organizations. *10th Annual Report to the Congress, Fiscal Year 1984.* Rockville, Md., DHHS, June 1985, p. 4.

more than 3 million members. The remaining 21 had their qualification revoked and have ceased operations.
- Of the 309 organizations receiving grant funds, 186 (60.2 percent) never reached operational status. These 186 organizations received $27,933,593 (19.3 percent) of the grant funds awarded; 135 of the 186 organizations received grant funds to study only the feasibility of establishing an HMO.

In addition, loans and loan guarantees were made to 109 qualified HMOs from 1975 through 1983, the last year in which new federal loans were issued. Of these, 103 received direct loan commitments totaling $205.3 million. Of the 109 organizations, 95 (87 percent) have been developed with grant funds provided under the HMO Act and amendments. Federal grants and loans totaled $363.8 million.[15] InterStudy, however, estimated that most of the money invested in HMOs—$1.2 billion from 1974 to 1980—was provided by the private sector.[16] It was the Reagan administration's policy that the government should serve as an advocate of the HMO concept, but that financial support must ultimately come from private companies.

NONFINANCIAL ASSISTANCE

In addition to limited financial support, the HMO Act provided for several other forms of assistance designed to aid HMO development. Congress felt that this kind of encouragement and stimulus was essential if HMOs were to have the opportunity to prove themselves in the competitive health care market.

Restrictive State Laws

First, the federal legislation superseded restrictive state laws to the extent that they impeded the development of HMOs in meeting the requirements of the act. Some existing state legal barriers related to physician control, open physician participation in HMOs, and the prohibition or restriction of group practice. Although this state law override was initially considered vital to the development of HMOs, federal officials realized the potential difficulties in enforcing such federal mandates on state lawmakers and officials. Thus, the federal Office of Health Maintenance Organizations sponsored educational programs and provided support to the states to help change restrictive state laws. The result was that most states enacted state HMO-enabling laws that

---

[15] Ibid., p. 5.

[16] Linda E. Demkovich. "Private Sector Moves in as Washington Ends Its Financial Assistance for HMOs." *National Journal*, (15):1787–1789, September 3, 1983.

allowed for HMO development; however, in many instances the laws were as, or more, stringent than the federal HMO Act in requiring developing HMOs to meet certain financial, management, health services delivery, underwriting, and marketing standards. By the mid-1980s a significant number of HMOs opted not to become federally qualified because, in many instances, state licensure was more rigorous than the qualification process.

Employees' Health Plans, Dual Choice, and Mandating

HMOs are given an opportunity to compete in the labor marketplace with other health insurance plans through a mandating process. This provision of the HMO Act requires that an employer with 25 or more workers, subject to the minimum wage provisions of the Fair Labor Standards Act, include in the company's health benefits plan (if it has one) the option of joining a federally qualified HMO in the area. This selection option is called dual (or multiple) choice.

Regulation for Quality Care Assurance

The assurance of quality care by HMOs is aided by the authority given to the secretary of Health and Human Services to continue to regulate HMOs that receive financial assistance or are federally qualified under the legislation.

RELATION TO MEDICARE AND MEDICAID

The law exempts HMOs from the definitional requirements of the act with respect to Medicare and Medicaid enrollees, for whom health care services continue to be those allowed under the two programs. The Social Security Administration, however, through the Medicare program, can contract only with HMOs qualified by the Public Health Service under the HMO Act; those contracts continue to be under the control of the Social Security Administration. Also, federal participation with HMOs under the Medicaid program was limited to contracts with qualified HMOs, excluding Neighborhood Health Centers, Migrant Projects, Appalachian Regional Commission Projects, and organizations with a contract in effect for several years. In 1985, with the passage of the Tax Equity and Fiscal Responsibility Act of 1982, the Federal Government was also authorized to contract with competitive medical plans and HMOs for the provision of Medicare Part A and B health services to program recipients. At that time, risk contracts with both qualified HMOs and "eligible" CMPs were placed under the control of the Health Care Financing Administration, DHHS.

EVALUATION OF THE HMO PROGRAM: QUALITY CARE ASSURANCE PROGRAMS AND PROGRAM OPERATION AND COMPLIANCE

P.L. 93-222 calls for research and evaluation programs on the effectiveness, administration, and enforcement of quality assurance programs for health care to be conducted by the secretary of Health and Human Services through the assistant secretary for health. The secretary also is directed to contract with an appropriate nonprofit private organization for an independent study of health care quality assurance programs. The study is to include the development of a set of basic principles, to be followed by an effective health care quality assurance system that will relate to such matters as the scope of the system, methods for assessing care, data requirements, and specifications for developing criteria and standards concerning desired outcomes of care. The organization selected must have a national reputation for objectivity in the conduct of studies for the Federal Government, expertise, and a history of interest and activity in health policy issues.

HMO QUALIFICATION

The HMO laws describe the standards that an HMO must meet to become a "qualified" HMO—the federal seal of approval. During the period from 1974 through 1981, when grants and loans were available, qualification, or a statement by a new HMO seeking federal funds that it would attempt to become qualified under the HMO law, allowed that organization to qualify for federal grant funds, loans, and loan guarantees. Most health plans have found that the major advantages of qualification include:

- Mandating of employers, which allows the plan to gain access to otherwise closed accounts and obtain a potential competitive edge on traditional health insurance programs
- A continuous process of review and evaluation of all aspects of the operation of the health plan—in effect, a management control process not unlike accreditation activities in other health services organizations
- The opportunity to obtain outside managerial advice and assistance from federal qualification reviewers expert in the operation of successful HMOs
- Approval by the Federal Government, signifying a certain level of performance by the qualified HMO that may assist employers in choosing among health plans

- The opportunity to contract with federal and state governments regarding health services to beneficiaries under Medicare and Medicaid; Native Americans; migrant workers; federal employees and their dependents covered under the Federal Employees Plan (FEP) of FEHBP, and other programs such as the Primus and NavCare programs of the Army and Navy; individuals covered under CHAMPUS; and individuals eligible for veterans' health benefits under Veterans Administration programs
- Positioning of the HMO for qualification to receive capitated payments from the Federal Government if and when federal social health insurance programs are expanded to include more individuals than under the current Medicare program

On the other hand, qualification is a long process, requiring complex reporting to the Federal Government as well as adherence to regulations (some of which have been modified through amendments to the HMO Act) that can put the operation at a competitive disadvantage to other health services. Disadvantages may include the following:

- The need to community rate—although the amendments to the HMO Act allow substantial flexibility—may seriously affect the HMO's ability to compete with a nonqualified plan that experience rates its premiums
- The lack of flexibility in the benefits packages that can be offered by qualified plans, and the HMO's inability to compete with plans that offer made-to-order benefits packages that may include substantial copays and deductibles as well as limited benefits, or to offer "triple-option" programs; recent amendments have also provided great flexibility to the HMO to offer less-comprehensive packages
- The potential for enrollment problems, especially adverse selection of the HMO by individuals in ill health, based on open enrollment requirements; the amendments to the act have mitigated the effect of this requirement if it threatens the HMO's financial viability
- The cost of the qualification process in both direct payments to the Federal Government for direct qualification activities and staff time spent on preparing qualification documents and the like, rather than on other HMO activities
- Under the risk-contracting process, insufficient payments to the HMO for Medicare recipients, which may not provide funds to cover all of the health services costs under the contract

In order to qualify, an application must be filed with the federal Health Care Financing Administration in Washington, D.C. Notification and deficiency letters are then sent to the HMO requesting information on areas needing further clarification or substantiation. Sites are visited by a group of national HMO officials, including legal, health care, management, marketing, and financial specialists. The team reports its findings to an HMO case officer, who reports his or her findings to the qualification officer. Ultimately, the division administrator for the DHHS Office of Prepaid Health Care approves or disapproves the HMO.

Amendments to Title XIII of the Public Health Service Act

The original act was amended in 1976, 1978, 1980, 1981, 1986, and 1988. Amendments and legislative acts that deal with other health-related topics also have affected qualified HMOs; these include the 1979 amendments to the National Health Planning and Resources Development Act (P.L. 97-79), the 1979 amendments to the Health Planning Act (P.L. 92-603), the Tax Equity and Fiscal Responsibility Act of 1982 (P.L. 97-248), and the Omnibus Budget Reconciliation Acts of 1986 through 1989, among others. The most important issues of these laws are:

- Changes in the process of mandating employers
- Modifications to the basic and supplemental benefits packages
- Use of community rating, changed to adjusted community rating and community rating by class
- Provision that allows HMOs to meet employer demands for rates that reflect the experience of their employees and dependents
- Authorization to allow the HMO greater flexibility in organizational structure and provider contracts
- Funding of grants through FY 1984
- Funding of loans through FY 1986
- Repeal of the original funding authorizations in 1986
- Repeal of the open enrollment requirement
- Authorization for the HMO to arrange for its physicians to assume all or part of the financial risk for basic health services on a prospective basis
- Repeal of the requirement for Health Systems Agency review of qualified HMO programs

Although these and other changes to the HMO Act are important, the 1988 amendments provided for major changes in premium-rating activities. Previously, HMOs were allowed to use only community rating or community rating by class. Bowing to employer pressures that premiums should be based in part on the utilization and cost experience of particular employers' employees and dependents, the act allows for HMOs to use "adjusted community rating." HMOs now can set rates at the beginning of the policy year based on the anticipated experience of members; premiums, however, cannot be adjusted at the end of the year based on actual experience, that is, retrospective experience rating is specifically forbidden. In this way, an HMO continues to be at risk for care in excess of premiums paid, and it must be prepared to disclose the rating formulas and the data on which the rates are based to employers.

The requirement that an employer with 25 or more employees must offer the option of choosing a federally qualified HMO program was interpreted as requiring contributions to HMOs equal to the highest contribution made to alternative health plans. For example, if the employer contributes $200 to a Blue Cross/Blue Shield premium for family coverage, a similar amount has to be available as the employer's contribution for the HMO's family package. The 1988 HMO Act amended this section to require that employer contributions for employees that enroll in the HMO program must not "financially discriminate" against those employees. It was felt that some HMOs had been "shadow pricing" by setting their premiums on what employers contributed to competing health plans rather than basing them on the costs of operation or community rating. This change allows employers to determine their contribution to HMO premiums on other than a dollar-for-dollar basis, but one that does not discriminate against any person enrolled in the HMO. Finally, the 1988 act specified the repeal of the dual choice mandate and the employer contributions section of the HMO Act seven years after its enactment, which would be October 24, 1995.

Were the HMO Laws Successful?

Title XIII of the Public Health Service Act was originally enacted to help solve three problems—the maldistribution of health resources, the escalation in health care costs, and the quality of care. Specifically, the act and its amendments served as a time-limited demonstration program to provide assistance in the development of HMOs. The HMO concept, as defined through the legislation, appeared to be an effective means of providing comprehensive health services efficiently and economically.

With regard to the maldistribution problem, Congress gave preference to funding HMO development in rural and medically underserved areas until that section of the act was amended in 1981. Although 20 percent of the funds were set aside for nonmetropolitan areas, approximately 13 percent of the total funds were awarded. Generally, there were a limited number of applications and an even more limited number of application approvals from rural areas. Several rural HMOs exist today, but they tend to be small, with limited financial success. Thus, the act has not had a major impact on the maldistribution problem.

Have HMOs had an effect on the escalation of health care costs, and have they contained costs? National health expenditures and the costs of health services continue to rise; national health expenditures as a percent of the U.S. gross national product rose from 7.4 percent in 1970 to 11.1 percent in 1987. Since only a small portion of the U.S. population with health insurance coverage has been enrolled in HMOs (from approximately 2 percent in 1970 to approximately 13 percent in 1989), it may be more useful to review the "savings" created by the HMO industry. According to the Group Health Association of America, the national association of HMOs, HMO monthly premiums increased less than 3 percent during 1986, while the medical care portion of the Consumer Price Index went up 7.5 percent, and all employers paid 7.7 percent more for health care per employee in 1986 than the year before. Also, conventional insurance products increased 11 percent between 1987 and 1988, while group model HMO premiums increased only 8 percent. By 1989, HMO premiums rose 16 percent, which was slightly less than the 16.9 percent increase in 1988 and higher than the growth in the medical care component of the Consumer Price Index for the same period. These substantial increases in premiums from 1986 through 1989 suggest that HMOs may have held premiums at an artificially low level prior to 1986; however, HMO premium increases generally were below the increases in indemnity premiums for the same period.

HMO inpatient utilization rates were substantially below the national average for 1987—394 days per 1,000 HMO members versus the national average of 809 days per 1,000 individuals under age 65. Persons over age 65 averaged 1,945 days per 1,000 in HMOs, compared to a national average of 3,030 days per 1,000 population. Overall, inpatient hospital days per 1,000 enrollees for the nation were approximately 70 percent higher than they were for the average established HMO. National discharge rates were some 40 percent higher, and a length of hospital stay was approximately 20 percent higher than in HMOs. Although these rates may represent variations in HMO practice style and the populations included in the HMO versus the national data, the differences are significant. This becomes even more important because physician visits per HMO enrollee per year were at the national rate—4.3 ambulatory encounters per HMO member and 4.4 visits per person nationally for the under age 65 population, and 9.1 ambulatory encounters for over age 65 HMO enrollees versus 8.1 physician visits for the over age 65 national population.[17] Thus,

---

[17] Group Health Association of America. "HMO Profile Examines Utilization Patterns." *HMO Managers Letter,* 5(11):6, June 20, 1988.

by passing the HMO Act, Congress has fostered cost containment—at least for approximately one-tenth of the population.

Have HMOs been instrumental in controlling the quality of health services? Two areas of inquiry are necessary to answer this question—one deals with the clinical or professional aspects of health services delivery while the other deals with patient satisfaction. Most studies of morbidity, mortality, and health outcomes suggest that HMOs are equal to or better than the traditional system in managing patient care and appropriate outcomes.[18] There continue to be questions, however, about physician incentives in HMOs to limit care, as evidenced by the passage of Sections 9312 and 9313 of the Medicare Quality Protection Act of 1986 and the Office of Prepaid Health Care's tightening of its interpretation of the 1973 HMO and 1985 CMP statutory language regarding quality assurance policies and standards.[19] In addition, the question of patient/enrollee satisfaction continually receives mixed answers. Overall, HMO consumers appear to be satisfied with the health services they are receiving, but HMOs continue to experience problems in the length of waiting time for appointments, parking arrangements, availability of hospitals, and continuity of care.[20] Title XIII probably has had little effect on the quality of health services provided in HMOs or in the traditional system; health outcome studies of HMO prototypes (prior to passage of the HMO Act) show results similar to those for current HMO activities.

Finally, did Title XIII provide assistance in developing HMOs? The answer is "yes," although the initial ambitious projections in 1972 of 450 HMOs by

---

[18] Shouldice. "Questioning the Quality of Health Services," pp. 8–11.

[19] Sections 9312 and 9313 of the Medicare Quality Improvement Act address the issue of quality assurance of services provided to recipients under Titles XVIII and XIX using incentive systems. Section 9312 provides the following amendment that is relevant to risk-sharing contracts with the Health Care Financing Administration. If an eligible organization with a risk-sharing contract fails to provide medically necessary services that are required to be provided to the individual as outlined in the contract, then that organization will be subject to a civil money penalty of not more than $10,000 in the event that the failure has affected the individual. Section 9313 provides the following relevant amendment to Section 1869(b)(1) of the Social Security Act: If a hospital or HMO knowingly makes a payment, directly or indirectly, to a physician as an inducement to reduce or limit services to individuals who are indigent (recipients under Titles XVIII and XIX) or just normal enrollees, these physicians and the health care entity will be subject to penalties of not more than $2,000 per individual described. Section 4016 of OBRA 1987, however, delayed the enactment of this amendment, prohibiting physician incentive arrangements with HMOs until January 1, 1990. Section 9313 also provides for the development of a strategy for quality review and assurance; the secretary shall arrange for a study to design a strategy for reviewing and assuring the quality of care for which payment may be made under Title XVIII of the Social Security Act.

[20] Shouldice and Singpurwalla, "Consumer Satisfaction and Quality of Health Services"; and Group Health Association of America, "HMO Fact Sheet," Washington, D.C., GHAA, May 1988, p. 4.

1973 and 1,700 by 1976, with an enrollment of 40 million, were way off target. The act was successful in bringing a large percentage of its grantees from development to successful operation. The greater success of the program, however, was its halo effect in generating interest among the private sector to invest in HMO development and operation and to create a competitive environment in the medical care industry, where HMOs, PPOs, and other alternative delivery systems provide the potential for helping solve the original three questions addressed by Congress in 1973.

Current Federal HMO Activity

As originally conceived, the HMO Act was a time-limited demonstration program to assist HMO growth; Congress did not intend for HMOs to be continually federally funded. Indeed, the federal role throughout the 1980s was that of a venture capital investor, spurring HMO growth through the distribution of initial supporting funds and the stimulation of private investment. Currently, the federal role is in the areas of qualification, compliance, and administration of the loan repayment program. The federal HMO strategy during the Reagan and Bush administrations called for doubling the current number of HMOs nationwide and tripling enrollment over 1980 levels. Described by the Bush administration as the Private Health Plan Option (PHPO), federal policy continues to place priorities on the development of capitated risk contracts with provider organizations that serve beneficiaries under federal programs. Generally, the three goals of the national HMO strategy through the 1980s were:[21]

1. To increase the number of HMOs so as to increase the public's access to comprehensive health services
2. To expand enrollment in existing HMOs and increase competition in the health care system
3. To maximize the cost-savings potential of HMOs

The federal role continues to include a review of the present legislation, with the objective of making revisions that will assist in expanding HMOs and their ability to be successful. Some members of Congress, as well as health industry leaders, feel that the current HMO legislation has fulfilled its purpose and is no longer needed; they speak of "sunsetting" the act by 1991, although most in the field feel that repeal of the HMO Act seems premature.

---

[21] U.S. Department of Health and Human Services, Health Care Financing Administration, Office of Health Maintenance Organizations. *HMO Governing Board Handbook,* Rockville, Md., DHHS, HCFA, OHMO, April 1981, p. 17.

Other HMO Enabling and Assistance Laws

Together with several existing laws, there are two major programs that enable enrollment in and assist with the planning, development, and operation of HMOs: the Federal Employees Health Benefits Program and Medicare and Medicaid.

P.L. 86-382—THE FEDERAL EMPLOYEES HEALTH BENEFITS ACT OF 1959

Federal employees and annuitants have had the option of electing a comprehensive medical plan to cover their health benefits since enactment of P.L. 86-382, the Federal Employees Health Benefits Act of 1959, which became effective July 1, 1960. Under this act, Federal Employees Plan beneficiaries can choose between a health service benefits plan (Blue Cross/Blue Shield), several indemnity benefit plans (historically, Aetna was the major plan), one of several employee organization plans, or an approved HMO, referred to as a "comprehensive medical plan." Generally, an employee must live within the service area of the HMO to be eligible for that option. The program is administered by the Office of Personnel Management (OPM), which has the authority to contract for and approve the various health plans, the benefits offered, and the rate-setting method to be used. Benefits are comprehensive, including inpatient, ambulatory, and supplemental benefits. Regarding rate setting, OPM allows experience rating, but has strict rules regarding costs used in the rating process.

In February 1990, there were approximately 10 million federal employees, dependents, and annuitants. More than 300 health benefits plans were offered. HMOs provided coverage to approximately 25 percent of the eligible enrollees and dependents. In comparison, in 1970, there were only 10 HMOs in the FEP, serving less than 4 percent of the federal workers.[22]

A study commissioned by the Office of Personnel Management in 1988 identified problems in the Federal Employees Health Benefits Program— especially fragmentation of the risk pool and lack of competition to enter and remain in the program. The fragmentation may be due to the proliferation of participating HMOs. According to the study, it is estimated that inefficiencies in the structure and operation of the FEHBP are costing the Federal Government nearly $500 million a year. These findings may suggest changes in contracting

---

[22] Group Health Association of America. "FEHBP Reform Review Underway." *HMO Managers Letter*, 5(9):1, May 23, 1988.

procedures with the health plans and the government, which could have a substantial impact on plans where the FEHBP represents their single largest source of enrollment. For example, 1990 proposals recommend streamlining the system by offering one plan only with two basic options—standard and high—with employees paying $10 every two weeks for individual coverage and $22 for family coverage under the standard plan.

MEDICARE AND MEDICAID

Medicare (Title XVIII); P.L. 92-603—The Social Security Amendments of 1972; and P.L. 97-248—The Tax Equity and Fiscal Responsibility Act of 1982

Medicare beneficiaries have been eligible to receive certain services from HMO organizations since the original Medicare act was passed in 1965. Under Section 1833(a) of the law, a prepayment organization that provides or arranges for the provision of medical and other health services could elect to be reimbursed on a reasonable-charge (fee-for-service) basis or it could deal directly with the Social Security Administration on a capitation basis (i.e., "direct dealing"). It is important to note that this authority was extended only to Part B, physician services, and not Part A, hospitalization.

The Social Security Administration established general guidelines for the type of plans it would approve under this program, encouraging the larger, well-established plans with a broad range of benefits to seek this mechanism. A liberal interpretation of prepaid group practice was made, however, which allowed great flexibility in payment. As of December 1975, there were 390,000 Medicare beneficiaries enrolled in 39 HMO plans, with the Social Security Administration paying approximately $90 million for services on their behalf during 1975.

Several important changes in the administration of Medicare were proposed in Alternative C to Medicare. Section 226 of P.L. 92-603, signed into law on October 30, 1972, provides the authority to contract with HMOs for covered services, using monthly capitation payments for services covered by both Parts A and B.

The Tax Equity and Fiscal Responsibility Act of 1982 authorized Medicare to pay organizations—including qualified HMOs and eligible CMPs—a prospective capitation for Medicare recipients who elected to enroll in the HMO or CMP. These risk-sharing contracts became available in February 1985. By late 1988, it was estimated that more than 1.82 million recipients were enrolled in risk-contract HMOs, with another 582,000 Medicare recipients enrolled in HMOs under federal cost contracts but receiving their care on a fee-for-service basis.

Medicaid (Title XIX); P.L. 92-603—The Social Security Amendments of 1972; and P.L. 97-25—The Omnibus Budget Reconciliation Act of 1981[23]

Medicaid is a federal/state public assistance program that has been implemented in all states and U.S. territories and possessions. The program is administered at the state and local levels within very broad guidelines established by DHHS's Rehabilitation Services Administration. The cost to the federal and state governments of funding Medicaid, the largest program providing medical assistance to the poor, has grown from a 1965 estimate of $250 million annually to more than $45 billion in 1987. Lawmakers envisioned that only 2.3 million individuals would be enrolled in the program at any given time, but by 1987, more than 23.0 million persons qualified for health services assistance. Because states share in these programs, approximately half of the costs are paid by the Federal Government. The escalating cost of the program (between 1986 and 1987, average annualized growth, adjusted for inflation, was 14.5 percent), compounded by high health care inflation, led federal policymakers to reevaluate the program and, ultimately, to allow states to explore innovative financing mechanisms as ways to cut Medicaid costs without reducing services covered under the program.

Payments to providers on a capitated basis have been explored by states to control costs and utilization. States are free to negotiate and implement Medicaid/HMO contracts as they desire. Because of unfamiliarity on the part of officials, indifference, and lack of provider groups considered acceptable by Title XIX state agencies, few contracts were signed prior to 1976. As of mid-1989, at least 180 HMOs had contracts with state Medicaid agencies.

Success in the use of capitated systems, including HMO experience in commercial settings and experimental Medicare risk contracting, led Congress to pass additional legislation in 1976, 1981, 1985, 1986, 1987, and 1988 promoting capitated risk contracting in the Medicaid program.[24] The state agrees to prepay a contracting entity a flat fixed amount per Medicaid recipient for a negotiated period of time. In exchange, the organization agrees to provide a negotiated range of services to the Medicaid members. Thus, the contractor/provider is "at risk" for costs that exceed payments by the state; this gives the contractor a strong incentive to control utilization and costs.

---

[23] This discussion is based on Robert G. Shouldice, "Medicaid Contracts and Capitation," *Medical Group Management*, 34(2):13–14, March/April 1987.

[24] 1976 HMO Amendments (P.L. 94-460); 1981 Omnibus Budget Reconciliation Act (OBRA—P.L. 97-25); 1985 Consolidated Budget Reconciliation Act (COBRA—P.L. 99-272); Omnibus Budget Reconciliation Act of 1986 (OBRA—P.L. 99-117, Section 9313); Omnibus Budget Reconciliation Act of 1987 (OBRA—P.L. 99-509, Section 4016); and Sixth Omnibus Budget Reconciliation Act of 1988 (SOBRA—P.L. 100-203).

Services required in the contract follow Medicaid (Title XIX) guidelines and are comprehensive in nature, like those of HMO commercial packages and competitive medical plans for Medicare recipients. States have the option of expanding covered services above the standard set of services to include care in intermediate facilities, dental care, pharmaceutical services, and eyeglasses. Many states prefer to contract with just one regional organization that can provide or arrange for the provision of all covered services; this concept is known as "geographic capitation."

The enabling legislation, especially the Omnibus Budget Reconciliation Act of 1981 (OBRA), has achieved its desired effect. Prior to OBRA, only 17 state Medicaid agencies, including the District of Columbia, had these contracts, covering only 1 percent of the Medicaid population. In 1988, 27 states had entered into such contracts, covering an estimated 8 percent of Medicaid recipients. As of June 30, 1989, there were 1.1 million Medicaid beneficiaries in 183 plans, of which 127 were federally or state qualified HMOs. OBRA provided for large reductions in the federal share of Medicaid program costs, as well as an expansion of alternative financing approaches, thus providing incentives to the states to develop cost-controlling approaches.

Medicare and Medicaid membership in these plans can be as high as, but cannot exceed, 75 percent of total plan membership. States may extend Medicaid eligibility for enrollees for up to six months, after which an individual's eligibility technically ends—thus resolving many of the administrative difficulties of managing a prepaid system that enrolls members whose eligibility can change monthly. States can also impose a six-month lock-in period on individuals, during which time their membership in a plan is guaranteed, provided that voluntary disenrollment is allowed during the first month of enrollment and that disenrollment is allowed thereafter upon showing good cause.

In addition, federal waivers of these rules are granted when the state can show such a waiver to be "efficient, cost-effective, and consistent with the objectives of the Medicaid program." Under the Consolidated Budget Reconciliation Act (COBRA), certain waivers can continue on request. One waiver allows new plans to have more than 75 percent of their membership in the Medicaid program or 50 percent combined Medicare and Medicaid enrollment. The Tax Equity and Fiscal Responsibility Act of 1982 allows for a three-year extension of the 75 percent waiver, provided that the plan shows that it is attempting to enroll commercial accounts. As of 1990, some 30 states had requested waivers under Section 2175 of OBRA.

State Medicaid agencies administer the program and can contract on a risk basis with several types of organizations, including HMOs, prepaid health plans (PHPs), and health-insuring organizations (HIOs). All HMO models, including the staff, group, network, and IPA models, are now represented with state contracts, but the medical group model has the lowest enrollment (approximately 6 percent of the total Medicaid population enrolled in plans, with enrollment in the other three models equally divided). PHPs do not qualify as HMOs but are (1) organizations that provide health care, have received grants of $100,000 or more from the Public Health Service since 1976, and will provide and/or arrange for the provision of a full range of services under Medicaid; (2) nonprofit primary care entities in rural areas; or (3) organizations that have had contracts with the state to provide services on a prepaid risk basis since 1970. HIOs do not provide services but act as service brokers for the state, meet the state insurance requirements, and are willing to contract to provide all or most acute care services to the Medicaid population on an at-risk basis.

The yearly capitation payment cannot exceed what the Federal Government estimates that the state would pay for those same services in the traditional fee-for-service system. In most cases, states have paid contracting organizations 90 to 95 percent of estimated fee-for-service costs. This approach is generally accepted in capitated medicine because it is felt that inpatient utilization will be reduced from the high fee-for-service rates to approximately 499 days per 1,000 enrollees (a rate higher than that of HMO commercial enrollees but less than the 600 days per 1,000 individuals in the traditional delivery system). Setting capitation rates, however, has been a difficult task for the states; the rates must demonstrate a savings over the traditional system and yet be high enough to interest potential contracting entities. Generally, historic "paid claims" data provide the basis for determining what agencies paid by county. Then the agency determines the adjusted average per capita cost (AAPCC), the average cost to the state for providing services to each Medicaid member of the specified population group within a specific geographic area. After additional adjustments by "rate cells," the agency will reduce the estimated fee-for-service costs through a program savings percentage, such as 5 percent, creating a final capitation rate of only 95 percent of the fee-for-service cost. States may also deduct a percentage of the capitation rate to cover their administrative expenses.

Like other federal and state program participation, the HMO must weigh the benefits of improving Medicaid payments and other advantages against the costs and problems inherent in these contracts. Advantages for HMOs that are already serving Medicaid patients *and* are involved with capitated systems with the government may include improved payment for services, a lock-in on a segment of the market, and a greater financial stability for the HMO. Conversely, there are concerns about developing a state contract: marketing and enrollment issues, use of appropriate management informations systems, and financial issues such as physician reimbursement and adverse risk-taking by the health plan. Marketing is usually handled through or approved by the state Medicaid agency, at least initially, an arrangement that may create awkward and potentially ineffective activities. Further, little is known about the Medicaid recipient's incentives to enroll or not enroll in the plan. Enrollment may be voluntary or mandatory, and questions of extending plan eligibility beyond Medicaid eligibility must be considered. Lock-in arrangements add more confusion to the issue. Management information systems and physician compensation questions are common to all HMOs and may or may not pose greater problems in Medicaid risk contracting.

Summary

The HMO philosophy has evolved over the past 80 years. It grew from a need to obtain adequate health care, usually when the traditional fee-for-service system could not cope with the demand. Although several plans began prior to 1929, the major growth of HMO organizations came after that date. Pre-1929 plans usually were developed around a group practice of physicians for particular groups of employees and were initiated by the employees themselves or by their employers. These group practices generally were formed as partnerships; early medical group practices include the Mayo Clinic, the Palo Alto and Ross-Loos medical clinics, the Bridge clinics, and the Western Clinic.

The Great Depression of 1929 was instrumental in changing the social structure of American life, including the financing and delivery of health care. Health insurance was introduced by the American Hospital Association in the form of Blue Cross plans to finance hospital care and thus to stabilize the critical financial plight of hospitals. Individuals were faced with serious financial problems and lack of access to acceptable medical care. Using the English and European cooperative society concepts as models, Americans joined together in a common effort; with strength and stability in numbers, health cooperatives began to appear.

The early cooperative philosophy stressed stability and security in group action—*assurance* of health care services rather than *insurance* against loss due to illness or accident. It was not until competitive pressures were felt from Blue Cross and Blue Shield and the private insurance companies that the prepaid health plans began to identify one of their objectives as an insurance function. The early cooperative experiments regarded the function of pooling individual resources for the good of the group as a method for controlling the cost of medical care and a way of including economics in health delivery. Over time, individual members would save money—their limited financial resources would go farther. The cooperatives were described as a socialized approach—not in the political sense of a federal social program but in terms of a group action approach of "self-help."

The passage of the Wagner Act hastened the expansion of labor unions and the resultant bargaining for health benefits by union employees. For the first time, many employers were forced to participate in financing health care for their employees and in developing new health care plans. Union- and employer-sponsored prepaid health plans appeared throughout the country. This interest in negotiable health benefits was heightened during World War II, when such benefits were used as a method of attracting employees from a limited civilian labor force. Employer and union awareness of prepaid health plans has influenced sound management principles in the provision of quality care to employees and the delivery of health care by all providers.

The early plans sought stability and quality care—a comprehensive rather than a piecework, fee-for-service approach to health care. The prepaid plans' objectives of quality and comprehensive care required that both consumers and providers hold joint and parallel objectives. This compromise approach between a totally federal socialized system and a totally fee-for-service solo practice system further required that the health system have controls to safeguard the interests of both vendor and patient. The cooperative's members needed total financial disclosure and quality care in exchange for prospective monthly payments. The physicians needed an environment where they could practice their profession without the financial constraints of a fee-for-service system and could demand a salary or retainer comparable to yearly fee-for-service income. The physicians also were interested in using joint action, with the objective of providing quality care—the thesis being that medical care is not only a long-term joint venture among providers but also between the providers and the health plan members. Ultimately, the interests of the medical group became the interests of its community.

By 1967, HMO activities were recognized by health care experts as a possible method for controlling the rapid increase in the cost and utilization of medical care. Federal Government interest in the HMO concept, beginning in 1968, was based on a recognition of three major health-related problems that may be partly solved by the use of HMOs. The first was maldistribution of health resources among geographic areas in the country and among selected socioeconomic groups. A second problem was the escalating cost of health care as a result of the increasing demand for services without concurrent increases in the supply of such services or large increases in the productivity of providers. The third problem was the inability of purchasers of care—the public as well as the Federal Government—to recognize and evaluate the quality of care rendered, as well as the difficulties experienced by providers in controlling the quality of care.

By the beginning of 1973, with the introduction of numerous bills, none of which were passed, the Nixon administration changed its forthright stand for HMOs to a time-limited demonstration approach. No long-term federal commitment was to be made for HMO activities. By December 1973, an HMO bill, S. 14, had been signed into law—P.L. 93-222, the Health Maintenance Organization Act of 1973, authorized the expenditure of $375 million over a five-year period. Additional amendments extended that authorization to the present, although grant activities terminated in 1981. Development assistance of $145 million in grants and $205.3 million in loans was provided to a limited number of HMO projects, with the ultimate goal of self-sufficiency. These demonstration projects were designed to help stimulate the interest of consumers and providers in the HMO concept and its potential advantages, and to interest private industry in investing in HMO development and operation.

One final word concerning the HMO laws: P.L. 93-222 and its amendments have certainly provided a far-reaching and innovative approach to traditional health delivery. It is forward looking in that it requires participating HMOs to provide ingenious financing mechanisms, it requires employers to provide the HMO option to their employees if a qualified HMO is available in their locality, and it identifies a comprehensive set of treatment and preventive health services. Some experts projected that the health industry would not be able to meet these challenges—especially the expanded benefits packages, which they say may not be competitive with the traditional BC/BS and indemnity programs currently available. It appears that the HMO strategy did work; today more than 32 million Americans are enrolled in 590 HMOs nationwide, and the federal HMO Act helped create substantial interest in and financial support of HMOs and other alternative delivery systems.

References

Casselman, P. H. *The Cooperative Movement and Some of Its Problems.* New York, The Philosophical Library, 1952.

Chase, Stuart. *The Story of Toad Lane.* Chicago, Ill., The Cooperative League of the U.S.A., 1969.

Committee on the Costs of Medical Care. *Medical Care for the American People.* Chicago, Ill., University of Chicago Press, 1933. (Reprint ed. Washington, D.C. Community Health Services, Health Services and Mental Health Administration, U.S. Department of Health, Education, and Welfare, 1970, pp. v–xiii, 103–144.)

Dorsey, Joseph L. "The Health Maintenance Organization Act of 1973 (P.L. 93-222) and Prepaid Group Practice Plans." *Medical Care,* XIII(1):1–9, January 1975.

Ford, James. *Co-operation in New England.* New York, Survey Associates, Inc., 1913.

Gintzig, Leon, and Robert G. Shouldice. "Prepaid Group Practice—A Comparative Study." Part I. Vols. 1–3. Washington, D.C., The George Washington University, 1971.

InterStudy. *National HMO Census 1987.* Excelsior, Minn., 1988.

Kress, John R., and James Singer. *HMO Handbook.* Gaithersburg, Md., Aspen Publishers, Inc., 1975, pp. 33–108.

MacColl, William A. *Group Practice and Prepayment of Medical Care*. Washington, D.C., Public Affairs Press, 1966, pp. 10–56.

McCaffree, Kenneth M. "How Organized Medical Programs Have Been Established: The Urban Cooperative Plan." *Proceedings of the 9th Group Health Institute*. Chicago, Ill., Group Health Association of America, 1969, pp. 31–34.

McLeod, Gordon K. "The Federal Role in Health Maintenance Organizations." In: *Health Maintenance Organizations, Proceedings of a Conference, 1972*. Denver, Colo., Medical Group Management Association, 1972, pp. 2–4.

Prussin, Jeffrey A. *HMO Legislation in 1973–74*. The Health Legislation Report Series, Vol. 11. Washington, D.C., Science and Health Publications, Inc., 1974.

Rafkind, Faith B. *Health Maintenance Organizations: Some Perspectives*. Chicago, Ill., Blue Cross Association, 1972.

Rorem, C. Rufus. *Private Group Clinics*. New York, Milbank Memorial Fund, 1971, pp. 115–118. (Reprint)

Roy, William R. *The Proposed Health Maintenance Organization Act of 1972*. Washington, D.C., Science and Health Communications Group, 1972, pp. 1–29, 162–257.

Schwartz, Jerome L. *Medical Plans and Health Care*. Springfield, Ill., Charles C Thomas, Publisher, 1968.

Statement of Frank C. Carlucci Before the Subcommittee on Public Health and Environment, Committee on Interstate and Foreign Commerce. March 6, 1973.

Strumpf, George B.; Frank H. Seubold; and Mildred B. Arrill. "Health Maintenance Organizations, 1971–1977: Issues and Answers." *Journal of Community Health*, 4(1):33–54, Fall 1978.

University of Chicago, Graduate Program in Hospital Administration, Center for Health Administration Studies, Graduate School of Business. *Health Maintenance Organization: A Reconfiguration of the Health Services System*. Proceedings of the Thirteenth Annual Symposium on Hospital Affairs. Chicago, Ill., 1971, pp. 2–10.

U.S. Congress, House of Representatives. *Health Maintenance Organization Amendments of 1976*. P.L. 94-460. October 8, 1976.

U.S. Congress, House of Representatives. *Health Maintenance Organization Amendments of 1981*. 97th Congress, 1st Session, May 19, 1981. Report No. 98-88

U.S. Congress, Senate. *Health Maintenance Organization Act of 1973*. P.L. 93-222. December 29, 1973.

U.S. Department of Health, Education, and Welfare. *A Report to the President on Medical Care Prices*. Washington, D.C., U.S. Government Printing Office, 1967.

3

PREFERRED PROVIDER ORGANIZATIONS[1]

The preferred provider organization (PPO) is another innovation in managed care. Like HMOs, PPOs are designed to contain health benefits costs and to promote the delivery of high-quality, medically appropriate health services to members. Unlike traditional HMOs, however, PPOs generally seek to retain a high degree of freedom for their members in selecting the providers of their choice for each episode of care.

PPOs are largely the result of two related socioeconomic phenomena. First, major purchasers of health care are struggling to control escalating health care expenses without reducing benefits or compromising the quality of care for their beneficiaries. Consequently, they are beginning to take advantage of their considerable buying power to negotiate discounts and other preferential terms with providers in an attempt to contain the rapidly rising costs of employees' health benefits. Recently, A. Foster Higgins and Company, Inc., a large health benefits consulting and actuarial firm, conducted a health benefits survey of 2,017 employers with more than 13 million covered lives. The results showed that in 1987, the average employer spent $1,985 dollars per employee for health benefits, representing approximately 10 percent of payroll costs. In unionized companies, the figure was $2,364 per employee.[2] Total costs for health care benefits increased to approximately $3,200 per employee in 1990, an increase

---

[1] This chapter was written with the assistance of Julia Cronin Hawley, Ph.D., Executive Director, Travelers Health Network, a PPO in the Baltimore, Md./Washington, D.C. region.

[2] A. Foster Higgins and Company, Inc. "Foster Higgins Health Care Benefits Survey." *Medical Benefits*, 5(4):1–2, February 29, 1988.

of more than 60 percent over 1987 costs.[3] In effect, if allowed to increase, employee health benefits costs could wipe out other corporate benefits within the next few years.

The second socioeconomic phenomenon promoting PPO growth is heightened competition among providers, resulting from a surplus of physicians, an oversupply of hospital beds, and the growth of HMOs. Consequently, providers have become increasingly willing to negotiate premiums with purchasers in exchange for the potential of increasing, or at least maintaining, their market share. The resulting contractual arrangements between purchasers and providers of health services are the essence of the preferred provider organization.

The PPO Concept

Since the PPO concept was introduced in the early 1980s, PPOs have proliferated rapidly in number and distribution. As shown in Figure 3-1, PPO development has accelerated most between 1984 and 1987. The field includes more than 800 PPOs covering 60 to 65 million people who are eligible for PPO benefits and participation by approximately 48 percent of the acute general hospitals and 46 percent of the practicing medical and osteopathic physicians in the United States. Their popularity may derive from the fact that PPOs promise something for everyone. They offer each of the major stakeholders in the health care system—employers, insurers, providers, and subscribers—the potential to enhance their respective competitive positions in the marketplace without requiring inordinate compromises. PPOs are especially appealing because they do not disrupt the traditional fee-for-service health care financing and delivery system.

PPOs offer employers the potential to contain escalating health benefits expenses without compromising quality or accessibility of care. For insurers, the PPO enticement lies in discounted reimbursement rates and utilization controls, which together translate into the likelihood of a favorable underwriting experience. For providers, PPOs hold the potential to channel patients into their practices. Furthermore, PPOs usually offer traditional fee-for-service reimbursement, albeit at a discount, and often provide expeditious claims payment, thereby improving providers' cash flow and minimizing administrative overhead. Finally, for subscribers, the PPO promise is relative freedom to select the provider of their choice for any episode of care, with the opportunity to

---

[3] Russell A. Jackson, "Foster Higgins Survey Finds Health Benefits Cost Rose 20% in 1989," *Health Care Competition Week*, 7(10):4, March 5, 1990; and A. Foster Higgins and Company, Inc., personal communication, July 1991.

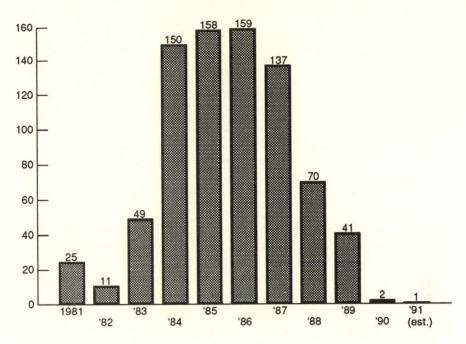

SOURCE: Edward Pickins, American Managed Care and Review Association. Personal Communication, June 11, 1991.

FIGURE 3-1   PPO development.

minimize out-of-pocket health care expenses by choosing designated preferred providers.

Are PPOs simply transitional managed care organizations that will evolve into HMOs? Or will PPOs continue to proliferate at a rapid rate and ultimately subsume a significant share of the traditional insurance market, to emerge as the dominant health care delivery and financing model in the 1990s? The answers to these and related questions are elusive because PPOs are so diverse in size, scope, sponsorship, and mission. The objective of this chapter is to provide a clear and rational overview of the key structural and functional features of PPOs.

Definition and Characteristics

Like HMOs, preferred provider organizations are somewhat difficult to define. In fact, the term preferred provider organization is, itself, something of a misnomer. PPOs rarely constitute formal organizations in the conventional sense.

Rather, they are brokered arrangements between providers and purchasers of health care services, the terms and conditions of which are specified by contract.

It may be more accurate to refer to this system of interrelationships as a preferred provider arrangement (PPA) rather than a preferred provider organization. Most of the literature on the subject uses the the latter designation. In the interest of consistency, this text will adhere to convention and use the term preferred provider organization or PPO throughout.

In generic terms, a preferred provider organization is described as a managed care arrangement in which a select, limited panel of health care providers contract to provide health care services, usually at a discount, to a defined population of patients.[4] Providers are induced to negotiate fees and submit to stringent utilization controls by the prospect of increased patient volume. Together, PPOs and PPAs are, therefore, contractual arrangements in which health providers agree to deliver health services to a defined patient population at established fees that may be discounted from usual and customary or reasonable charges and to allow utilization and quality reviews of their medical practices.[5] Purchasers (usually employers), in turn, offer health insurance benefits coverage to a defined group of beneficiaries, with a free choice of providers and economic incentives (such as reduced deductibles or copayments) to use designated preferred providers.

Managed care arrangements are designed to contain escalating health benefits costs without compromising the quality or accessibility of care. The typical PPO approaches this ideal in several ways. First, it selects and contracts with providers who are sensitive to the issue of escalating health benefits costs. Second, it negotiates substantial rate concessions from providers in exchange for their designation as preferred providers. Third, it conducts or arranges for systematic utilization management. Fourth, it provides a means of controlling employers' health benefits costs through benefits package designs that incorporate substantial economic incentives to use preferred providers.

As depicted in Figure 3-2, there are three major constituencies represented in preferred provider arrangements: the providers of health care services, the purchasers of those services, and the patients as ultimate users of the systems.

---

[4] Michael John Tichon. "PPOs: Definition and Background." In: *Attorneys and Physicians Examine Preferred Provider Organizations.* Edited by J. Mark Waxman, J.D. Washington, D.C., National Health Lawyers Association, 1984, p. 4.

[5] Pam Politser. "PPOs: Physicians Competing with HMOs." *Bulletin of the American College of Surgeons, 71*(5):24, May 1986.

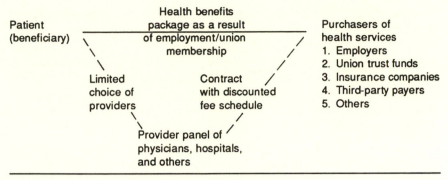

FIGURE 3-2 Preferred provider arrangement.

PROVIDERS

PPO provider panels usually include both a professional and an institutional component. The professional component is composed of physicians representing various medical and surgical specialties, augmented in some cases by selected nonphysician care givers, such as psychologists, podiatrists, and dentists. The mainstay of the institutional component is acute care hospitals. As PPOs grow in size and sophistication, however, it is becoming increasingly common to include other types of institutions on the panel, such as home health agencies, hospices, long-term care facilities, pharmacies, laboratories, and various ancillary care providers.

PURCHASERS

The purchasers of health care services in a PPO generally fall into primary and secondary categories. Primary purchasers include commercial insurance companies; third-party claims administrators; self-administered, self-funded employer groups; and union trust funds (including Taft-Hartley Health and Welfare Funds). These primary purchasers contract with PPO providers, either directly or through a PPO acting as a broker, for professional medical services at a negotiated price. The primary purchaser, with the assistance of the broker, designs, rates, and underwrites a PPO health insurance benefits plan option or options and subsequently offers the option(s) to its own employees and to secondary purchasers, such as other employers or union groups. The specific configuration of benefits varies considerably from plan to plan, but most PPO benefits packages have one key characteristic in common: they offer end users, or beneficiaries, freedom of choice in selecting a health care provider for any covered service, but provide substantial economic incentives to choose only preferred providers.

TABLE 3-1   Percentage of PPO Eligibles from Self-Insured Groups and Small Groups

Sponsor	From self-insured groups (percent)	From small groups* (percent)
Hospitals	74	15
Physicians	55	34
Blue Cross/Blue Shield	31	41
Commercial Insurers	37	27
Investor Owned	56	46

*Groups with fewer than 100 covered individuals.

SOURCE: Gregory de Lissovoy, Thomas Rice, Jon Gabel, and Heidi J. Gelzer. "Preferred Provider Organizations One Year Later." *Inquiry, 24*(2):132, Summer 1987.

One of the most important group of clients for the PPO is self-insured employers. These employers have shown, by becoming "self-insured" (that is, by taking direct control of the financing and benefits and claims administration of this employee fringe benefit), that they are interested not only in containing the costs of their employee/dependents health benefits package, but also in demonstrating this commitment through involvement with PPOs. PPO growth has not been confined to self-insured employers only. In most major urban areas, the majority of large employers offer PPOs; small employers searching for affordable insurance products are offering PPOs as well. Table 3-1 suggests that most PPO sponsors are active with self-insured and small groups.

PATIENTS (BENEFICIARIES)

The patient, as ultimate user of the system, may choose at the point of service from among any physician included on the PPO panel or, for that matter, any available physician in the community, for each episode of care. This is known as a "point-of-service" option. No prior or initial (at enrollment in the PPO) provider selection is necessary. This characteristic of PPOs creates a two-tiered benefits structure; when patients use designated preferred providers, their out-of-pocket expenses are reduced. A basic indemnity level of coverage, however, is provided for covered services rendered by non-PPO providers, but coinsurance and deductibles usually apply and the patient is responsible for any amounts that the provider bills in excess of the PPO maximum allowable payment. Thus, there is a relatively small but psychologically important financial incentive for the patient to choose panel physicians; this may be viewed as a partial lock-in of patients. Contrasted with HMOs that tend to create a total lock-in of enrollees in the HMO system, PPO enrollees have greater flexibility in the choice of physicians since the financial consequence of choosing an out-of-panel physician is significantly less than in an HMO, where the patient would have to pay the entire fee of an out-of-HMO-plan physician.

This also compares with the total lock-in used by exclusive provider organizations (EPOs). Like HMOs, EPOs require health plan members to use only the providers under contract, with no choice available if the enrollee wishes to avoid payment for services; the enrollee can use out-of-plan providers but must bear the total cost of their services. Two major advantages to the employer of using an EPO are simplified benefits administration and the ability to accurately determine potential savings, since both the treatment costs and the number of enrollees using exclusive providers and nonpreferred providers are known. Because PPOs do not require a total lock-in, employers may find it difficult to determine potential savings.

The Generic PPO Model

The generic PPO model, presented in Figure 3-3, provides the basic PPO components and interrelationships. In the arrangement shown, the PPO is independent of the buyers and sellers of health care services; it simply acts as a broker, mediating arrangements between the contracting parties. The PPO contracts with a select group of hospitals and physicians to deliver health care services at discounted rates. It subsequently markets the services of this provider panel to insurers. Insurers develop a PPO health benefits package with economic incentives for subscribers to use preferred providers. They also establish PPO claims payment mechanisms, underwrite the insurance risk, and market the benefits plan to employers.

Employers purchase the health insurance plan on behalf of their employees (beneficiaries or subscribers) and covered dependents in exchange for premiums paid to the insurance company. Employees and their covered dependents, referred to collectively as subscribers or members, use the benefits plan to pay for their medical care.

Although many PPOs do not adhere strictly to this generic model in terms of sponsorship and structure, most share at least the following common characteristics:[6]

- A panel of preferred providers (physicians, hospitals, and others), selected or self-appointed on the basis of quality and efficiency, whose number may be limited or unlimited

---

[6] Adapted from Dale H. Cowan, M.D., J.D. *Preferred Provider Organizations: Planning, Structure, and Operation.* Gaithersburg, Md., Aspen Publishers, Inc., 1984, p. 10.

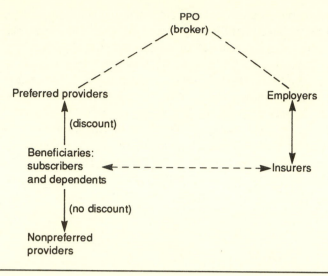

FIGURE 3-3   The generic PPO model.

- Negotiated contracts between purchasers and providers governing the delivery and financing of health care services
- Reimbursement arrangements based on negotiated fee schedules, usually reflecting a discount, with no assumption of insurance risk by providers
- Systematic utilization management and a management information system for tracking and reporting utilization and claims data, operating quality assurance programs, and having the capability to complete provider profiling
- Claims administration, including authorization to treat, examination and payment of claims, adjudication of disputed claims, and claims cost control
- PPO benefits packages, offering subscribers some flexibility in choice of provider, with economic incentives to use only preferred providers
- Client services, including marketing, eligibility verification, a provider referral process, and a consumer grievance procedure
- Provider relations that include physician and hospital selection processes, contract management, and a grievance appeal process
- Frequently, but not always, promotion of primary care physicians (gatekeepers) as the entry point into the system of services

Each of these features is explored in greater detail later in this chapter.

PPO Sponsorship

Perhaps the most accurate predictor of the nature, scope, design, and level of success of a particular PPO is its sponsorship. PPO sponsors include providers, insurance companies, investors, third-party administrators (TPAs), IPA/HMOs, and self-insured employers. Each of these sponsors approaches the PPO business with slightly different motives, objectives, and management capabilities. Table 3-2 reflects the distribution of PPOs by type of sponsorship.

It is interesting to note that in 1986, providers were the principal sponsors of PPOs; 50 percent of the 506 PPOs were sponsored by physicians, hospitals, or physician-hospital joint ventures. By 1990, insurance organizations had taken the lead, sponsoring 246 or 30 percent of the 814 PPOs nationally. Together with Blue Cross and Blue Shield, commercial insurance carriers sponsored 160 plans in 1986, or 31 percent of the total; by 1990, the number of plans they sponsored (along with PARTNERS health plans) had more than doubled, reaching 336, or 41 percent of the total. These data suggest that the Blues and commercial carriers are involved in vigorous PPO development, possibly to protect a previously strong market share that is being jeopardized by the marketing activities of HMOs and provider-sponsored PPOs. In 1990, 40.8 million persons were eligible to use PPOs, a 147 percent increase over 1986. During that year 16.5 million persons were eligible, which is nearly three times the 1985 number (5.75 million), and up from 1.3 million in December 1984.[7]

Provider sponsorship and support of PPOs is driven by three major factors: first, the desire to retain or acquire a large, privately insured patient base in the face of increasing competition; second, the determination to maintain a traditional, fee-for-service system of financing and delivering health care; and third, a strong motivation to retain provider control over the allocation of health care resources.

Insurers sponsor PPOs because they offer a cost-effective alternative to HMOs. They require little start-up capital, are relatively easy to integrate into existing benefit structures and administrative systems, are accepted readily by employers and subscribers, and offer the potential to generate favorable claims experience for fully or partially underwritten business. Other reasons that insurers sponsor PPOs include pressure from employers and other large group health insurance purchasers and the perception that failure to start a PPO will leave the insurer at a considerable competitive disadvantage in the

---

[7] Gregory de Lissovoy, Thomas Rice, Jon Gabel, and Heidi J. Gelzer, "Preferred Provider Organizations One Year Later," *Inquiry,* 24(2):128–129, Summer 1987; American Managed Care and Review Association, *Directory of Preferred Provider Organizations and the Industry Report on PPO Development,* Washington, D.C., AMCRA, 1990; and Russell A. Jackson, "Providers Losing Their Advantage in PPO Sponsorship," *Health Care Competition Week,* 7(10):3, March 5, 1990.

TABLE 3-2 Distribution of PPOs by Type of Sponsor, 1986 and 1990

Sponsor	1986 Number	1986 Percent	1990 Number	1990 Percent	% Change
Other Insurance Carrier	100	20	246	30	146
Physician/Hospital	99	20	114	14	15
Hospital	59	12	78	10	32
Physician	92	18	72	9	− 22
Blue Cross and Blue Shield	60	11	68	8	13
Investors	31	6	52	6	68
Third-Party Administrator	24	5	26	3	8
HMO	16	3	25	3	56
PARTNERS Health Plans	—	—	22	3	—
Pharmacy PPO	—	—	22	3	—
Self-Insured Employer	9	2	19	2	111
Dental PPO	—	—	15	2	—
Others	16	3	55	7	244
Total	506	100	814	100	60.9

SOURCE: American Medical Care and Review Association, *Directory of Preferred Provider Organizations and the Industry Report on PPO Development,* Washington, D.C., AMCRA, 1986; and American Managed Care and Review Association, *Directory of Preferred Provider Organizations and the Industry Report on PPO Development,* Washington, D.C., AMCRA, 1990.

future. Investors view PPOs as entrepreneurial opportunities with the potential for a high margin of profitability. HMOs and TPAs, on the other hand, use PPOs as a diversification strategy to enhance market share and capitalize on expertise and systems already in place for their core businesses. Self-insured employers sponsor PPOs for the same reasons as other insurers and employers: to manage the costs associated with financing and delivering health care services to their beneficiaries without compromising accessibility or quality of care. In summary, purchasers and providers of health care services sponsor PPOs for two main reasons. The first is heightened competition fueled by the escalation of health benefits costs, the alleged over-supply of physicians and hospital beds, and the proliferation of HMOs and related managed care systems. The second reason is less tangible than the first, but no less compelling: the fear of missing out on a health care financing and delivery innovation that has been touted as the "wave of the future" and that may provide a fresh edge over the competition.

The above characteristics of PPOs are summarized in Table 3-3 and compared to HMOs. Although there are several similarities between the two alternative delivery systems, there are also substantial differences—especially with regard to federal and state regulation of the HMO activities, limits on consumer choice of providers, insurance risk assumed by providers, and level of capital for start-up. Table 3-3 also indicates that in PPOs there is

TABLE 3-3 Comparison of HMO and PPO Characteristics

Basic Characteristics	HMOs	PPOs
1. Regulated premiums	Yes	No; subject to employer's indemnity insurance methodology
2. Fixed premiums	Yes	Yes; subject to variable out-of-pocket costs
3. Employee cost sharing		
Premium	Yes/No	Yes/No
Deductibles	No	Yes/No
Copayments	No/Limited	Limited/Significant
4. Development and provision of physician/hospital network	Yes	Yes
5. Regulatory requirements for basic medical services	Yes	Yes; subject to state oversight
6. Provider credentialing	Yes	Yes
7. Negotiated fee arrangements/ performance incentives between employers/insurers and participating physicians	No	Yes
8. Provider contracts/agreements	Yes; capitation and discounted fee-for-services	Yes; discounted fee-for-services
9. Utilization review/quality assurance process	Yes	Yes
10. Data collection necessary to evaluate provider performance	Yes	Yes
11. Employee/consumer choice of doctors/hospital	No; limited	Yes; unlimited, but with penalty if preferred provider not used
12. System for member complaints	Yes	Yes
13. Potential to negotiate different services and financing arrangements	Not possible; limited	Broad flexibility
14. Risk assumption by providers	Yes	No
15. Claims administration	Not relevant	Optional
16. Start-up capital	Substantial	Low
17. Premium rating	Modified community	Experience-rating normal

SOURCE: Adapted from Donald G. Lightfoot, "Preferred Provider Organization Concepts and Arrangements," *Risk Management*, *32*(11):30, November 1985, courtesy of *Risk Management*.

a negotiated fee arrangement as well as negotiated performance incentives between employers/insurers and panel physicians (number 7); in contrast, fee arrangements, efficiency incentives, and capitation levels in HMO systems are negotiated between the physicians, usually practicing in groups, and the HMO as the "insurer." The HMO then negotiates with employers to provide their employees with health insurance coverage. A useful method of differentiating between these two alternative delivery systems may be to consider the incentives in the PPO system as a way to improve the provider panel's productivity (more output from one input), while HMO incentives create an environment where the providers must become more efficient (the manner in which all inputs are combined to produce the final output).

Organizational Form

Structure will vary with each PPO and will depend on who is sponsoring it, the PPO's goals, the legal and political climate in the geographic area, and the scope of activities to be undertaken. The most popular organizational form is the corporation—either for-profit or not-for-profit; the corporate form generally insulates the principals from personal liability for the corporation's acts and omissions, thus limiting the general business liability of the PPO. Other main structural issues include the arrangement of the PPO's functional areas, the composition of the board of directors, the function of the various PPO committees, and the complex network of contracts among the parties to the PPO, including payers, physicians, hospitals, beneficiaries, and outside organizations that process claims or perform other administrative activities.[8] The typical functional areas and relationships are displayed in Figure 3-4. Note that this organizational chart reflects the board of directors as the ultimate governing authority for the PPO. In a carrier-sponsored PPO, where the PPO is organized as a line of business rather than a separate corporate entity, governance is provided by the sponsoring agency itself.

Most PPOs are managed under the direction of a chief executive officer (CEO) or executive director. Depending on the size and complexity of the PPO, the CEO may be supported by a chief operating officer (COO), who would manage the total day-to-day operations of the plan. Although titles and organizational structure vary from PPO to PPO, the functional components that are necessary for successful plan performance fall into four major categories: medical management and provider relations; finance, rating, and underwriting; marketing and member services; and operations and claims administration.

---

[8] Jeffrey B. Schwartz. "The Preferred Provider Organization as an Alternative Delivery System." *The Journal of Legal Medicine*, 6(1):152, 1985.

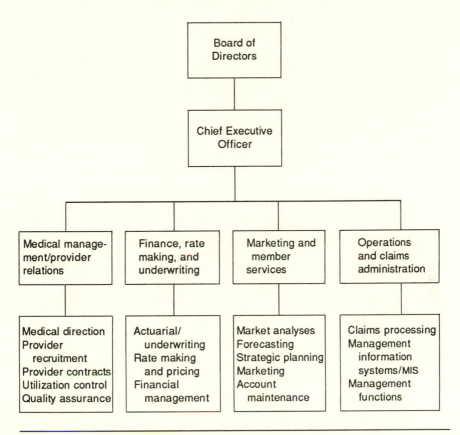

FIGURE 3-4   Typical PPO organizational chart.

Medical management is the key function that differentiates a PPO from an indemnity-type insurance plan. PPOs control health care costs through two mechanisms: discounts, which lower the unit cost of health care services rendered to PPO members, and utilization management, which attempts to control the volume and intensity of medical services. The medical management component of the PPO is responsible for representing the PPO to the provider community, recruiting providers, managing provider contracts to ensure compliance with contract terms, adjudicating provider complaints, monitoring the utilization of health care services, and ensuring that only medically necessary, high-quality care is rendered to PPO members. The medical management team usually consists of a medical director; a staff of registered nurses, who perform first-line utilization review; a provider relations staff; and appropriate administrative support.

Financial management in a PPO involves two distinct functions: developing the underwriting and pricing strategies for the PPO product, and managing the financial aspects of the PPO's business operations, such as tracking revenues and expenses, preparing budgets, and compiling reports and financial statements. The composition and size of a PPO's financial team depend, to a great extent, on plan sponsorship. Carrier-sponsored PPOs tend to use existing, in-house, corporate staff to perform actuarial and underwriting functions and, to a lesser extent, routine business financial functions. Provider-sponsored PPOs frequently retain consultants for actuarial and product-pricing work, but hire dedicated in-house staff to manage the financial operations of the plan.

The configuration of marketing and member services functions also varies from PPO to PPO. Some use the sponsoring organization's sales staff to market the plan. Others use only dedicated on-site PPO sales and service staff in the interest of stimulating product enthusiasm and loyalty and promoting accountability for the products' sales success. Regardless of whether the PPOs sell only PPO products or an array of other insurance products as well, it is imperative for the PPO to develop an incentive system that will reward not only new sales, but also the retention of old cases. In addition, the successful PPO must have a marketing strategy for selling its product to clients directly or through brokers and agents.

The final functional component is PPO operations, including claim processing and management information systems. The ultimate success of a PPO is contingent, in part, on its ability to pay claims quickly and accurately. Equally important is the PPO's capability to compile internal management reports to support rational decision making in areas of medical management, product design and pricing, marketing strategy, and tactical and strategic business planning. The PPO also must be capable of providing clients with meaningful account-specific reports of their company's utilization and claims experience, ideally, compared to the aggregate experience of clients similar in size, location, and industry code.

History and Evolution

Although PPOs, in their present form, are a product of the 1980s, the concept was used in the states of Washington and Oregon as early as 1911; insurance carriers negotiated both inpatient and outpatient discounted rates for patient-covered services under the newly enacted worker's compensation laws. In the late 1930s, the California Physicians' Service (CPS) was marketing medical services directly to purchasers. Under this arrangement, participating physicians agreed to accept the CPS payment as full reimbursement for covered group members.[9] Similar arrangements were developed by BC/BS and Medicare/Medicaid and continue today in their traditional participating provider contracts.

The PPO concept moved forward in the 1930s with the establishment of Blue Cross plans, which covered the cost of hospital care. The concept was expanded further with the development of Blue Shield plans in the 1940s to encompass physician services. Blue Shield agreed, as a condition of participation, to accept the plan's reimbursement as payment in full for covered services rendered to subscribers, with the exception of any copayments dictated by the subscriber's benefits package.[10]

By the 1950s, the Foundation for Medical Care in California began using reimbursement structures for its physician members, based on the concept of usual, customary, and reasonable (UCR) fees. About the same time, more and more employers began providing their employees with health insurance coverage as a fringe benefit. Generous employer-sponsored health benefits plans were becoming the norm rather than the exception. Finally, in the mid-1960s, the U.S. government established Medicare and Medicaid, extending health insurance coverage to America's aged and poor. This proliferation of health insurance coverage, characterized by a third-party payer system that insulated both providers and subscribers from the economic reality of health care costs, was a major factor in the rampant inflation of health costs in the 1970s and 1980s.

The present PPO movement began in California and Colorado in the early 1980s. One of the first steps was the creation of exclusive provider organizations/arrangements between the Medi-Cal program and cost-efficient hospitals for the provision of care to California's Medi-Cal participants. In Colorado, PPOs evolved from an environment that included a growing population, a surplus of physicians and hospital beds, and an unusually high number of self-insured employers who were interested in health services cost containment. Private sector insurers in California soon followed suit and developed PPOs under the auspices of the newly enacted PPO-enabling legislation.[11]

The PPO phenomenon spread rapidly eastward and, according to the American Medical Care and Review Association, in 1988, there were operational PPOs in 44 states, the District of Columbia, and Puerto Rico.[12] The distribution of PPOs by region is reflected in Table 3-4. As of January 1990, there were 814

---

[9] S. Brian Barger, David G. Hillman, and H. Randall Garland. *The PPO Handbook*. Gaithersburg, Md., Aspen Publishers, Inc., 1985, p. 4.

[10] Ibid., p. 11.

[11] Ibid., p. 12.

[12] American Medical Care and Review Association. *Directory of Preferred Provider Organizations and the Industry Report on PPO Development*. Washington, D.C., AMCRA, 1988, pp. f–j.

TABLE 3-4   Distribution and Percent Change of PPOs by Region as of December 1985, June 1988, and January 1990

Region	December 1985		June 1988			January 1990		
	No. of PPOs	% of Total	No. of PPOs	% of Total	1985–1988 % Change	No. of PPOs	% of Total	1988–1990 % Change
Midwest	63	18	146	22	131.7	186	23	27.4
Northeast	71	21	141	21	98.6	192	24	36.2
Southeast	79	23	153	23	93.7	189	23	23.5
West	130	38	220	34	69.2	247	30	12.3
Total	343	100	660	100	92.4	814	100	23.3

SOURCE: Extrapolated from Clearinghouse on Business Coalitions for Health Action, *What Employers Should Know About PPOs*, Washington, D.C., U.S. Chamber of Commerce, 1986, p. 39; and American Managed Care and Review Association, *Directory of Preferred Provider Organizations and the Industry Report on PPO Development*, Washington, D.C., AMCRA, 1990, p. j.

operational or developing PPOs in the country, with 23 percent in the Midwest, 24 percent in the Northeast, 23 percent in the Southeast, and 30 percent in the West. Of the 247 PPOs in the West, 48 percent are located in California. Also by 1991, more than 500 PPOs made PPO benefits available to approximately 60 to 65 million eligible Americans, a figure 20 percent higher than the number of people enrolled in the nation's HMOs.[13]

Provider Selection, Contracting, and Practice Patterns

A key characteristic of PPOs is a panel of preferred providers, selected or self-appointed on the basis of quality and efficiency. To a large extent, a PPO's marketability and financial viability is determined by the size, composition, distribution, and reputation of the physicians and hospitals on its preferred provider panel. And, the long-term financial success of a PPO depends on the preferred providers' capability and willingness to provide quality, cost-efficient care to PPO members while controlling unnecessary utilization.

The provider panel must be sufficiently large, comprehensive, geographically diffuse, convenient, and accessible in order to attract major purchasers. At the same time, the panel must be small enough to enable member providers to increase their patient volume significantly as a result of PPO participation. Furthermore, the panel's size must not invite antitrust allegations, such as those

---

[13] Jackson, "Providers Losing Their Advantage in PPO Sponsorship"; and A. Foster Higgins and Company, Inc., personal communication, July 1991.

described later in the legal issues section of this chapter. Consequently, most PPOs subject their preferred providers to a rigorous credentialing process. A PPO can achieve success in the marketplace only if its physicians and hospitals project a robust quality image, both individually and in the aggregate.

At the outset, a PPO must negotiate favorable rates with providers, usually in the form of discounted fees. Careful monitoring of services is necessary, because providers can easily make up revenues they may have lost through discounting their services by simply increasing the volume of services that they provide to PPO subscribers. Without utilization controls or comprehensive cost management programs, increased utilization will offset price discounts, but it could lead to financial disaster for the PPO and its purchasers. Thus, utilization management that monitors and evaluates the type, level, and amount of care provided is more important to the employer purchaser in achieving cost savings than price discounts.

Ideally, only providers with a proven history of cost consciousness and cost efficiency should be recruited for the provider panel. Unfortunately, meaningful historical data on the efficiency of providers are very difficult to obtain. Even in instances where such data are available, analysis and generalizability of the data can present problems. Many PPOs circumvent these problems by recruiting panel providers who meet all their other selection criteria and who express a strong commitment to cost efficiency when caring for PPO members, especially when expensive hospital and specialist care are involved. These PPOs typically include provisions in their contracts to discipline or terminate providers who fail to meet cost-efficiency standards over the long run.

The philosophical approach used by PPOs to select their panel of physicians and hospitals is largely contingent on the sponsorship of the PPO. As a general rule, if the PPO sponsor is assuming the underwriting risk, as is usually the case with insurance companies and self-funded employers, the cost-efficiency criteria for physician participation tend to be more stringent. On the other hand, if the sponsor does not assume the underwriting risk and the principal impetus to start the PPO is to increase the sponsor's market share, as is the case with most provider-sponsored PPOs, much less emphasis may be placed on cost efficiency as a condition of participation. For these PPOs, preexisting alliances may constitute a more important qualifying criterion than demonstrated cost consciousness. This fundamental difference in a sponsor's orientation can be critical in determining the ultimate success or failure of the PPO.

Regardless of a PPO's sponsorship, the pragmatics of the provider selection and contracting process generally involve the following steps: strategic planning, development of the provider selection criteria, and development of the contracting methodology. Strategic planning is a critical first step. Ideally, planning a PPO's provider selection and contracting strategy begins with a clear delineation of the PPO's overall mission, goals, and objectives. Special consideration must be given to any legal, regulatory, and political constraints that could affect provider recruitment. Strategic objectives for provider selection and contracting can then be developed and prioritized. Finally, a specific provider selection and contracting plan, consistent with the PPO's overall business objectives and time frames, can be drafted. The plan should specify the size, specialty composition, scope, and distribution of the proposed PPO provider panel.

The next step is development of the provider selection criteria. In lieu of using stringent, objective performance criteria, most PPOs select physicians on the basis of indirect measures of quality and efficiency, such as:[14]

- Professional credentials and board status
- Provider's specialty
- Malpractice record
- Privileges at a PPO hospital
- Geographic location and facilities
- Capability and willingness to provide services to PPO subscribers
- Acceptance of the PPO payment schedule
- Agreement to cooperate with PPO utilization management activities

The approach to hospital selection is usually somewhat more quantitative. Historical data often are available on hospital performance in such areas as average cost per day or per admission, occupancy rates, average lengths of stay, case mix, and morbidity and mortality rates. Analysis of these data provides a baseline for comparing the relative efficiency of various hospitals and establishing a reasonable point of departure for negotiating rates and services. In addition, PPOs usually require their contracting hospitals to meet specified criteria, which may include:

- Reputation for quality
- Accreditation and Medicare certification of the care organization by the Joint Commission on Accreditation
- Clean malpractice history
- Demonstrated cost efficiency
- Broad range of services
- Highly reputable medical staff
- Desire to become a preferred provider

---

[14] Adapted from Cowan. *Preferred Provider Organizations*, p. 144.

- Capability to serve PPO members
- Agreement on negotiated discount, where permitted by law
- Agreement to comply with utilization review and PPO procedures

As in the case of physician recruitment, the acceptance of a hospital by the PPO's provider panel is usually contingent on a hospital's expressed interest in participating, its ability to meet or exceed objective selection criteria, its agreement to accept all terms and conditions of the contract, and an available slot on the provider panel.

The third and final step in the provider selection and contracting process involves the development of a contracting methodology. Contracting methods generally fall into three categories: general offerings, solicitation of bids, and direct negotiations. In a general offering, the contract terms are specified in advance and offered to all eligible providers. Through a self-selection process, interested providers join the PPO on the basis of their ability to meet or exceed the selection criteria and their willingness to accept the contract terms as offered.

Bid solicitations usually involve the development and dissemination of a request for proposal or request for contract (RFP or RFC) by the PPO. Interested providers prepare and submit proposals in response to the RFP, outlining their capabilities and proposed terms. Proposals, or bids, are then evaluated, using specific objective criteria that are developed in advance by the PPO. The winning proposals are either accepted as submitted or are subject to subsequent negotiations between the PPO and the bidders.

Under the direct-negotiated contract model, the PPO targets a specific provider or providers for inclusion on the panel. The PPO approaches the provider to explore its interest in participating. If the provider is interested, both parties typically enter into direct negotiations, which continue until mutually agreeable terms are reached or further discussions are deemed futile.

Reimbursement and Risk Sharing [15]

Provider reimbursement arrangements usually include discounts and involve no assumption of insurance risk by providers. PPOs aim to reduce health care costs by negotiating favorable rates with preferred providers and reducing the volume of medically unnecessary and highly discretionary health care services.

---

[15] This section draws on material provided in Clearinghouse on Business Coalitions for Health Action, *What Employers Should Know About PPOs*, Washington, D.C., U.S. Chamber of Commerce, 1986, pp. 43–47.

Provider payment strategies and techniques that PPOs use to control the unit price of health care are described in the sections that follow.

PHYSICIANS

Although reimbursement methodologies vary among plans, payment to providers is based either on discounts against traditional fee-for-service schedules or on full or partial capitation payments, although the latter approach is rarely used. Discounted fee schedules are achieved by applying a set percentage discount to fee schedules; by applying a discount to the usual, customary, and reasonable (UCR) fees; or by applying a discount to fee schedules created by using relative value scales.

Regarding the UCR approach to physician reimbursement, the fee paid to the provider is based on a negotiated percentage (usually 70 to 90 percent) of the payers' claims profiles for usual, customary, and reasonable rates in a given geographic area. Although it may appear that physicians provide services at a discounted rate, the use of the 70th to 90th percentile may actually increase some physicians' fees over the payment levels of other traditional payers, such as Blue Shield and Medicare. This method of reimbursement encourages physicians to increase their fees so that UCR levels also rise.

A second approach to reimbursing physicians is based on relative value scales. Relative values reflect the complexity and intensity of services performed in various medical and surgical specialties and are expressed in relative value units. Units are subsequently multiplied by a conversion factor, expressed in dollars, to compute the appropriate payment level for any given service. The dollar value of the conversion factor is usually established by the PPO sponsor and, to account for a discount over traditional fees, the conversion factor is usually somewhat lower than what generally would be used in traditional fee-for-service reimbursement.

A third approach to physician reimbursement is payment on a full or partial capitation basis. The PPO negotiates a per person amount to be paid to the providers early in the month and generally before services are necessary. Providers are then required to provide all services required by the enrollees without additional PPO payments. In effect, the providers are risking loss if the capitation payment is not sufficient to cover all the costs of care for enrollees. Currently, reimbursement of PPO physicians based on provider risk is rarely used; by definition, use of a capitation payment placing physicians at-risk would imply the creation of an HMO rather than a PPO.

Regardless of the reimbursement methodology used, most PPOs attempt to negotiate payment levels that are between 5 and 25 percent below the fees that providers charge their non-PPO patients. In addition, PPOs usually limit the annual increase in physician fees to the Consumer Price Index or the Medical Price Index.

HOSPITALS

In principle, PPO hospital reimbursement strategies are similar to those used for reimbursing physicians. As with physician fees, PPOs generally strive for a 5 to 25 percent discount from the hospitals' usual charges, and a ceiling often is applied on the annual rate of increase. Hospital reimbursement typically is based on first dollar discounts, volume discounts, or fee schedules. First dollar arrangements involve an agreed-upon percentage discount on each dollar of hospital charges. Discounts are applied to a base schedule of charges that are developed by the hospital prior to negotiation. This method is most effective in achieving hospital cost savings when applied in conjunction with strict utilization controls.

In volume discount arrangements, the hospital gives discounts after the employer directs a certain volume of business to the hospital. Volume is measured by patient days, admissions, or dollars billed. Because the hospital provides a discount only after the agreed-upon level of volume is reached, this approach is most attractive to hospitals. Similar to first dollar arrangements, this method is very effective in achieving cost savings when strict utilization controls are applied.

The fee schedule arrangement is favored by many PPOs because of its administrative simplicity. The hospital is paid a set amount for each unit, usually per diem or per case, although multitiered per diem and case-mix reimbursement are also typical. In the per diem arrangement, a hospital is reimbursed a set amount for each day of inpatient care regardless of the specific service rendered. The per diem rate is based on the hospital's current average per diem rate. To minimize their risk, hospitals may also negotiate a multitiered per diem that offers the hospital services at specific per diems. Accordingly, intensive care may be reimbursed at the per diem rate of $1,500 while medical/surgical is reimbursed at an $800 per diem rate. The disadvantage to this approach is the lack of incentive for hospitals to provide care at the least intensive level of service.

The third type of fee schedule arrangement involves reimbursement on the basis of case mix or diagnostic-related groupings (DRGs). Most hospitals already have administrative systems in place to bill by DRG. This method of reimbursement allows the PPO to streamline claims administration, reduce associated processing costs, and control underwriting risks. Because this method of reimbursement may often be related to unnecessary inpatient admissions, strong preadmission review should be applied.

UNDERWRITING RISK

Although risk assumption by providers is rare, a few PPOs incorporate limited risk-sharing models. More PPOs will evolve into shared-risk arrangements in the future, with the blurring of clear definitions between PPOs and HMOs. At present, risk sharing typically involves a holdback arrangement, where 5 to 25 percent of providers' fees are withheld and placed in escrow. If the PPO's utilization experience, especially hospital care, is more favorable than targeted expectations, withhold amounts are returned to the providers, usually with interest, plus a percent of the surplus resulting from the better-than-expected utilization performance. If, on the other hand, utilization experience falls below targeted expectations, all or part of the withhold amounts revert to the PPO, in accordance with the terms of the risk-sharing agreement, and are used by the PPO to defray the higher-than-expected health services costs. Provider liability seldom exceeds the withhold amount; the remainder of the downside risk is borne by the PPO.

Utilization and Management Information Systems

Price discounts are only half of the cost-containment equation. Of equal importance is the need to reduce or eliminate claims for health care services that are not medically necessary and, at the same time, to ensure that the care rendered to PPO members is acceptable quantitatively and qualitatively. Accordingly, utilization review includes the length of stay, discharge practices, services ordered and provided, and appropriateness of admissions.

PPO utilization management programs are conceived and conducted either internally or through contracts with insurance carriers or independent agencies. A few PPOs delegate review responsibitity to their participating providers. But PPO utilization management programs share some common characteristics: (1) most programs are administered on a day-to-day basis by registered nurses, with direct physician oversight; (2) most programs use objective medical criteria, as well as the clinical experience of reviewers, to make medical necessity determinations; (3) many PPOs use manual systems to conduct utilization management activities, although automated systems are becoming increasingly common; (4) many PPOs impose substantial penalties for failure to comply with utilization management protocols, often 50 to 100 percent of the bill; and (5) most PPO utilization management systems incorporate grievance and appeal mechanisms to adjudicate disputes arising from utilization management.

TABLE 3-5   Prototype for a Comprehensive PPO Utilization Management Program

Type of Service	Method of Review	Scope of Review
Inpatient care	Preadmission review	Scheduled admissions
	Admission review	Nonscheduled admissions
	Concurrent review	All admissions
	Discharge planning	All admissions
	Second opinion consult	Selected procedures
	Hospital bill audit	Claims over $15,000
Outpatient care	Retrospective review	Quality/cost outliers
	Provider profiles	Quality/cost outliers
	Second opinion consult	Selected procedures
Catastrophic care	Admission review	Selected diagnosis
	Discharge planning	All catastrophic cases
	Post-discharge care	All catastrophic cases

SOURCE: Adapted from Linda L. Kloss, "Quality Review and Utilization Management," In: *The New Healthcare Market: A Guide to PPOs for Purchasers, Payors, and Providers,* Edited by Peter Boland, Homewood, Ill., Dow Jones-Irwin, 1985, pp. 686–687.

An effective PPO utilization management program typically encompasses a review of inpatient care, outpatient care, and catastrophic care. The first priority is review of hospital care, which accounts for almost two-thirds of a PPO's claims expense. The next priority often is given to catastrophic cases from designated diagnostic categories such as spinal cord injuries, closed head injuries, severe multiple traumas, acquired immune deficiency syndrome, low birth weight, neonates, and respirator-dependent adults and children. Aggressive management of these and related cases may save the PPO a great deal of money and substantially improve the quality of life for the member. The third priority is usually given to the review of outpatient, office-based in-plan care.

A prototype of a comprehensive PPO utilization management program is outlined in Table 3-5. Typically, hospital care is subject to intense prospective, concurrent, and retrospective review. Preadmission authorization is required for all scheduled hospital admissions. Nonscheduled admissions are reviewed as well, usually within one working day. Both preadmission and admission reviews include the assignment of an expected length of stay. After admission, each case is reviewed concurrently at logical intervals throughout the hospital stay, and additional inpatient days are authorized as appropriate. Discharge planning, an integral part of the utilization management process, begins as soon as possible so as to facilitate discharge with appropriate support services.

Hospital bill audits are conducted routinely for claims in excess of $15,000. These audits verify the accuracy of the hospital bill and ensure that the PPO pays only for medically necessary, covered services that were actually rendered to the patient.

Potentially catastrophic cases are reviewed as soon as possible after admission and are followed aggressively throughout the acute phase of hospitalization. Discharge planning is initiated at the earliest possible time, and creative solutions—sometimes involving extracontractual benefits—are explored in the interest of restoring maximum function and releasing the member to his/her home or to a less-acute facility at the earliest appropriate time. Long-term follow-up after discharge is ongoing, and the usual retrospective reviews and bill audits apply.

Emergency room visits and out-of-plan care are reviewed retrospectively, but prior to payment, on a per-claim basis as the claim is entered into the automated claims processing system for payment. Questionable claims are earmarked for manual review. If the services rendered were not authorized or are determined to be not medically necessary, the claim is rejected and the member is responsible for payment of the bill. Referrals to out-of-plan specialists are not captured on the system and are always subject to manual review. In-plan specialist referrals are also subject to review and usually are conducted on a random or exception basis.

Studies reported by de Lissovoy et al.[16] suggest that PPOs have become highly sophisticated in their utilization management efforts, including the application of stringent measures against providers who are viewed as overusers of services. They found that almost all PPOs require preadmission certification and concurrent review of hospital admissions and care, except when the hospital is paid according to DRGs. Retrospective reviews, however, typically are not used because plans favor "online" review as most effective in controlling use. Second opinion consultations continue to be used even though many experts now feel that they are not effective in utilization management. It may be that many employers still insist that second opinions be included in PPO contracts. Health services managers have found that there were very few instances when the second opinion differed from the original; in situations where third opinions were authorized and sought, when the second opinion differed from the first, the final opinion usually corroborated the first. Thus, the process did not eliminate unnecessary services; in fact, it added to the cost of care.

Regarding physician office services, the PPO attempts to provide retrospective reviews on a random basis and to create individual profiles of physician

---

[16] de Lissovoy, Rice, Gabel, and Gelzer. "Preferred Provider Organizations One Year Later," p. 131.

activities. According to de Lissovoy et al., almost half the PPOs are using physician profiling that entails the collection of all expenditures relating to an enrollee's episode of care and the assignment of these costs to a responsible PPO physician. Over time, it is then possible to compare physicians with one another to determine those who may be out of line with normally accepted volume of service and costs to the PPO. Actions then may be taken to deal with those physicians not practicing within generally accepted norms, including discussions with the physician, educational efforts to change the physician's behavior, or termination of the physician's preferred provider relationship with the plan. Additionally, in PPOs where "gatekeeper" physicians are capitated or receive a retainer for case management activities, there appear to be utilization control activities at the basic and primary level. Again, de Lissovoy et al. found that 36 percent of investor-sponsored plans and 20 percent of insurer-sponsored plans used the gatekeeper concept. Primary gatekeeping, however, was rare with provider-sponsored programs, which emphasize freedom of choice.

A good automated management information system (MIS), especially for outpatient care, where the sheer volume of claims makes manual review prohibitively labor intensive, increases the effectiveness of utilization review. The MIS must provide accurate, timely feedback to providers and purchasers (e.g., employers and others) through simple, focused, and accurate reports that can be used by PPO managers, providers, and employers who are vitally interested in knowing whether savings have occurred. Employers must be able to identify changes created by the PPO in employee/dependent utilization patterns. They need to know how health resources are being managed by the PPO and to compare the use by and costs of beneficiaries under the PPO with all beneficiaries covered by their health benefits program.

Unfortunately, many PPOs do not have the capability to provide reports that provide more than a summary of utilization activity. To be effective, the MIS must provide data on actual *changes in utilization* as well as *savings*. For employers, utilization review ideally should permit an analysis of changes in the use of both inpatient and outpatient services, including hospital days per 1,000 members, physician visits per member, outpatient surgery per member, average length of hospital stays, numbers of patient days, and so on. Regarding savings, the MIS should create reports of PPO savings based on the difference between "covered charges" and "PPO covered charges." At present, many health plans inaccurately calculate savings on the difference between "billed charges" and "PPO covered charges," with inflated savings resulting. Billed charges may include services (or charges) that are not eligible for payment under the PPO agreement. The MIS should also capture and report the employee use patterns of preferred and nonpreferred providers.

Employers' savings can be adequately delineated only by determining the "per capita costs or savings" of PPO member use rather than employers' overall health benefits costs. Overall costs mask increased volume of services (e.g., frequency or intensity of service use). Per capita costs can be calculated by using the following formula (but notice that this method requires a defined population to serve as a denominator).[17]

$$\text{Per Capita Savings} = \frac{\begin{array}{c}\text{Treatment costs of}\\ \text{PPO enrollees not}\\ \text{using preferred}\\ \text{providers}\end{array}}{\begin{array}{c}\text{Number of PPO}\\ \text{enrollees not using}\\ \text{preferred providers}\end{array}} - \frac{\begin{array}{c}\text{Treatment costs of}\\ \text{PPO enrollees}\\ \text{using preferred}\\ \text{providers}\end{array}}{\begin{array}{c}\text{Number of PPO}\\ \text{enrollees using}\\ \text{preferred providers}\end{array}}$$

Some PPOs do not keep accurate dependent counts, but rely on the number of covered employees multiplied by a standard dependent factor, usually between 2.5 and 3.0. Calculation of per capita experience in these circumstances is extremely difficult. Because PPO members are not "locked-in" or restricted in the use of preferred providers, it is necessary to identify the population using the PPO versus the population using services of providers outside the system. Thus, it may be difficult to judge whether the PPO is saving money for participating employers or merely offering lower prices but recouping its loss on volume.

PPO Benefits Packages

Preferred provider arrangements offer a health services benefits package to employees or union members and their dependents (see Figure 3-2). Employers and other purchasers develop and offer these benefits packages, providing members with a choice of provider, along with substantial economic incentives to select and use only preferred providers. There is no standard PPO benefits package. In fact, employers using preferred provider arrangements offer a broad array of benefit options, ranging from traditional, indemnity-type coverage to comprehensive, HMO-type benefits with coverage for wellness and prevention services.

Many PPO benefits packages incorporate deductibles and coinsurance to keep premiums affordable and to discourage unnecessary or marginal utilization of health care services. A deductible is a fixed amount that a member must pay before benefits become payable by the employer. If a per-admission deductible for inpatient hospital care is set at $200, a member is responsible for payment of the first $200 of claims incurred for each hospital stay. The

---

[17] Peter Boland. "The Illusion of Discounts in the Health Care Market." *Health Affairs*, 4(2):95, Summer 1985.

health benefits plan would generally cover the remainder, less any coinsurance. A coinsurance provision may require the member to then pay part of the remaining medical bill, usually a fixed percentage such as 20 percent of the total remaining after the deductible is met. For example, an inpatient stay may cost $3,000. After applying the $200 deductible ($3,000 − $200 = $2,800) and a coinsurance of 20 percent of the total remaining after the application of the deductible ($2,800 × 20% = $560), the member's share would be $760 ($200 + $560 = $760) and the health plan would pay the remaining $2,240. Deductibles are often criticized as being counterproductive to cost containment, because they provide a perverse incentive to overutilize once the deductible amount has been satisfied; thus, the coinsurance is used to counterbalance that incentive.

PPO benefits packages may reduce or eliminate members' out-of-pocket costs when members use preferred providers. By the same token, benefits packages impose substantial deductibles and/or copayments as disincentives to using nonpreferred providers. PPO benefits plans can be structured either as incentive or disincentive arrangements. In incentive plans, the payment level for using nonpreferred providers is kept at the standard indemnity insurance level, say 80 percent. The payment level for preferred providers is increased beyond the indemnity level, say 90 percent, thus rewarding members for using preferred providers by covering their services at a higher-than-normal reimbursement rate; however, no penalties are assessed for using nonpreferred providers since coverage for their services remains at the usual indemnity rate. Incentive plans are particularly attractive to employers wishing to make a transition from traditional indemnity insurance coverage to managed care, without reducing benefits.

Disincentive plans also offer a two-tiered benefit, with services by preferred providers covered at a higher rate than those provided by nonpreferred providers. The preferred provider reimbursement level, however, typically is set at the standard indemnity rate, say 80 percent, while the nonpreferred provider coverage is established below the standard indemnity rate, say 70 percent, or even less where permitted by state law. Although disincentive plans offer greater cost-containment potential than incentive plans, they may create human relations problems, for obvious reasons. In both incentive and disincentive plans, benefits may be reduced even further if members fail to follow prescribed utilization management procedures, such as preadmission authorization for nonemergency hospital care. An example of the variance in coverage levels for using preferred versus nonpreferred providers in a typical PPO benefits package is summarized in Table 3-6.

In the typical PPO benefits package, coverage for medically necessary health care services rendered by a preferred provider is provided at 90 percent after the calendar year deductible has been met. The same services provided by a nonpreferred provider are covered at only 80 percent after the $200 calendar year deductible has been met and a hospital deductible of $200 per

TABLE 3-6   Variance in Coverage Levels for Use of Preferred versus Nonpreferred Providers in a Typical PPO Benefits Package

Coverage Issue	Preferred Provider	Nonpreferred Provider
Calendar year deductible	$200	$200
Per admission deductible	0	200
Coinsurance	10%	20%
Utilization review noncompliance penalty	50%	50%

admission is imposed. If a member fails to follow the prescribed utilization management procedures governing nonemergency care, benefits are reduced by 50 percent. Utilization management penalties usually apply whether a preferred or nonpreferred provider is used.

Table 3-7 shows the reimbursement options available to members of a typical PPO, with an example of a total claims expense of $5,500 for the delivery of surgery services.

Total claims expense for the episode of care described in the example is $5,500; however, the preferred hospital claim is reduced by 15 percent to reflect the negotiated discount from charges. Assuming that the hospitalization was medically necessary and the required preadmission authorization was obtained, the preferred hospital claim is covered at 90 percent after the calendar year deductible has been met. Total out-of-pocket liability for the member using the preferred provider is $647.50.

TABLE 3-7   Sample PPO Hospital Payment Liability Options

Payment Issue	Preferred Provider	Nonpreferred Provider
Hospital charge	$5,500	$5,500
Discount (15 percent)	<825>	0
Adjusted charge	4,675	5,500
Annual deductible	<200>	<200>
Admission deductible	0	<200>
Claim minus deductible	4,475	5,100
Coinsurance	× 90%	× 80%
Plan pays	4,027.50	4,080
Member pays (deductibles + coinsurance)	647.50	1,420

The nonpreferred hospital claim also is subject to the $200 annual calendar-year deductible. In addition, the member must pay a $200 per-admission deductible. Since no hospital discounts apply, the base charge is also higher. Computing the two deductibles and the 80 percent coinsurance level, the member's payment liability at the nonpreferred hospital is $1,420, or more than double the out-of-pocket costs for the same service performed at a preferred hospital. It should be noted that if the utilization management protocol had not been followed, the payment would be reduced by 50 percent in either case.

Legal and Regulatory Issues

PPOs face three major types of legal and regulatory concerns: antitrust issues; state regulations, including statutes pertaining to corporations and insurance activities; and matters pertaining to professional and corporate liability. Antitrust issues can be subdivided further into price fixing, monopoly, group boycotts, and a concerted effort not to deal (unwillingness by one party to an agreement to resolve differences and issues). Price fixing, a per se violation of federal antitrust laws, occurs any time there is an agreement between two or more competitors with the intent to directly or indirectly control prices, use uniform discounts, or share pricing information. Violations occur whether the agreed-upon price is above or below prevailing market prices.[18] While antitrust issues are of concern to PPOs in general, they are particularly troublesome for provider-sponsored PPOs where fee setting is not handled by a separate administrative entity.[19]

Monopoly is a concern when a PPO includes so many providers that its market share is determined to be anticompetitive. While there are no established guidelines on what constitutes the combined allowable market share for a PPO under antitrust laws, conventional wisdom dictates that PPOs with

---

[18] Douglas L. Elden, J.D., LL.M. and Richard A. Hinden, J.D., "Legal Issues in Creating PPOs," In: *The New Healthcare Market: A Guide to PPOs for Purchasers, Payors, and Providers*, Edited by Peter Boland, Homewood, Ill., Dow Jones-Irwin, 1985, pp. 811–821; and J. Mark Waxman and Phillip A. Proger, "Preferred Provider Organizations: A Pro-Competitive Alternative or an Antitrust Liability?" In: *Attorneys and Physicians Examine Preferred Provider Organizations*, Edited by J. Mark Waxman, J.D., Washington, D.C., National Health Lawyers Association, 1984, pp. 69–70.

[19] Thomas C. Fox and Anne W. Weisman. "Introduction." In: *Attorneys and Physicians Examine Preferred Provider Organizations*. Edited by J. Mark Waxman, J.D., Washington, D.C., National Health Lawyers Association, 1984, p. xiv.

fewer than 20 percent of the providers in any given market are unlikely to be challenged.[20]

Concerted refusals to deal, or group boycotts, also are prohibited by the antitrust laws. While it is permissible for individual buyers and sellers to unilaterally refrain from dealing with certain parties, it is an antitrust violation when buyers or sellers agree, collectively, not to do business with other buyers or sellers in the marketplace.[21] To avoid the allegation of refusing to deal, PPOs are well served to use objective criteria as the basis of their decisions to contract or not to contract with certain parties.

There has been considerable movement among state legislatures to pass PPO-enabling legislation or to amend existing insurance laws to create a more favorable climate for PPOs. Unfortunately, there is little consistency in this new legislation from state to state. This lack of uniformity is especially problematic for PPOs that operate across state lines. In states where there are no clear legislative guidelines governing PPOs, the task of asserting jurisdiction over PPOs usually falls to a state's insurance commissioner, even though many PPOs do not assume risk in the conventional insurance sense.

The final set of legal concerns with which PPOs must cope includes corporate and professional liability. PPO corporate liability relates, principally, to the fulfillment of the duties and responsibilities set forth in various contracts with providers, insurers, employers, and members. Professional liability, on the other hand, relates to the professional health care providers' responsibilities to provide proper medical care, prevent avoidable injury, and protect patients' confidentiality.[22] In addition, recent court rulings, such as *Wickline vs. State of California,* have promoted serious concern about the substantial liability that PPOs may be assuming by virtue of their quality assurance and utilization review activities.[23]

Second Generation PPOs

Before and during the early and middle 1980s, the health services industry was dominated and controlled by health services providers and, to a much

---

[20] Richard C. Warmer, Bertrand M. Cooper, and Christopher W. Savage. "Antitrust Considerations Relating to PPOs." In: *The New Healthcare Market: A Guide to PPOs for Purchasers, Payors, and Providers.* Edited by Peter Boland. Homewood, Ill., Dow Jones-Irwin, 1985, p. 869.

[21] Elden and Hinden. "Legal Issues in Creating PPOs," p. 817.

[22] Ibid, p. 837.

[23] Ibid, p. 838; and Jeffery W. Lemkin and J. Peter Rich, "PPOs: Utilization Review," In: *Attorneys and Physicians Examine Preferred Provider Organizations,* Edited by J. Mark Waxman, J.D., Washington, D.C., National Health Lawyers Association, 1984, p. 54.

lesser extent, by purchasers of care. Health services of the 1990s appear to be much more purchaser driven, with the Federal Government, insurers, and business taking a stronger role in directing and mandating health services benefits packages, quality assurance mechanisms, utilization control, and overall direction of the industry. To meet these conditions PPOs and HMOs are moving toward more sophisticated and complex arrangements that might be called "second generation." According to Peter Boland,[24] five major trends are evolving as the market shifts from first to second generation PPOs.

1. Hybrid organizations are emerging that make it difficult to differentiate among IPA model HMOs, PPOs, and managed care fee-for-service health plans.

2. Internal administrative controls, such as provider selection standards and credentialing, utilization review procedures, and information systems, are replacing discounts as the most effective strategy for achieving long-term cost savings.

3. Program flexibility is accommodating health benefits design and "carve-outs" for particular specialty services such as mental health care and dental coverage.

4. Quality assurance is becoming the single most important delivery system feature, because it is the key to ensuring appropriate treatment, cost-effective services, and targeted cost control.

5. Second generation PPOs are taking on more characteristics of a mature health services industry by offering a comprehensive mix of services, integrated product lines, clearly defined distribution channels, and financial stability.

These trends have appeared in several major metropolitan areas, with changes in organizational form making it even more difficult to distinguish between different managed care arrangements. The outcome, however, will be companies that achieve the objectives of purchasers of health care—quality assurance; control of excessive use; more emphasis on identification and use of the "best" providers; flexibility to tailor benefits packages to clients, including the use of "triple options" by the same plan; and a range of low-risk- to high-risk-sharing arrangements. All of these changes will eventually produce a stable and mature managed care market. Indications that this is occurring include the growth achieved by PPOs and HMOs during the 1980s and their move to become the dominant health plans in the health insurance market. It is also seen in the many mergers, buy-outs, and acquisitions by larger plans of smaller, less-stable firms, and the growth of multifirm, multistate, and multimodel corporations.

---

[24] Peter Boland. "Trends in Second Generation PPOs." *Health Affairs,* 6(4):75, Winter 1987.

Finally, this maturity is seen in the movement of some firms from nonprofit to for-profit status, and the drop of shareholder returns to lower but more normal levels.

Summary

Preferred provider organizations are a product of the complex and competitive health care marketplace of the 1980s. Rampant health cost inflation has driven major purchasers of health care services to exercise their considerable buying power to negotiate preferential rates with providers in an effort to keep health insurance affordable. Providers of health care services, on the other hand, threatened by rising competition and shrinking market shares, have demonstrated willingness to negotiate with purchasers on the basis of price and to control utilization in return for the potential of increased market share. The resulting contractual arrangements between purchasers and providers are the essence of the preferred provider organization.

The generic preferred provider organization might be defined as a managed care arrangement in which the professional services of a select panel of health care providers are marketed, typically at a discount, to purchasers of health care services who, in turn, offer health insurance benefits, with free choice of provider and economic incentives to use preferred providers, to a defined group of subscribers.

PPOs are highly diverse in sponsorship, size, scope, and mission, and generally share a number of basic features, including a panel of preferred providers, negotiated contracts between purchasers and providers, discounted fee schedules, utilization management, claims administration, and benefits packages that allow members flexibility in the choice of providers.

Sponsorship of PPOs includes providers, Blue Cross/Blue Shield and commercial carriers, investors from outside the health services industry, and others. Sponsorship by insurers and providers seems to be motivated by their desire to retain or acquire a large privately insured market base in the face of increasing competition from other managed care organizations such as HMOs. It appears to be an attempt on the part of providers to retain the traditional fee-for-service payment system. Insurers sponsor PPOs not only because they are a cost-effective alternative to HMOs but because of pressure from employers and other large group health insurance purchasers to contain rising health benefits costs.

Similarities as well as differences are observed between PPOs and HMOs. Similarities include employee cost-sharing of premiums, development of a network of providers and credentialing of providers, utilization and quality review, consumer and provider complaint systems, and so on. Differences are particularly noted in the areas of HMO federal and state regulation, HMO capitation that places physicians at-risk (while not generally used by PPOs), and a complete lock-in of members in the HMO, while only a partial lock-in is apparent in PPOs.

Growth in PPOs has been significant since their development in the early 1980s. It is estimated that there are more than 800 PPOs in operation, with PPO benefits available to approximately 60 to 65 million Americans. As PPOs continue to grow in strength and number, there has been a tendency for their organizational structures and processes to move from simple, first-generation models to more complex and sophisticated second-generation products that tend to blur the differentiating characteristics of PPOs, HMOs, and fee-for-service managed care insurance products. These changes will continue to occur as the PPO and managed care markets continue to mature. Greater numbers of hybrid models are emerging to meet the objectives of purchasers (employers, unions, government, etc.), while providers continue to lose their ability to control these systems and ultimately their future.

References

American Managed Care and Review Association. *Directory of Preferred Provider Organizations and the Industry Report on PPO Development*. Washington, D.C., AMCRA, 1990.

American Medical Association. *A Physician's Guide to Preferred Provider Organizations*. Chicago, Ill., AMA, 1983.

American Medical Care and Review Association. *Directory of Preferred Provider Organizations and the Industry Report on PPO Development*. Washington, D.C., AMCRA , 1988.

Barger, S. Brian; David G. Hillman; and H. Randall Garland. *The PPO Handbook*. Gaithersburg, Md., Aspen Publishers, Inc., 1985.

_____. *Preferred Provider Organizations: Their Status, Development and Future*. Gaithersburg, Md., Aspen Publishers, Inc., 1985.

Boland, Peter. "Questioning Assumptions About Preferred Provider Arrangements." *Inquiry*, 22(2):132–141, Summer 1985.

_____, ed. *The New Healthcare Market: A Guide to PPOs for Purchasers, Payors, and Providers*. Homewood, Ill., Dow Jones-Irwin, 1985.

_____. "Trends in Second Generation PPOs." *Health Affairs*, 6(4):75–81, Winter 1987.

Carlova, John. "What's Hiding in that PPO Contract?" *Medical Economics*, 61(16):66–71, August 6, 1984.

Clearinghouse on Business Coalitions for Health Action. *What Employers Should Know About PPOs*. Washington, D.C., U.S. Chamber of Commerce, 1986.

Cowan, Dale H., M.D., J.D. *Preferred Provider Organizations: Planning, Structure, and Operation*. Gaithersburg, Md., Aspen Publishers, Inc., 1984.

de Lissovoy, Gregory; Thomas Rice; Don Ermann; and Jon Gabel. "Preferred Provider Organizations: Today's Models and Tomorrow's Prospects." *Inquiry, 23*(1):7–14, Spring 1986.

de Lissovoy, Gregory; Thomas Rice; Jon Gabel; and Heidi J. Gelzer. "Preferred Provider Organizations One Year Later." *Inquiry, 24*(2):127–135, Summer 1987.

Demkovich, Linda E. "Controlling Costs at General Motors." *Health Affairs, 5*(3):58–67, Fall 1986.

Eastaugh, Steve R. "Differential Cost Analysis: Judging a PPO's Feasibility." *Healthcare Financial Management, 40*(5):44–51, May 1986.

Ellwood, Paul M., Jr., "But What About Quality?" *Health Affairs, 5*(1):135–140, Spring 1986.

Fielding, Jonathan E. *Corporate Health Management.* Reading, Mass., Addison-Wesley, 1984.

Fine, Max W. "Introduction." *A Primer for HMO Managers.* Washington, D.C., Group Health Association of America, March 1986.

Fox, Peter D., and Maren D. Anderson. "Hybrid HMOs, PPOs: The New Focus." *Business and Health, 3*(4):20–33, March 1, 1986.

Goodspeed, Ronald B., and Norbert Goldfield. "Quality Assurance in a Preferred Provider Organization." *Journal of Ambulatory Care Management, 10*(2):8–16, May 1987.

Johns, Lucy; Maren D. Anderson; and Robert A. Derzon. "Selective Contracting in California: Experience in the Second Year." *Inquiry, 22*(4):335–347, Winter 1985.

Koch, N., et al. "Group Practice and PPOs: Meeting the Quality Challenge." *Quality Review Bulletin, 15*(11):358–361, November 1989.

Kraft, Jeffrey G. "Preferred Provider Organizations. Part 2: Addressing the Legal Issues." *Healthcare Financial Management, 37*(8):10–16, August 1983.

Lemkin, Jeffrey W., and J. Peter Rich. "Hospital Sponsored PPOs: A Practical Guide to Structural and Organizational Options." *Healthcare Financial Management, 37*(12): 80–86, December 1983.

Millikan, Diane L. "HMOs and PPOs: How Do They Stack Up?" *Medical Group Management, 33*(4):32–34, July/August 1986.

O'Gara, Nellie, and Kevin Hickey. "Marketing the Preferred Provider Organization." *Hospitals, 58*(12):75–78, December 1984.

Rice, Thomas, et al. "The State of PPOs: Results from a National Survey." *Health Affairs, 4*(4):25–40, Winter 1985.

Strumwasser, Ira, et al. "The Triple Option Choice: Self-selection Bias in Traditional Coverage, HMOs, and PPOs." *Inquiry, 26*(4):432–441, Winter 1989.

Tibbitts, Samuel J., and Allen J. Manzano. *Preferred Provider Organizations, An Executive Guide.* Chicago, Ill., Pluribus Press, Inc., 1984.

Waxman, J. Mark, J. D., ed. *Attorneys and Physicians Examine Preferred Provider Organiza-tions.* Washington, D.C., National Health Lawyers Association, 1984.

4

ORGANIZATIONAL STRUCTURE OF HMOs

Health maintenance organizations (HMOs) are characterized by flexibility in both composition and organizational form. This flexibility in organizational structure, created in the process of adapting to local viewpoints and requirements, is, in part, the underlying basis for the strength and tenacity of HMOs. The HMO legislation describes the functions and types of services that should be incorporated in the HMO. The law also allows for flexibility in the *provider* arrangement. Health services may be rendered by a group or staff of physicians, through an individual practice association (IPA), or any combination of these provider arrangements. The 1988 HMO amendments provide even greater flexibility to the corporate structure, methods of delivering primary physician services, pricing strategies, and benefits design.

Major organizational arrangements that have been successfully used by HMOs are categorized and reviewed in this chapter. Two important issues should be kept in mind. First, although Title XIII of the Public Health Service Act and its amendments, as well as state HMO enabling laws, define specific organizational requirements, the organizational forms continue to evolve as the field changes, and possible amendments reflect the changing nature of these health plans. Many experts predict that Title XIII will be repealed within the next few years; the process of meeting federal regulations, of fitting the HMO to federally mandated organizational arrangements and definitions, and of becoming a qualified HMO would no longer be key issues. Of greater importance may be the need to meet accreditation standards by one of the independent health organization accrediting bodies. Regardless of possible changes in federal regulations, however, the discussion here will include the major structural models that currently are in use, as well as those that are evolving—especially the hybrid arrangements such as open-ended HMOs.

Second, the successful HMOs have evolved and are surviving in their own unique settings; to follow one model explicitly, without regard to particular environment, demography, competitive setting, and community needs, would be misleading. Thus, it will be useful to become familiar with the many structural forms that are available so that, when developing an HMO or going through a corporate reorganization, one may choose those elements that best suit the individual project.

The term "organizational structure" is defined here as the method by which the HMO components or elements can be arranged, established, or ordered to achieve a functioning and successful health delivery system. General management theory suggests that the *purpose* of organization is summarized by two principles—the unity of objective and efficiency. These principles suggest that the HMO's organizational structure must facilitate an individual's contribution toward the attainment of the HMO's objectives. The principle of efficiency requires that an HMO's structure makes possible the accomplishment of organizational objectives by employees with minimum unsought consequences or cost. In addition, two other characteristics are associated with the organizational structure—authority and delegation, and departmentalization. Authority is the cement of the organization, and delegation is the primary line of communication. They are the means by which coordination of HMO units can be furthered. Departmentalization is the framework of the organization in the sense of activity groupings. The organizational structure should reflect a classification of the tasks required of HMO personnel and should assist in their coordination by creating a system of related roles. The flow of authority and of departmentalization is included in the review of organizational models that follows.

HMO Sponsors and Owners

Like other health services organizations, HMOs are controlled by a board of trustees (in a not-for-profit organization) or board of directors (in a for-profit or proprietary organization). This primary policy- and decision-making body is accountable and responsible for all activities of the HMO. As fiduciaries, board members hold in "high trust" the assets of the HMO—for society in not-for-profit plans or the stockholders in for-profit HMOs—and, therefore, are accountable to these groups for their actions or the actions of all other HMO personnel. The board delegates to a manager—the HMO executive director— the authority for day-to-day management. Although the executive director is held responsible for the activities of the HMO, the board cannot escape the ultimate responsibility and accountability for such activities.

The differentiation between the *sponsors* of the HMO and its *policymaking body,* which represents the owners, should be clearly defined. It is necessary that there be an organization (for our purpose, defined as the sponsor) that can be held responsible for the developing HMO or for the reorganization of an existing health services corporation. For developing health plans, it is necessary, therefore, to identify the decision-making body that is established once the HMO legal entity is formed. The models that follow are described from the perspective of the legal organizational entities, the owners, and the sponsoring organizations.

According to DHHS's Office of Health Maintenance Organizations, during the initial years of Title XIII, 44.2 percent of all applications for federal grants were received from consumer-sponsored organizations (see Table 4-1). Another 36.2 percent of the applications were received from provider sponsors—physicians, hospitals, and medical schools—while only a relatively small percentage of the applications and actual grant awards were sponsored by public or private organizations (5.8 and 13.1 percent, respectively). Most of the grant awards went to consumer-sponsored HMOs (47.5 percent) and to provider-sponsored plans (41.9 percent). By 1984, sponsoring organizations of federally qualified HMOs had moved from consumers and providers to the private sector. As shown in Table 4-1, approximately 36.8 percent of all federally qualified HMOs were sponsored by private firms—one of the ultimate goals of Title XIII. Notice, however, that approximately 31.5 percent were sponsored by consumers and some 31.2 percent by provider organizations.

TABLE 4-1 HMO Sponsors of Federal Grants: 1975 and 1984

Sponsors	1975				1984	
	Number of Applications	% of Total	Number of Awards	% of Total	Number of Federally Qualified HMOs	% of Total
Public	22	5.8	5	2.8	2	0.8
Consumer	169	44.2	85	47.5	83	31.5
Private	50	13.1	14	7.8	98	36.8
Providers:						
Physicians	81	21.2	48	26.8	58	21.8
Hospitals	48	12.6	21	11.7	20	7.5
Medical schools	9	2.4	6	3.4	5	1.9
Total	138	36.2	75	41.9	83	31.2
Other	3	0.8	–	–	–	–
Total	382	100.1	179	100.0	266	100.3

SOURCE: U.S. Department of Health, Education, and Welfare, Health Resources and Services Administration, Office of Health Maintenance Organizations, *HMO Program Status Report,* Rockville, Md., DHEW, 1976, p. 61; and U.S. Department of Health and Human Services, Health Resources and Services Administration, Bureau of Health Maintenance Organizations, Office of Health Maintenance Organizations, *10th Annual Report to the Congress, Fiscal Year 1984,* Rockville, Md., DHHS, June 1985, pp. 25–158.

TABLE 4-2   Health Plans of 42 National HMO Firms by Type of Sponsor: 1986

Type of Sponsor	Number of HMOs	Total HMOs (%)	Membership	Total Members (%)
HMOs	131	42.2	11,227,523	71.9
Insurers	95	30.6	2,452,403	15.7
Multihospital companies	29	9.4	642,225	4.1
Joint insurer-hospital company firms	31	10.0	713,204	4.6
Corporations and consulting firms	24	7.7	571,344	3.7
Total	310	99.9	15,606,699	100.0

SOURCE: InterStudy. *National HMO Firms, 1986.* Excelsior, Minn., 1987, pp. 24–26.

Over the years, sponsoring organizations have included universities, medical schools, cities, industries, consumer groups, associations, insurance companies, Blue Cross/Blue Shield, hospitals, physicians, and neighborhood health centers. Reasons for sponsorship include goals to improve the availability of health services in their community, to make available an alternative to the traditional system, to control the rising costs to employers of their health insurance benefits packages for employees, to meet the competition and to control a segment of the market, and to foster personal entrepreneurial motives. Individual HMO advocates may be called on to serve as board members with the newly established HMO entity. Initially, in almost every case, the sponsor assumes the risk for the overall performance of the new HMO, influences its contractual arrangements with providers, and is directly involved in the day-to-day management decisions made by the HMO.

As the HMO industry has matured, multicorporate, multistate firms have sponsored and now own and/or operate many health plans in various states. Table 4-2 reviews 1986 data concerning these national firms, which include the Kaiser Foundation Health Plan, Maxicare Health Plan, CIGNA Healthplan, and the like. Recently, health plans have been sponsored increasingly by existing HMOs, which expand by establishing or purchasing developing HMOs in areas where the parent HMO is not currently operating health plans. For example, this would include the development of Kaiser Foundation Health Plans in areas east of the Mississippi River, in Cleveland, Ohio, Washington, D.C., Baltimore, Maryland, the New York City area, and so on. These HMO-sponsored health plans also account for the greatest number of enrollees—approximately 72 percent of all enrollment in national HMO firms. Insurers, however, are also

TABLE 4-3   Ownership of HMOs, 1987 and 1989

	1987		1989	
Type of Ownership	Number of HMOs	Total (%)	Number of HMOs	Total (%)
Multistate (national)				
HMO firm	51	27.1	37	11.1
Hospital(s)	20	10.7	83	25.0
Physicians	12	6.4		
Self-owned (independent				
HMO ownership)	48	25.5	89	26.8
Blue Cross/Blue Shield	19	10.1	55	16.6
Other Insurers	17	9.0	58	17.5
Other	21	11.2	10	3.0
Total	188	100.0	332	100.0

SOURCE: Group Health Association of America, *1987 Survey of HMO Industry Trends,* Washington, D.C., GHAA, 1987, pp. 15–16, 24; and Marsha Gold and Dennis Hodges, *HMO Industry Profile, Volume 1: Benefits, Premiums and Market Structure in 1989,* Washington, D.C., Group Health Association of America, 1990, p. 40. Note that these figures represent only a sample of all HMOs—188 of the total 662 plans, or approximately 28.4 percent in 1987 and 31.9 percent in 1989.

sponsoring multistate HMOs; Table 4-2 suggests that approximately 30 percent of all national HMO sponsorship is by insuring organizations, accounting for approximately 16 percent of the total national firm membership. This conclusion suggests that existing, successful HMOs will continue to grow and will probably expand and evolve into national firms. To meet this competition from the national HMOs, large insurers such as CIGNA, Prudential, and John Hancock will have to become even more involved in HMOs, and their HMOs will also continue to expand nationally. Multihospital corporations such as Henry Ford Health Care Corporation and hospitals in joint venture with insurance companies (Equicor and Partners National Health Plans) will continue to play somewhat lesser roles in sponsoring HMOs in multiple states. Interestingly, physicians, either in group plans or individually, are not national HMO sponsors of health plans and will probably not play a leading role in either future HMO sponsorship or ownership.

Although "national" or "multistate" ownership of HMOs is the predominant ownership status, independent ownership is also currently as important. Table 4-3 shows the results of Group Health Association's 1987 and 1989 surveys of the HMO industry. Of the 188 HMOs in the 1987 sample, multistate, national HMO firms owned 27.1 percent of all HMOs, but by 1989 the percentage had dropped to 11.1 percent (from a sample of 332 HMOs). Independent or self-owned HMOs accounted for 25.5 percent of the total in 1987 and 26.8 percent in 1989. Hospitals and physicians together increased their ownership from 17.1 percent in 1987 to 25 percent in 1989. In 1987 insurers (including Blue Cross andBlue Shield) owned 19.1 percent, but increased their holdings to 34.1 percent in 1989. These data, compared with the sponsor information, suggest that HMO sponsors also tend to become the ultimate owners of HMOs. There has been an increasing tendency, however, for newer, smaller, and less-successful plans to be purchased by the larger, national, and provider-sponsored HMO firms. For example, in 1987, 13 percent of the HMOs owned by multistate firms had been in operation 16 years or more, 23 percent had been in operation from 8 to 15 years, and approximately 64 percent had been in operation for 7 years or less[1] This ownership trend will probably continue. In the recent past, however, some of the large multistate plans, especially Maxicare, have experienced significant financial stress because of their quick growth, the purchase of small plans with financial problems of their own, and the inability to cope with the management of national activities. The difficulties of these large conglomerates may slow multiplan growth through the early 1990s.

HMO Models

Based initially on the Federal Government's classification system, three organizational HMO models were created—staff, group, and individual (or independent) practice association (IPA).[2] The HMO industry has added at least two additional models, which are based on the initial three: the "network" and "hybrid" models. On close inspection, it is likely that particular health plans will fit into one of the five models. Note that the three federally defined models are based on the method by which (1) physicians are paid for their services and (2) their services are provided.

THE STAFF MODEL

The staff model HMO provides the entire administration of the health plan as well as the direct and actual application of physician services. In effect, the HMO provides both the administrative and medical functions of the health

---

[1] Group Health Association of America, *1987 Survey of HMO Industry Trends*, Washington, D.C., GHAA, 1987, p. 16; and Marsha Gold and Dennis Hodges, *HMO Industry Profile. Volume 1: Benefits, Premiums and Market Structure in 1989*, Washington, D.C., Group Health Association of America, 1990, p. 40.

[2] The managed care industry uses both independent practice association and individual practice association. In this book, individual practice association or IPA will be used to describe this HMO model.

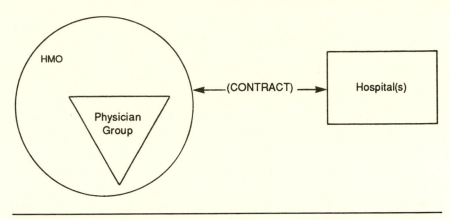

FIGURE 4-1   Closed-panel/staff model HMO.

plan.[3] As such, the HMO employs its own physicians (or contracts with staff physicians) to provide services to health plan enrollees.[4] These relationships are shown in Figure 4-1. In effect, the staff model uses a *closed panel* of physicians, that is, only salaried physicians provide services, with nonplan community physicians excluded from participation in the health plan.

Organizational Form

As depicted in Figure 4-2, the staff model HMO employs physicians to provide medical services to health plan members. The HMO medical staff includes a medical director who is responsible for the overall quality and quantity of the medical services that are provided by the HMO and individual salaried physicians. The HMO also employs specialists whose services are in constant demand, while less frequently used specialists may be on contract or on a referral panel. Hospital services may be provided through an agreement or formal contract with local hospitals. In this regard, HMO staff physicians must first be credentialed by the hospital before staff admitting privileges will be extended to them. Other services, such as long-term care, pharmaceuticals, dental services, and the like, may also be provided by staff professionals or through contracts and agreements with local organizations.

---

[3] U.S. Department of Health and Human Services, Health Care Financing Administration, Office of Health Maintenance Organizations. *Guide to the Development of Health Maintenance Organizations.* Rockville, Md., DHHS, 1982, p. III-17. DHHS Publication No. (PHS) 82-50178

[4] Ibid.

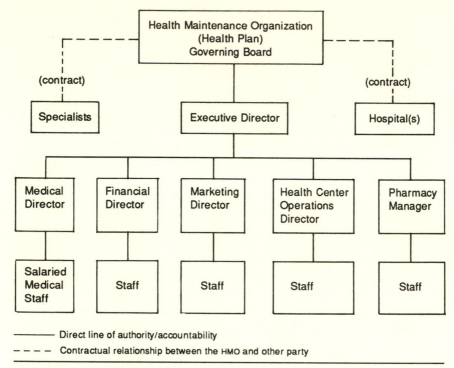

FIGURE 4-2   Organizational structure of a staff model HMO.

Figure 4-2 also identifies the general functional areas of HMO operations, including medical services delivery, finance, marketing, and health center operations (which will be discussed in later chapters). Hospital and pharmacy services also may be arranged or provided directly by the HMO. Health plans find that operation of a pharmacy provides additional income that helps maintain the competitive posture of the HMO. Also, the provision of pharmacy services in the health plan center is convenient for the HMO's membership.

Conversely, only a few HMOs actually own and/or operate their own hospitals; these include the Kaiser Foundation Health Plans, Group Health Cooperative of Puget Sound, and Health Insurance Plan of Greater New York— none of which are staff model HMOs.

Contractual Relationships

The contracts between physician staff and the health plan are much less complex than in other models. The plan hires medical staff—usually primary care providers and some specialists—support staff, and ancillary providers, creating an employer/employee relationship. Physician contracts must describe the duties of the physician, responsibilities of the HMO, and the physician's compensation and responsibilities as a patient manager. The contract may delineate any limitations restricting the physician from entering into contracts with other HMOs or establishing a separate fee-for-service practice; it may also describe those HMO policies and procedures that the physician must abide by, such as approvals and record keeping for referrals.[5]

Most staff model HMOs contract with area specialists whose services are not needed by the HMO as frequently as the services of the primary care physicians. It would not be economical to hire these specialists on a full-time basis, since they generally command a much higher income than primary providers. Specialist contracts stipulate that the HMO will reimburse the physician at a specified rate for providing referral services. The specialist is an independent contractor; the number of HMO patients he or she accepts may be limited either by the amount of time agreed upon to devote to HMO members or by the number of members the physician will be expected to treat. In addition to HMO patients, the physician may maintain a fee-for-service practice. Payment to independent specialists may be on the basis of fee-for-time; capitation; discounted fee-for-service; full charges, based on the physician's or HMO's fee-schedule; or retainer, in which case the physician agrees to a set payment for treating up to a stipulated number of patients or cases over a specified period of time.

The staff model HMO pays its physician employees a salary, based on the prevailing community fee-for-service incomes of physicians with equivalent education, training, and experience. The salaries paid to HMO staff physicians, however, are generally somewhat below their fee-for-service counterparts. In return for lower pay, not only is compensation guaranteed, regardless of the number of patients treated, but the staff physician does not have to pay overhead expenses, does not have to take the normal risks of operating a small business, does not have to manage the practice as a private business, does not have to market the practice, and is relieved of the duties of collecting fees from patients or their insurance companies. Hopefully, the staff physician will identify strongly with the best concepts and interests of the HMO, especially in controlling utilization at appropriate levels while striving to provide quality care. This particular principle is like that found in most prestigious multispecialty group practices, such as the Mayo Clinic and the Cleveland Clinic. These groups also employ salaried physicians at relatively low average annual salaries (at Mayo the average physician salary was approximately $130,000 in

---

[5] Ibid.

1988),[6] who have strong organizational loyalty and commitment and with low turnover (again, at Mayo, physician turnover was only 1.5 percent in 1990).

Risks and Incentives

Staff model HMOs tend to use fewer risk-sharing arrangements and provide fewer financial incentives than do group and IPA models. Staff model HMO financial incentives to control costs usually take the form of end-of-the-year bonuses that are paid to physicians who have stayed within the organization's established budget and utilization goals, or merit bonuses based on annual individual and departmental performance reviews. These bonuses, rewards, and other perquisites may be cash payments or benefits such as the availability of low-interest loans.

Staff model HMO physicians are at financial risk for the cost of care only to the extent that over-utilization might affect their bonuses and other rewards. Therefore, while it may appear that these plans find it difficult to effectively control utilization, this is not always the case. Utilization data provided in Chapter 8, Table 8-2, for 1986 through 1989 suggest that staff model HMOs experience an average number of physician encounters for under age 65 members as well as over age 65 enrollees. More importantly, under age 65 enrollees in staff model HMOs appear to use less than the average number of hospitals days. One might conclude that, of all the plans, staff model HMOs provide the weakest physician incentives to control utilization, but they also require the least amount of risk assumption by physicians.

When utilization is effectively controlled by staff model HMO physicians, as is the case for physician services and hospital use by their under age 65 enrollment, several reasons can be given for this success. Employed staff physicians are subject to the HMO's policies regarding referrals and service utilization. Internal utilization review committees monitor physicians' practice patterns to ensure that referrals are kept at a minimum and that expensive tests are ordered only when medically necessary and when alternatives are not available. Physicians who are chronic abusers are subject to the disciplinary actions initiated by the plan's medical director. Also, certain psychological factors may work to control physicians' utilization, because they recognize that maintaining their salary depends on the financial success of the HMO. Success depends on the delivery of high-quality, yet cost-effective, health care

---

[6]Milt Freudenheim. "Mayo Clinic Prescription: Growth." *The New York Times.* Monday, July 4, 1988, p. 1; Business Section, p. 31.

to plan members. Finally, staff physicians frequently develop a team or group identity found in a true multispecialty medical group practice. These collegial and professional relationships become part of the HMO's corporate culture and result in a minimum of unnecessary costs while providing a high level of quality services and maintaining enrollee satisfaction.

Advantages and Disadvantages of the Staff Model

The staff model is the least legally, organizationally, and administratively complex of all HMO models, creating both advantages and disadvantages. It affords executive management maximum control over employee physicians' utilization patterns. All services operate through one legal entity, reducing administrative burdens and simplifying service coordination. Because the HMO is the provider entity, however, it must have its own facilities and equipment, as well as a facilities management team. These facilities must be in place before members enroll, which requires high levels of start-up capital. It is this need for start-up capital that often precludes the development of a staff model even when market analyses indicate that, given the situation, such a model would be best and probably the most successful.

Staff models are open to considerable legal liability for negligence by employee physicians. In network and IPA models, stringent physician monitoring, accompanied by a well-drafted contract, may reduce or limit the HMO's liability for negligence by associated physicians. Under the principle of agency, however, the staff model HMO will be liable for its employees' torts so long as these employees act within the scope of their employment.

Accurately projected cost and enrollment estimates are important for all HMOs, but they are imperative for staff models, which run the risk of overestimating enrollment, hiring too many physicians, and having fixed costs that are too high.[7]

For the employee physician, the staff model offers many advantages, such as no physician overhead expenses, guaranteed salary, and more limited office hours than in private practice.[8] Many physicians, however, desire more autonomy than is afforded them through the staff model. To increase autonomy and decision-making power within the health plan, staff model physicians

---

[7] Roger W. Birnbaum. *An HMO Management Primer for the National HMO Management Fellowship Program II*. Washington, D.C., Group Health Association of America, 1985, p. 12.

[8] David B. Nash. "HMO Practice: Advantages and Disadvantages." *Physician's Management,* 25(5):245–257, May 1985.

TABLE 4-4 HMOs by Model, Enrollment, and Percentage of Total Operational Plans: 1985, 1987, 1989, and 1990

Model	1985				1987				1989				1990			
	Plans	%	Enroll-ment (000)	%	Plans	%	Enroll-ment (000)	%	Plans	%	Enroll-ment (000)	%	Plans	%	Enroll-ment (000)	%
Staff	66	13.5	3,200.3	14.2	63	8.9	3,316.4	10.7	66	10.6	3,564.5	10.4	64	10.5	4,147.9	11.5
Group	93	19.0	7,570.5	33.5	92	13.0	8,729.9	28.1	85	13.6	9,558.0	28.0	77	12.6	10,182.9	28.2
IPA	243	49.6	6,846.2	30.3	439	62.1	12,661.7	40.8	386	62.0	14,955.4	43.9	371	60.8	15,896.4	44.0
Network	88	18.0	4,989.4	22.0	113	16.0	6,316.4	16.0	86	13.8	6,047.3	17.7	98	16.1	5,909.1	16.4
Total operational HMOs in U.S.	490	100.1		100.0	707	100.0		100.0	623	100.0		100.0	610	100.0		100.1
Under development	43	–		–	30	–		–	1				4	–		–
U.S. Total	533		22,606.4		737		31,024.4		624		34,125.2		614		36,136.3	

SOURCES: Marion Merrell Dow, Inc., *Marion Managed Care Digest. HMO Edition*, Kansas City, Mo., 1988, pp. 5, 6; _____, *Marion Managed Care Digest. HMO Edition*, Kansas City, Mo., 1989, p. 5; _____, *Marion Managed Care Digest. HMO Edition*, Kansas City, Mo., 1990, p. 5; and _____, *Marion Merrell Dow Managed Care Digest. Update Edition*, Kansas City, Mo., 1990, pp. 3, 6, 11. Reprinted Courtesy of Marion Merrell Dow, Inc.

frequently establish their own union for collective bargaining purposes.[9] When this occurs, management may lose much of the control that makes the staff model attractive.

For many reasons, staff models control a dwindling share of the HMO market, as shown in Table 4-4. These include high start-up costs and the reluctance of practicing physicians to give up established practices and their independence to become employees. Employers are beginning to favor other models that they admit may or may not control costs as well but give their employees more freedom in selecting a physician.[10] Staff models are also more difficult to market than some of the other models; many customers feel that they project an unappealing "clinic" atmosphere.[11]

THE GROUP MODEL[12]

The group model HMO is an organized prepaid health care system that contracts with one or more independent, multispecialty medical group practices to provide health services. As shown in Figure 4-3, this model HMO delivers medical services through the use of a medical group practice in the classic sense—a partnership or corporation that has three or more physician groups formally organized to deliver medical services; pools income; shares supplies, equipment, and personnel; and distributes net income according to a pre-arranged formula. Most medical group practices that become involved with a group model HMO will treat prepaid members along with their traditional fee-for-service patients.

This model is known as a closed-panel HMO because, like the staff model, only those physicians who are included in the participating medical group(s) are eligible to provide services to health plan members. Thus, the health plan is closed to all physicians who are not members of the medical group(s).

As shown in Table 4-4, the number of group model HMOs remained stable during the period 1985 through 1989, although, in relation to the total number

---

[9] Dustin L. Mackie and Douglas K. Decker, *Group and IPA HMOs*, Gaithersburg, Md., Aspen Publishers, Inc., 1981, p. 110; Harold S. Luft, *Health Maintenance Organizations: Dimensions of Performance*, New York, John Wiley and Sons, 1981, pp. 13, 350–351; and J. Riffer, "Physician Unions Fight Loss of Control," *Hospitals, 60*(2):82, January 20, 1986. An example of physician unionization and the problems that such unionization can cause is illustrated by the physician strike at Group Health Association of America in Washington, D.C. in the winter of 1986.

[10] "IPAs Can Expand Their Market Easier." (Editorial.) *Health Services Information, 12*(26):5, June 24, 1985.

[11] S. Alan Savitz and Paul R. Roberts. "Some Notes on the Development of an IPA Model HMO." *Journal of Ambulatory Care Management, 9*(2):33–53, May 1986.

[12] This discussion draws on Robert G. Shouldice, "HMOs: Four Models Profiled," *Medical Group Management, 33*(3):9, May/June 1986.

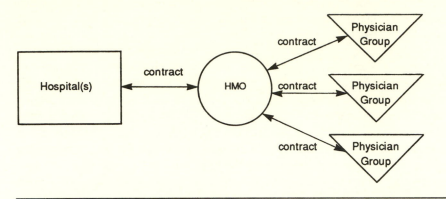

FIGURE 4-3   Typical group model HMO.

of enrollees, this model dropped from 19 percent in 1985 to 13.6 percent in 1989. There was a moderate increase in total enrollment in group model HMOs from 1985 to 1989 to approximately 9.6 million members. The model showing the greatest growth in both number of plans and enrollment, however, is the IPA model. Overall growth in operational HMO health plans between 1985 and 1990 was approximately 15.4 percent, while growth in enrollment during this same period was approximately 60 percent.

There are several approaches to developing a group model HMO. These variations are discussed in the sections that follow.

Contractual Group Model

In this model, two separate companies, a group practice and an HMO, develop a contract describing the rights and responsibilities of each party. Included are issues of utilization control, medical review and audit, services to be provided, and methods of payment for services. Control of the group's medical practices, patterns, and financial destiny are at stake in these contracts. The medical group physicians agree to treat health plan patients exclusively. In this situation, the medical group is considered a "captive group," whose sole existence is for service delivery to the HMO's members. Occasionally, the HMO is instrumental in the group practice's development; the plan may recruit its physicians and provide management services to the group even though the group is a separate legal entity.[13] The Permanente Clinics of the Kaiser

---

[13] Peter R. Kongstvedt. *The Managed Health Care Handbook.* Gaithersburg, Md., Aspen Publishers, Inc., 1989, p. 15.

Foundation Health Plan are examples of captive group practices providing services exclusively to the HMO.

Independent Group Model

In other, less common situations, a well-established medical group may agree to deliver medical care to enrollees of the HMO along with its usual fee-for-service business. In some instances, the medical group may have sponsored or may even own the HMO, but unlike the captive group model, the contractual relations created between the two organizations allow these group practices to act independently of the HMO, continuing their traditional practices as well as serving HMO members. Thus, these arrangements are called independent group model HMOs.[14] Examples of such arrangements include Peak Health and the Colorado Springs Medical Center in Colorado and the Geisinger Health Plan and the Geisinger Clinic in central Pennsylvania. Some of these groups have found that the growth of the HMO business has been so great that the HMO wields tremendous control over the independent medical group. As some group practice managers have said, "the tail wags the dog."

Integrated Group Model

A third variation occurs when an existing medical group develops, owns, and operates its own HMO as another line of business in conjunction with its existing activities. The term "integrated" defines this approach since the HMO is totally integrated within the other activities of the multispecialty medical group—as a department or a division. Historically, this approach was used by the early prepaid group practice plans such as the Ross-Loos medical group, the Western Clinic, and the Palo Alto Medical Clinic. Today, however, one seldom observes the integrated medical group model HMO. With HMOs showing major growth, acceptable returns to owners, and control of risk, it is obvious that being an owner/provider is better for physicians than just being a provider. Substantial control over the group's destiny weighs in the balance, and group ownership of the HMO strengthens the group's ability to help manage its own financial and medical affairs over the long term. Physician involvement in sponsoring and owning HMOs, however, is becoming ever more limited.

HMO developers and the large multistate, national HMO firms have penetrated all major markets and are moving swiftly to capture the secondary targets—small towns and communities surrounding the large metropolitan areas. What remains for physician groups may be a 5 to 30 percent token position of

---

[14] Ibid.

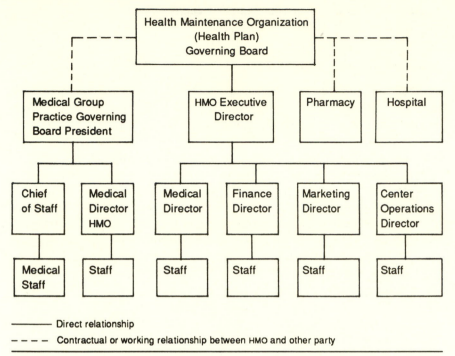

FIGURE 4-4 Organizational structure of a contractual group model HMO *not* established/owned by the medical group practice: health center (clinic) operations under HMO management.

ownership in any new HMOs. This seems hardly enough to sway board policy to join or not join in HMO activities. But partial ownership at least allows the physicians to share in profits and risks, provide opportunities for initial and ongoing capitalization, and create a voice in policy formation. It tends to bring to the HMO board table, as well as to the examining table, some commonality of purpose and understanding between the HMO and the medical group.

Organizational Structure

Figures 4-4, 4-5, and 4-6 provide the structure of contractual and integrated group model HMOs. Note that Figures 4-4 and 4-5 depict contractual arrangements between HMOs and affiliated medical groups. In Figure 4-4, the medical group is in control of its own professional (physician) operations and the HMO manages health center operations (facilities). Figure 4-5 identifies a clinic

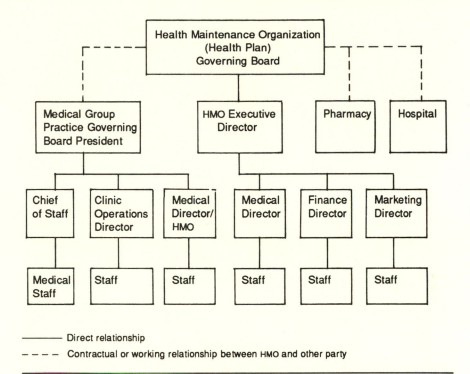

---------- Direct relationship

– – – – Contractual or working relationship between HMO and other party

FIGURE 4-5 **Example of a contractual group model HMO *not* established/ owned by the medical group practice: health center (clinic) operations under medical group practice management.**

operations director, usually described as a clinic manager or administrator. In addition, the medical group identifies a medical director who manages the group's medical affairs as they relate to HMO patients. Figure 4-5 suggests an approach where both the group practice and health center operations are under the management of the medical group practice. But, notice that the medical group has a need to appoint a medical director responsible for HMO activities. In both figures, the medical director of the medical group has a close working relationship with a medical director counterpart in the HMO structure. Finally, Figure 4-6 represents an integrated medical group with the HMO as a department. Health plan functions, especially marketing and financial/actuarial activities, are added to the usual medical group practice functions (nursing, business office, finance, and clinic operations). Because of the unique nature of HMO financial affairs, a separate functional area is created, but with direct working relationships with other clinic financial employees.

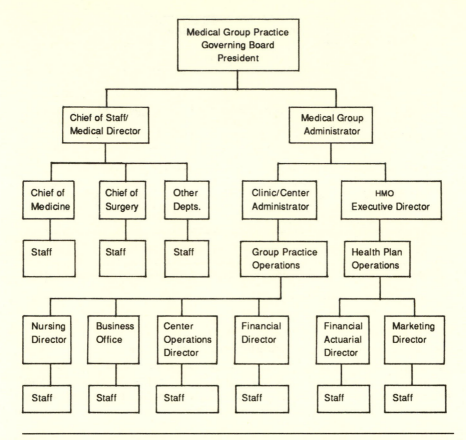

FIGURE 4-6   Organizational structure of a group model HMO sponsored/ owned by a medical group: an integrated group model.

Capitation

The HMO pays the medical group for its services from premiums and other revenues. These payments are made on a full or discounted fee-for-service, fee-for-time, or capitated basis, usually the latter. Since capitated payments to the group are radically different from traditional fee-for-service (FFS) payments, the physicians now must understand the new incentives that will force changes in their practice patterns but will give the physicians a broader variety of medical service alternatives which are not available under traditional FFS insurance plans. Because there will be both FFS income and capitated payments (in all but the captive group models), the group's current income-sharing formula may no longer be an equitable method for distributing the surplus from operations. The objectives of the HMO are to ensure that the services defined in the benefits package are available when enrollees require them and, thus, to develop relationships with medical groups for delivering needed services. The HMO also will attempt to spread the risks of required medical services to other organizations. By negotiating a capitation contract with the medical group that includes more than just primary physician services, the HMO transfers a substantial amount of its risks to the group. Conversely, the medical group's objective should be to negotiate a capitation level that assures sufficient funds to cover the costs of operation and allows for a profit or surplus from its business. By accepting a capitation for services it cannot provide itself, the medical group may be taking an undue risk of loss, since it becomes the group's responsibility to arrange and pay for such services by outside-the-group providers, usually at full FFS rates. Negotiating a capitation with the HMO is the key to creating acceptable levels of payment for the medical group.

Group Model Advantages and Disadvantages

The major advantages of the group model HMO are those associated with an organized multispecialty group practice—the economies of scale associated with moderately sized medical groups, the sharing of resources by group members, the management of patient care through utilization of a unit medical record, the perceived high quality of medical services provided by medical groups, the ability of physicians to practice medicine rather than spend some of their time with practice management activities, the greater application of physician extenders in medical groups than in other practice settings, and so on. Most important, shared medical charts and physician involvement in decision making produce more efficient and probably more effective medical behavior.[15]

The major criticism of the group model HMO and the staff arrangement relates to the use of the closed panel of physician providers. Traditional health plans suggest that HMOs provide no, or only a limited, choice of physicians—that is, enrollees are locked into a system with little choice of primary physicians and limited health center locations. Administrators of group and staff model HMOs recognize these potential problems in developing their strategic planning efforts. For example, most HMOs will not embark on a marketing effort until appropriate physician office locations and acceptable numbers of primary physicians have been procured. And, as new members enroll with the HMO, they are provided with some, although limited, choice

[15] Raymond Fink. "Organizational Imperatives—What Motivates Providers?" *Bulletin of the New York Academy of Medicine, 63*(1):40, January–February 1987.

of provider locations as well as a choice among two or three primary care physicians. Members are also given the opportunity to change sites and primary physicians, who then become their "family" or managing physicians. Ultimately, the growth of both the staff and group model HMOs will be limited by their ability to expand delivery sites, especially if the HMO must shoulder the capital costs of such expansion.

The group model HMO is an excellent compromise in health plan organization. It utilizes existing medical groups that maintain high standards of practice and are stable organizations, existing within a very competitive environment. Group practices are increasing in number and size and are relatively efficient methods of providing medical services. Utilization data suggest that group models generally fall within the average of all HMOs regarding physician encounters and hospital days per 1,000 members. Overall, HMOs utilizing medical groups have some of the lowest operational costs of all the models. Many researchers suggest that the reduced use of hospital care in HMOs occurs because of the multispecialty group practices that are utilized in the HMO industry.[16] In the final analysis, then, the group model HMO may contain costs more effectively than other models and may be able to pass these cost savings along to employers and subscribers through lower premiums than those charged by competing health plans.

THE INDIVIDUAL PRACTICE ASSOCIATION (IPA) MODEL

The individual practice association model HMOs provide physician services through a contract with an association of physicians, usually a separate legal entity, formed by an investor or group of investors that acts as the physicians' management organization (and bargaining agent). The IPA receives payments (usually capitations) from the health plan and arranges to have its physician members provide services; it then pays the physicians on a negotiated fee-for-service or capitation basis.[17] Physicians who enter into written service agreements with the IPA become IPA participating members, maintaining their own offices and practices instead of using a centralized facility owned by the HMO or a multispecialty group practice with shared staff, equipment, and medical records. They agree to provide services to HMO members along with their established non-HMO practices; practice patterns remain similar for both classes of patients, with the physician maintaining medical records for all patients and generally managing his/her private practice.

---

[16] Ibid, pp. 34–35.

[17] Payment in IPAs has traditionally been on a discounted fee-for-service basis, including a percentage "withhold" of the fees as a reserve against deficits. These issues are addressed in Chapters 6 and 11 as risk sharing.

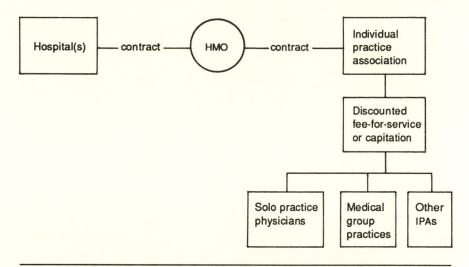

FIGURE 4-7   Open panel/individual practice association HMO.

Multispecialty medical groups, even though this model is predominately organized around solo practices, also become members of the IPA, agreeing to provide services to HMO enrollees along with their other patients. In addition, the IPA that is party to the contract with the health plan may, itself, contract with one or more associations of physicians in independent practice. These relationships are presented in Figure 4-7.

Open-Panel Model and Foundations for Medical Care

Unlike the staff and group model HMOs, the IPA model is described as an open-panel arrangement, because membership in the IPA is "open" to any physician in the community that meets the IPA's credentialing procedures. In the past, credentialing was almost automatic; if physicians were members of the local medical society and were willing to pay a small membership fee, they were routinely approved for membership. More recently, because of the great potential for malpractice suits against HMOs and IPAs, initial and annual reviews have become more important.

At this point, it might be useful to provide a historical basis for closed- versus open-panel models. In 1954, California physicians who were not affiliated with the closed-panel Kaiser Foundation Health Plan joined together to protect the fee-for-service solo practices that were being threatened by the expansion of the Kaiser-Permanente system. The organization that evolved was

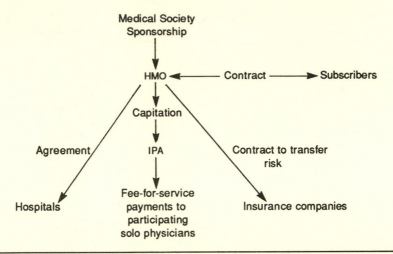

FIGURE 4-8 **Early individual practice association/Foundation for Medical Care model HMO.**

the Foundation for Medical Care (FMC) of San Joaquin Valley, California.[18] This arrangement, also known as a prepaid individual practice plan, was the precursor to the current IPA model HMO. It was usually sponsored and organized by county or state medical societies, and membership was open to all physicians who were members of the society. As a health plan, the FMC developed a package of comprehensive medical service benefits and guaranteed health services by contracting with various physicians in the local medical society and with hospitals and insurance companies (see Figure 4-8). The principal objectives of the FMC were to ensure accessibility of care through sponsorship of a prepaid health insurance program and to carefully monitor the quality of services, the appropriateness of delivery point, and the reasonableness of its costs. Although incorporating some of the most attractive features of prepaid health plans (that is, comprehensive benefits packages, quality and peer review, utilization control through claims review, etc.), FMCs still maintained the private practice of medicine *without* accepting risk in the manner that today's HMOs utilize. Risk was either limited by contract or subcontracted to insurance companies, although comprehensive FMCs had the capability of sharing a small portion of the underwriting risk (with the participating physicians receiving reduced fees if the premium did not cover

[18] William C. McMorran. "A Good Hard Look at IPAs." *Health Management Quarterly*, 9(4):9–11, Fall 1987.

the services provided). The majority of the risk, however, was transferred to the fiscal intermediary.

The FMC approach that used these concepts became the basis for the IPA model described in the HMO Act of 1973. Like other HMO models, the act allows the IPA model HMO to pass risk to providers and to obtain reinsurance through outside insurance carriers. Initially, the federally qualified IPA model HMO used two separate organizations, as shown in Figure 4-8—one was the HMO or health plan and the other was the IPA. As a medical management organization engaged in arranging for the coordinated delivery of all or part of the health services to members enrolled in the HMO, the IPA enters into service arrangements with individuals licensed to provide health services. The agreement describes the services to be provided to HMO members and the level of compensation and method of payment to physicians. An HMO member may, however, reasonably expect the individual practitioner or the IPA to provide all contracted-for benefits, but because the member's agreement is with the HMO and not directly with the IPA or the physicians, it is the HMO that bears direct responsibility to its members for all benefits covered under the agreement.

By the late 1970s, federally qualified IPA model HMOs began to bring together under one umbrella both the health plan management functions and the IPA medical management functions, as shown in Figure 4-9. Even though they continue to be separate corporations or partnerships, in practice the boards and staff of the two organizations are the same people, and payment of the capitation is a paper transaction between the two companies. In effect, the

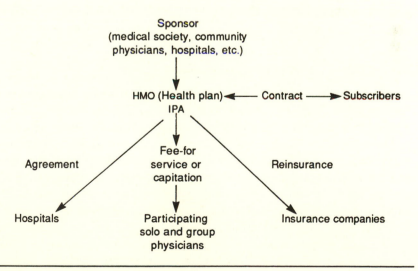

FIGURE 4-9 Modified IPA model HMO.

HMO and IPA operate as one organization, with the same company objectives and motives. Most IPA model HMOs that originally were sponsored by providers currently are organizationally arranged in this fashion.

The latest permutation of the IPA model HMO is one in which the IPA structure disappears completely and the HMO contracts directly with the individual physician providers; it is still considered an IPA model HMO, because the HMO is contracting with individual physicians rather than employing them or contracting with a medical group practice. Fitting newly developing HMOs into these categories is becoming more difficult. As pointed out in Chapter 3 on PPOs, there is a blurring of definitions of the HMO models and other managed care companies like PPOs and CMPs. By understanding the concepts included in each of the existing arrangements, one is able to understand the structures of the newly emerging forms.

Contractual Issues

In most IPA situations, the HMO contracts with the separate legal entity, the IPA. In turn, the IPA develops provider agreements and, through them, contracts with independent physicians. Major issues addressed in this contract deal with the services to be provided by the physician; the procedures for determining certification, authorization for referral, and hospital admission; utilization control and peer review; physician compensation; and the level of insurance the physician will be required to carry. The matter of coordinating benefits, copayments, and other enrollee contract issues may be addressed. Conditions and procedures for credentialing and terminating a physician are also clearly defined. Finally, the contract clearly specifies the method by which the physician compensation levels will be renegotiated in future periods.

Gatekeeper; Physician as Case Manager

Originally, HMOs signed participating agreements with any and all physicians who wanted to join with the IPA, and based payment for services on the fee schedules of usual and customary physician charges. Practice and referral patterns followed existing and traditional arrangements. The outcome was major financial problems experienced by both the health plan and the IPA. The lesson learned was that an IPA model HMO must, like other HMO models, choose managers and doctors that recognize the need for control. Methods were needed that would help physicians understand that they were spending their own money, because most participating physicians were also stockholders in the IPA. Thus, IPAs began selectively choosing participating physicians, initiating the concept of the gatekeeper or managing physician. Under this scheme, the patient has unlimited access to the primary care physician but must obtain a referral from that physician in order to receive health services from specialists, whose fees are generally higher.

By using this approach, IPAs move from a straight fee-for-service payment scheme to either a discounted fee schedule with a 10 to 20 percent withhold of fees as a reserve for cost overruns, or a capitation approach. In either situation, two different gatekeeper approaches may be used.

First, the capitation or discounted fees to the primary physician include only primary services, with specialists paid either through fees-for-service or a second capitation. Referrals of enrollees to participating specialists by the primary physician are based on the patient's need for such service; the primary physician has no financial stake in limiting the referrals. Under such an arrangement, there exists the possibility of inappropriate and excessive referrals.

A second approach is to place the primary care doctors at risk for the cost of specialists' care, that is, to make capitation payments or pay discounted fees with a withhold, to the primary physician for both primary and specialty services. In this situation, the primary physician as gatekeeper is in control of all referrals, because there is an added financial incentive to appropriately control referrals. Some experts suggest that this gatekeeper approach effectively controls utilization, but it may also limit necessary referrals. Compensating the primary physician on a capitation basis for both primary and specialty services may change the natural fee-for-service relations between primary and specialty physicians; instead of the specialist maintaining the higher level of respect, prestige, status, and influence, the primary gatekeeper has the clout to control the activities of the specialist. This change in roles may adversely affect the working relationships between these physicians. Even with some of the resulting adverse effects, it is estimated that more than 70 percent of all IPA model HMOs are of the gatekeeper type.[19]

Compensation

As noted, most HMOs compensate the IPA on a capitation basis. The HMO defines the type and amount of services that are to be delivered to enrollees and then rates these services, based on risks and generally accepted underwriting rules. Budgeted amounts are grouped into funds or pools for primary care, specialty care, hospitalization, pharmaceuticals, and so on. The capitation is, therefore, the HMO's estimate of costs per member per month for physician services and would be drawn from the physician's pool. Likewise, the IPA

---

[19] Merian Kirchner. "Can IPAs Save Small Practices?" *Medical Economics,* 62(15):180, July 22, 1985.

should estimate its level of risk before agreeing to the capitation offered by the health plan, although this seldom occurs. Then, the IPA compensates its physician members either through a fee schedule and fee-for-service (the classic model), a capitation, or a combination of fee-for-service and capitation.

In the classic IPA model, the participating physicians bill the IPA for services provided to health plan enrollees assigned to them. The IPA processes these fee-for-service claims, and payment is made to the physicians based on the IPA's fee schedule. Frequently described as "negotiated," the fees may be discounted from the physician's usual and customary charges; they are usually described as the lower of billed charges or a fee screen that is developed by the HMO or IPA, which identifies the maximum allowable IPA fees. Patients are free to visit any primary or specialty physician on the IPA's panel. Thus, the characteristic of traditional private practice is maintained while adding the prepaid component.

In the capitation approach, the primary care physician receives either a capitation based on the primary pool only or one based on both the primary and specialty pools together. While a primary care capitation limits physician payments to primary services, the physician continues to have the responsibility for managing all the care of HMO members in his or her practice and, in fact, may be paid a small "management fee" for his/her efforts. The full medical capitation, which could include primary and specialty services as well as emergency room fees, adds a financial incentive to the physician's other professional and ethical inducements to appropriately manage patient care. Specialists may likewise be paid a capitation for their services, although discounted fee-for-service is usually used with specialists whose services are infrequently needed.

Utilization, Peer Review, and Quality Assurance

Typically, IPAs collect data on each physician's average billings per patient and compare them against other fees for the same specialty area and against an acceptable range predetermined by health plan and IPA representatives. Any physician whose billings are above the allowed range is penalized by forfeiting part or all of his/her withhold, although individual IPAs vary in their treatment of deviations from the median range. For instance, broad ranges may be used to allow for individual variations. When deviations occur, they are examined individually to determine whether the physician has an unusually difficult case load.

Since much of the success of managed care health plans depends on the practice behavior of physicians, IPA model HMOs, where the physicians are at risk, are given incentives not only to control costs but also to lower quality—to underutilize. There are several ways that this problem is addressed. First, to the extent possible, the IPA evaluates each physician's utilization record before he or she becomes a provider in the system and uses selection criteria that may be more strict than those used for granting hospital privileges.[20] Once a physician joins the panel, evaluation of utilization is ongoing. In the event that a physician fails to eliminate inefficient practices, the provider contract contains provisions for terminating the relationship. Second, the initial health plan/physician relationship can be structured to avoid unwanted physician incentives. For instance, individual physicians may be allowed to receive no more than 20 percent of the savings from their actions, except for primary care.[21] Third, the health plan can use an outside organization, such as a professional review organization (PRO), to review the actual delivery of services, or DHHS's Office of Prepaid Health Care, to qualify the HMO or to certify it for Medicare risk contracting.

Evidence suggests that IPAs have gradually reduced hospital use. For instance, in 1981, IPA hospital use was 529 days per 1,000 members; by 1984, this figure dropped to 424 days per 1,000 members. In 1989, the figure for non-Medicare participants was 372.8 days per 1,000 members. In 1985, IPA rates were 15 percent higher than those for group model HMOs and 8 percent higher than those for staff model HMOs, but by 1989, IPAs were 12.3 percent higher than group models and 6.8 percent higher than staff models.[22] Although IPA models are still above the average for all HMOs in the United States, the success of IPAs in reducing hospital use is attributed to the combination of physician financial incentives, careful physician selection, and effective utilization review.

Summary of IPA Issues; Closed- versus Open-Panel HMOs

Heightened interest in open-panel IPA model HMOs has intensified interest in the value of these structures versus the closed-group or staff models. Obviously, the panel type chosen has great impact on the actual delivery element, marketing strategies, and, ultimately, the competitive position of the health plan.

---

[20] Savitz and Roberts. "Some Notes on the Development of an IPA Model HMO."

[21] W. Pete Welch. "IPAs Emerge on the HMO Forefront." *Business and Health*, 5(4):15, February 1988.

[22] Kirchner, "Can IPAs Save Small Practices?," p. 176; Fink, "Organizational Imperatives," p. 39; Marion Merrell Dow, Inc., *Marion Managed Care Digest. HMO Edition*, Kansas City, Mo., MMD, 1988, p. 24; and _____, *Marion Merrell Dow Managed Care Digest. HMO Edition*, Kansas City, Mo., MMD, 1990, pp. 24–25.

THE NETWORK MODEL

The fourth HMO model, the network shown in Figure 4-10, contracts with two or more separate medical groups and/or IPAs. It is also possible for each group to participate in more than one HMO, unless the medical group signs an exclusive contract with the HMO. From the HMO's perspective, it may contract with only a limited number of medical groups and, thus, will have characteristics similar to a closed-panel plan. Conversely, by contracting with IPAs and any physician that meets eligibility criteria, the network HMO is an open-panel plan. Each medical group and IPA in the network receives compensation from the HMO in the form of capitation for those HMO members who have selected the medical group or IPA physician as a provider. Each medical group and IPA physician provides its own facilities, equipment, medical records, and support staff.[23]

There are variations on this arrangement also. Probably the most common is the staff model HMO, which contracts with outside medical groups as a means of expansion; being composed of both staff model and group model characteristics, it becomes a network model.[24]

Administration and Contractual Relations

The HMO, its affiliated IPAs, and medical groups that are part of the network are separate legal entities. The health plan and the providers negotiate separate contracts that meet the needs of each party. Frequently, it is the provider's responsibility to contract with specialists, either on a fee-for-service or capitation basis. Further, like staff and group models, it is the HMO's responsibility to arrange for inpatient services, usually through hospital agreements. But such agreements will be limited by existing staff privileges of the participating physicians. Occasionally HMOs develop hospital agreements that allow the individual group practice physicians to automatically apply for hospital privileges if they are not already available; obviously, each physician must meet the credentialing process of the hospital to be admitted to the staff.

The network HMO is responsible for plan marketing, premium collections, and all other health plan activities. It has its own medical director, who is responsible for ensuring that all affiliated physicians meet established HMO

---

[23] U.S. Department of Health and Human Services, Bureau of Health Maintenance Organizations, Division of Analysis and Technical Assistance. *Guide for Fee-for-Service Medical Groups on Affiliation with Health Maintenance Organizations.* Rockville, Md., DHHS, March 1983, p. 12.

[24] The IPA designation of network model HMOs is significant only in relation to the mandatory dual/multiple-choice provision of the federal HMO Act, which states that the existence of one staff, one group, *and* one IPA model HMO in a given locality may mandate dual/multiple-choice offerings by employers having at least 25 employees.

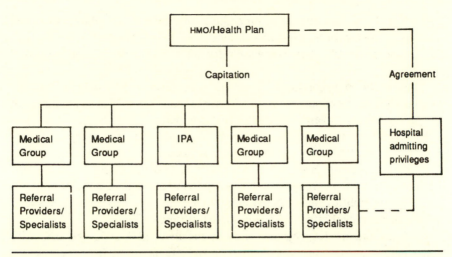

FIGURE 4-10 Network model HMO.

credentials and that all medical groups and IPAs have proper utilization review and quality assurance committees. Additional responsibilities of the HMO medical director include the resolution of medical issues that surface through consumer grievance procedures and any other medical issues brought to the HMO by the individual medical directors of affiliated medical groups.

Physician payments for service, risk arrangements, and incentives to control costs in the network model are the same as in the group model. In almost all cases, the medical group or IPA will be at full risk for referrals.[25] Incentives to control costs, therefore, will be based on the performance of each group or IPA provider, with the performance of the providers as a whole being an HMO-wide indicator of successful operation.

Advantages and Disadvantages of the Network Model

From a health plan's management perspective, the network model has a significant advantage over the traditional group model. By contracting with several delivery points, the HMO, at little cost, greatly increases its service area and its target population. The increased geographic reach outweighs the model's drawback of greater complexity in the administration of a system composed of several separate, independent medical providers. This problem is overcome through sophisticated computerized management information

[25] U.S. Department of Health and Human Service. *Guide for Fee-for-Service Medical Groups on Affiliation with Health Maintenance Organizations*, p. 47.

systems and standard operating procedures that require preauthorization and concurrent review of hospitalized patients, the use of the gatekeeper concept, full capitation, timely claim submission for services outside the capitation, and so on.

The ability to negotiate with several unaffiliated providers allows the health plan to develop the most favorable conditions. Contrast this with the group model, where the HMO-affiliated medical groups may also have close affiliations themselves—like the Permanente Clinics serving the Kaiser Foundation Health Plan—and may be able to form a strong bargaining position through joint effort. Even when there are strong intergroup relationships, however, the medical groups and IPAs are autonomous and, because of internal-to-the-group politics, may not be able to develop a united front that would enable them to deal effectively with the health plan.

The network model may also present the medical groups and IPAs with some unique cost-saving opportunities. Providers involved in a network can join together to form purchasing units or can establish service agreements with each other. But, most importantly, they may be able to form a negotiating unit that could help develop favorable contracts with the health plan, if a way is found to subordinate the petty, individual political issues of each group to the broader issues of all the groups.

HYBRID AND OPEN-ENDED HMOs[26]

During the the mid- and late 1980s, the HMO field experienced rapid changes in the organizational structure, benefits packages, marketing activities, relationships with providers and consumers, and the health plans' activities with their competition. Medical groups serving HMO enrollees have been allowed to collect higher copayments, and the HMOs have placed copayments on more services for certain groups of enrollees. In addition, providers involved in both HMO and PPO contracts have been asked to be placed "at-risk" in their preferred provider agreements. Some groups have even been asked to provide services to different classes of enrollees under multiple arrangements with the same managed care organization. Changes have occurred because HMOs and PPOs are competing more aggressively with each other, as well as with the traditional health insurance/delivery system. The following dramatic changes are taking place in the health services industry.[27]

---

[26] Adapted from Robert G. Shouldice, "New Hybrid HMO/PPO Models and Benefit Packages," *Medical Group Management Journal*, 35(5):12–14, September/October 1988.

[27] Adapted from Peter Boland, "Trends in Second Generation PPOs," *Health Affairs*, 6(4):75, Winter 1987.

1. *Players and Organizational Structures*

   - Health services are being purchaser driven, with the Federal Government and insurers, including HMOs, taking a stronger role in directing and mandating health services benefits packages, quality assurance mechanisms, utilization control, and the overall direction of the industry.
   - The domination and control of the industry by providers have diminished as purchasers have assumed these roles.
   - PPOs and HMOs are moving toward more sophisticated and complex arrangements that might be termed "second generation."
   - With the market shifts, hybrid organizations are emerging that blur the differences among IPA model HMOs, PPOs, and managed care fee-for-service indemnity health plans.

2. *Administration*

   - Discounts, as the major characteristic of PPOs, are being replaced by internal administrative controls (including provider selection standards and credentialing, utilization review procedures, and information systems) as the most effective strategy for achieving long-term cost savings for employers. Discounts, however, continue to be used along with these additional administrative activities.

3. *Benefits and Products*

   - HMOs are developing multiple-option products that allow them to compete more effectively with PPOs and traditional systems and that provide substantial administrative advantages to employers.
   - HMOs are also developing "minimum benefits" health insurance packages that are more like the Blue Cross/Blue Shield products of the 1960s than the comprehensive benefits packages required under the HMO Act.
   - Both HMOs and PPOs are initiating innovative health benefits designs that allow for "carve-outs" of optional services such as mental health care and dental coverage.

4. *Risks*

   - Low-risk- and high-risk-sharing arrangements in the same HMO are becoming available to employers and providers.
   - Some second-generation PPOs are adding a risk-taking component to their products; these insurance risk activities may be underwritten by outside indemnity insurance companies and may include risk sharing with the PPO's physicians.

5. *Quality*

- Quality assurance (QA) has become the single most important issue in programs that use provider incentives to control program
  costs. Even in programs such as nonrisk PPOs, QA is the key to
  ensuring appropriate treatment, cost-effective services, and targeted
  cost control.

The most significant development has been the movement by HMOs to offer
other than comprehensive benefits packages, namely, "open-ended HMOs" and
hybrid products. When InterStudy first described this activity in December
1986, only four HMOs were offering such services. By 1990, 14.6 percent of
all HMOs offered open-ended products; enrollment in these plans was 857,995,
an increase of 39.2 percent over 1989.

Arrangements for offering open-ended HMO products vary significantly,
depending on state regulatory requirements, but the costs of providing these
services outside the HMO are generally covered through a separate agreement
with an insurance company. This arrangement allows the HMO to compete with
traditional indemnity insurers by offering standard, comprehensive indemnity
policies and products that include benefits with large copayments or deductibles and limits on the dollar amount of coverage. Open-ended HMOs allow
members to receive services outside the HMO's provider network without
referral authorization. Hybrid HMOs, in addition, are regulated by state insurance departments as insurance products and included only two plans in 1990—
CIGNA FlexCare, with 426,572 members, and Prudential Plus, with 960,000
members. In several states, these arrangements currently are not allowed;
however, the 1988 HMO amendments do allow qualified HMOs to develop both
multiple insuring arrangements and nonfederally qualified health plans under
the HMO corporate umbrella.

Hybrid and open-ended HMOs modify the total lock-in of members, which
has been the most significant barrier to HMO enrollment. Open-ended arrangements are clearly the most important issues for HMOs that are accustomed to
closed panels of physicians (group and staff model HMOs), where utilization
control is the highest priority for a successful system. The HMO may perform
utilization review and quality assessment of the services included in the
indemnity segment of its plan, even though these benefits are covered by a
separate outside insurance company. Finally, the choice by HMO enrollees of the
HMO product rather than the indemnity option may depend on several factors—
the enrollee's previous experience with the HMO, a continuing relationship with
a particular physician, and the cost differential between using the HMO and the
indemnity plan, among others.

LINKAGES IN THE HMO INDUSTRY [28]

Joint ventures, networks and alliances, management agreements and contracts, franchises, syndicating, mergers, and acquisitions are occurring frequently in the managed care field. These management configurations, often successful in other industries and commerce, hold significant promise for the HMO and PPO systems, which are under incessant scrutiny and currently experiencing dynamic and driving changes. HMOs are keenly aware that they need to contain rising costs and premiums by creating acceptable linkages that will strengthen control of their market position. These new alliances may assure quality provider elements and make it easier for these alternative delivery systems to enter more fully into the major national employer market.

Organizational Arrangements—Horizontal and Vertical Integration

The multiorganizational arrangements described in the next several paragraphs can be categorized as either horizontally or vertically integrated. Horizontal integration suggests that the new arrangement consists of like kinds of organizations—all staff model HMOs or all single-specialty medical groups. Many multicorporate, multistate HMO firms have grown in this fashion; such growth may occur through acquisitions and mergers. The strength of the horizontal integration approach is rapid growth in one area: development and management of one "specialty" area such as IPA model HMOs.

Conversely, the vertically integrated arrangement would include "all levels of production" (services and financing). This latter type of organization might tie HMOs in with hospitals, multispecialty medical groups, solo super-specialty physicians, indemnity insurance companies, and the like. Most of the current hospital-based, investor co-owned operations are vertical organizations. These firms tie together capitated, indemnity, and even service plans with the providers of care at all levels (primary, secondary, and tertiary). Acquisitions and mergers are used to develop vertically, but the use of syndicating, franchises, and joint ventures will become commonplace as special services are developed—services that are unique, one-of-a-kind, and from a "sole-source provider." These arrangements will become local centers of excellence, owned and/or managed through large multistate corporations.

In the following listing, descriptions are provided of possible types of arrangements. Franchises are distinguished as an *organizational concept* that is sold to another group or individual. Syndicating is *programmatic,* usually

---

[28] Adapted from Joe E. Strange and Robert G. Shouldice, "Defining New Linkages in the HMO Industry: The Changing Market," *Hospital Topics,* 65(3):12–16, May/June 1987.

for advertising a marketing program that does not require a new building or the outlay of capital expenditures. Marketing networks are *shared systems,* which HMOs have been using for several years.

1. *Joint Venture:* The most common arrangement in the HMO industry, a joint venture is a legally enforceable agreement between two or more organizations—at least one of which is an entity already in operation as a going concern—for the purpose of conducting a new business or providing a new (not necessarily novel) service and/or product.[29] Such arrangements might include associate equity owners who take an active role in the formation and operation of the business. The advantages of forming a joint venture include reduced capital expenditures, improved technology transfer, rapid commercialization of new services like HMOs, achievement of economies of scale, and potential risk reduction. Joint ventures also allow HMOs to retain corporate autonomy while realizing the gains from cooperation on a specific project—perhaps in a new geographic location removed from its market area. Disadvantages of this type of organizational/financial arrangement may include disputes over procedures, disagreements between smaller health plans and their larger partner(s) over the pace of expansion, and the possibility that problems may emerge when a joint venture project is split from a firm's operations. Sometimes antitrust issues can arise, and care should be taken to examine all problems surrounding an antitrust issue.

2. *HMO Management Agreements and Contracts:* These are contractual agreements between independent HMOs and national health care management firms, through which the independent HMOs purchase administrative or other types of management and/or health care skills from the national firm without merging, syndicating, or franchising. Complete legal autonomy is maintained; no new firm is created. This arrangement is frequently used by fee-for-service medical groups that seek to enter the HMO arena but do not have the requisite HMO management capabilities. Although national HMO firms have managed local HMOs, most prefer an equity position in the local HMO as a condition of the management agreement. The feeling is that equity creates incentives for the success of both parties.

3. *Mergers:* Mergers are the union of two or more independent health care groups. Within the HMO arena, mergers historically tended to result in the absorption of small HMOs by large national organizations. Today, however, it is

---

[29] Neal F. Bermas. "Joint Ventures in Ambulatory Care." *Journal of Ambulatory Care Management,* 8(4):79–87, November 1985. *See also* Epstein, Becker, Borsody and Green, PC. "Joint Ventures, Level I, Introduction to Joint Ventures, Seminar Outline." Washington, D.C., May 14, 1985, p. 1.

not unusual for two or more small HMOs to merge in an effort to effect strong competition for a national chain that is trying to establish a foothold in the community.

4. *Acquisitions:* HMOs are establishing health care networks through the purchase of either similar or dissimilar health care delivery systems so as to provide their patients with more comprehensive and often less-expensive care. Through these acquisitions the HMO gains decentralization, convenience for its members, and an alternative to more expensive referrals.

5. *Franchises:* InterStudy has examined the presence of national HMO firms and found that approximately two-thirds of all prepaid health plans started in 1985 were developed by national HMO chains, while the remaining were independently started. As of January 1989, 60 percent of all HMOs were linked (by ownership or operation) to national firms, and national firms attracted 71 percent of the total HMO enrollment of 35.3 million members.[30] National chains such as Kaiser Foundation Health Plan, Inc., CIGNA, Prudential Health Care Plans, and others are able to provide management services and economies of scale that have traditionally made large organizations more competitive. Now, the same advantages that are enjoyed by these chains are available to individual entrepreneurs in the health care field through franchising. This option provides an alternative for physicians who are uncomfortable with the concept of being an employee of a large chain or becoming involved in the business aspects of a medical practice. Franchising offers freedom from corporate bureaucracy and efficiency through economies of scale.

A franchise is a right or license that is granted to an individual or group to market a company's goods or services in a particular territory. This alternative may be feasible when a national health services organization markets unique or one-of-a-kind health care packages to HMOs and licenses independent HMOs to sell the health services package in a particular location. The license includes the purchase of the national firm's trademarks, health care products such as unique benefits packages or programs for special groups such as farmers, unique marketing programs for subgroups in the target population, and management information and other systems required to administratively manage the health services packages franchised to the HMO. The HMO generally would pay a fee for this privilege, plus a royalty on gross premiums or some other measurement of success.

---

[30] Maureen Shadle, Lynn R. Gruber, and Mary M. Hunter, *1989 National Managed Care Firms,* Excelsior, Minn., InterStudy, December 1989, p. i; and Lynn R. Gruber, Maureen Shadle, Michelle Porter, and Patricia Ball, *The InterStudy Edge: Volume 2,* Excelsior, Minn., InterStudy, 1990, pp. 7, 16, 19.

Health services franchises are usually organizational concepts; they have been successful in providing ambulatory care (minor emergency centers, for example), dental care, optometry, and home care services throughout the United States.[31]

The advantages of franchising include not having to worry about marketing design and the creation of advertising strategies, trademarks, sources of supplies, design of health facilities, and actual setting-up of the operation. These arrangements bring with them the franchiser's expertise; proven systems; less financial risk; potential for higher patient volume; higher profitability; monitored and verifiable cost-effective, quality medical care; and the potential for enhanced medical group equity. In other industries, franchising is quicker, easier, safer, more profitable, more valuable, and less expensive than operating independently; however, most health care franchises offer standard HMO products and services where variances are not acceptable. The franchiser usually prefers uniformity in its franchises because this permits greater control and, usually, greater success with a proven product, service, or strategy. Many franchisers are very precise and demand that the franchise be operated in a specific manner; their reputation is at stake. Experimentation is not allowed. Also, health care franchises may be more complex than other types of franchises because of the various licensing criteria for medical personnel, clinic site, and equipment, as well as continuing education, special training needs, quality of care requirements, and peer and utilization reviews. Health services franchises, therefore, must grow slowly, because finding and training franchisees, and then making sure that the service is uniform, are much more difficult and complex than in other fields (for example, the fast food industry). Federal and state franchising regulations also must be carefully reviewed and considered. Although the Federal Trade Commission has promulgated uniform franchising rules and regulations, these rules must be adopted by each state, and variations frequently occur in state laws.

6. *Syndicating:* A syndication is a business concern that sells materials for publication in a number of newspapers or periodicals simultaneously or a group of persons or concerns who unite to carry out a particular transaction. Health care applications of syndicating have occurred with marketing and advertising programs, although many other applications are possible, especially in the HMO area. Syndicated advertising plans generally are developed by an advertising agency, a hospital, or other group that is able to develop a generic, rather than a specific, program. Syndicated plans should be distinguished from corporate advertising plans, which are used by large national health care firms.

---

[31] Edward L. Dixon. *1986 Franchise Annual Handbook and Directory.* Lewiston, N.Y., Info Press, Inc., 1986.

Multihospital systems such as Kaiser and CIGNA develop and test-market brand name advertising, but such programs usually are available only to the affiliates of the corporate entity.

Syndicated advertising is a response to the health service industry's need for low-cost yet effective advertising. While other industries are spending approximately 5 percent of total revenues on advertising, health services providers currently spend only 1 to 3 percent of their operating budgets on marketing programs, of which advertising is only one part. HMO managers are finding that their advertising expenses are higher than other health care industry components; indeed, HMO advertising costs are approaching other industries' costs and are increasing at an accelerated rate because of heightened competition from other local HMOs. Syndicated advertising may be one solution to HMO cost control without losing the competitive edge.

7. *Marketing Networks:* Marketing networks in the HMO industry have developed so as to provide comprehensive health service benefits packages to employees of companies or corporations that have multistate or regional operations; major marketers of health care (Prucare, HMO-USA) contract with independent HMOs to provide health care to the employees of those organizations. Each HMO manager should be aware of the unique arrangements that have been identified as essential for a successful network by employers that were surveyed. These include:[32]

- The provision of single account executives, uniform benefits, and authorized/standardized administrative functions (rated as the most important network arrangement)
- The use of flexible rates
- The ability to participate in selected parts of the entire network
- The ability to exist in states where there are variations in laws affecting networks
- The availability of an HMO network that meets the employer's specifications

HMO-USA has developed its own list of characteristics, which it believes are critical to an effective network.[33]

---

[32] National Industry Council for HMO Development. *HMO Network Study.* Washington, D.C., Bobkat Healthworks, Inc., March 1985, p. 9.

[33] Virgil March. Minutes of a Meeting of the National Industry Council for HMO Development, San Antonio, Texas, October 30–31, 1984, p. 2.

- Central accountability
- Single account control
- Specified level of benefits
- Flexible billing and enrollment
- Away-from-home care
- Coordination of HMO services with company health or medical programs
- Employee transfers

In light of these characteristics, it is evident that networking can be as beneficial to the HMO that is eager to expand and open new markets as it is to the industry needing regional/national group coverage and the syndicates that offer specific health care packages. Independent HMOs that are willing to join forces to compete with national chains can successfully beat the corporate challenge through careful and thorough market research.

8. *Alliances/Consortia:* This arrangement can be described as the affiliation/agreement and close association of two or more health services organizations for a common objective(s). Generally, the organizations involved have similarities in their characteristics, structures, and organizational objectives (e.g., all are community general hospitals, all are multispecialty medical group practices, all serve patients in the southeastern United States, all are HMOs, etc.). Usually, the initial "partners" become equal owners in a separate umbrella corporation, with board members of the new corporation drawn from the participating organizations. These alliances/consortia are established to develop, own, and operate health care enterprises, but generally the umbrella corporation markets, serves payers, and negotiates and administers preferred and exclusive provider contracts with third-party payers. They are useful in negotiating and dealing with contract health care such as governments, unions, HMOs and PPOs, self-insured employers, and insurance companies.

Vulnerability of Independent HMOs to Linkages

Linking, whether it be by joint venture, network, acquisition, franchise, syndicating, or the like, is becoming the management strategy to protect existing markets and to establish a broader competitive base. Well-established, credible HMOs that are located in large or growing metropolitan areas presently are the most vulnerable for these linkages, because they offer the prospective venturer an established patient base and require minimum expense for expansion. These organizations are often targeted by national health care chains as prospective business affiliates.

As the number of national linkages continues to grow, smaller, independent HMOs will be faced with some difficult decisions, for example, to venture with a chain and maintain some independence, or compete independently. Maybe it would be best to merge, sign a management agreement, or simply let the larger chain acquire them. Would it be best to establish a franchise or to syndicate with the corporation, or should they link with other local independents and become a strong competitive adversary? A growing suspicion within the health care industry is that it will be very difficult for independent health care organizations to exist without a linkage. If this suspicion is confirmed, independent HMOs must position themselves to meet the challenges ahead. Rules and methodologies for strategic market positioning are still being developed for health care linkages. Indeed, MaxiCare, the largest linked private HMO, developed major management and fiscal problems in 1988, and by March of 1989 had filed for bankruptcy.

When confronted with deciding whether or not to develop a link with another organization, the HMO manager should consider these new options from the standpoint of financial and economic issues, medical and business management activities, maintenance of quality care, consumer and marketing concerns, and survival past the near term. New management configurations will be instrumental in shaping the future of health care—configurations that will allow the HMO to have a competitive edge. Purchasers will demand increased services for lower costs, and patients will demand higher quality and reduced premiums. The source for the development of new organizational structures that meet these requirements may likely be one of the eight discussed on pages 124–128.

Summary

One of the major characteristics of HMOs is flexibility in organizational form, structure, and sponsorship. These structures are described by Title XIII of the Social Security Act and include staff, group, and IPA model HMOs. The HMO field has added additional models—network, hybrid, and open ended. It is useful to become familiar with these models so as to be more capable of understanding their operation and management and to choose the organizational elements that best fit the setting of a developing HMO or one undergoing corporate reorganization. HMOs are sponsored by any number of organizations; they help establish the HMO and develop its legal entity. The new organization then becomes responsible for HMO activities through its policymaking body—its board of trustees, if not-for-profit, or its board of directors, if for-profit.

Over the years, HMOs have been sponsored by many different groups, including universities, medical schools, cities, industries, consumer groups, associations, insurance companies, Blue Cross/Blue Shield, hospitals, and neighborhood health centers. According to the Office of Prepaid Health Care, DHHS, which manages Title XIII grant funds, almost half of all grant applications were received from consumer-sponsored organizations, but by the time grant funds had expired, only about a third of the newly developing health plans were consumer-sponsored while another third were sponsored by private organizations. Most recently, the HMO industry has reflected a change in the development of HMOs, with multicorporate, multistate HMO firms accounting for more than 70 percent of total enrollment. Because of the financial difficulties of some multistate plans, especially MaxiCare, there may be a slowing in the growth of large conglomerate health plans.

The three basic federally defined HMO models are based on the method by which physicians are paid for their services and practice arrangements. The staff model HMO is characterized by an HMO entity that provides both administration of the health plan and the direct application of physician services by salaried physicians. Because only employed physicians are eligible to provide services to HMO members, this model is called a closed-panel plan, where other community physicians are excluded from participation in the plan. The HMO entity provides the usual health plan functions, such as medical services delivery, finance, marketing, and health plan operations. Hospital, pharmacy, and other services are arranged through agreements and contracts with outside-the-plan organizations. Physicians are paid through a salary and bonus arrangement; the latter is based on annual individual and departmental performance reviews and is usually tied to the overall performance of the health plan in managing members' services. Thus, physicians are at-risk to the extent that overutilization might affect their bonuses.

The second model, the group HMO, is also described as a closed-panel practice. It contracts with one or more independent, multispecialty medical group practices; only those physicians will provide services to HMO members. The medical groups are compensated through a capitation for either primary services only or for both primary and specialty services; the physicians are placed at-risk in that the capitation may not be sufficient to cover all the contracted-for services for HMO members. Thus, there is an incentive for the physician to manage patient care effectively. This model appears to be the most efficient, perhaps because of its use of organized multispecialty group practices, combined with the strong incentives created by capitation payments. The major criticism of this and the staff model HMOs relates to the closed panel—that enrollees are locked into a system with little choice of primary physicians and limited health center locations.

The IPA model provides service through a contract with an association of physicians known as the individual practice association, or through contracts with "individual" providers, which include independent medical group practices. The IPA receives a capitation payment from the HMO and pays the providers on a discounted fee-for-service and/or capitation basis, which may also include a withhold that could be used to offset losses from over-utilization. After utilization over a period of time is reviewed, a part or all of the withhold may be returned to the physicians. Because of patient management and utilization concerns in early IPA model HMOs, many IPAs now use the gatekeeper or case-manager approach, where the patient has unlimited access to the primary physician but must obtain a referral from that physician to receive specialty health services. In effect, the primary care physician becomes the manager of patient care for enrollees included in his/her practice. Data suggest that the gatekeeper approach is effective in controlling unnecessary utilization; however, many specialists resent this intrusion of their former practice prerogatives.

A fourth HMO model, the network, is similar to the medical group model except that the HMO contracts with two or more separate medical groups or IPAs. Moreover, it is possible for the medical groups and IPAs to contract with more than one HMO. Compensation to these providers is in the form of a capitation payment; the physicians are responsible for all physician services described in the provider agreement. The health plan itself is responsible for plan marketing, premium collections, and all other plan activities. Usually, both the health plan and the provider panels have medical directors who are responsible for medical management activities.

Finally, to accommodate the quickly changing structures, the managed care field has developed hybrid and open-ended HMOs—organizations that allow for the characteristics of both HMOs and PPOs as well as indemnity insurance programs in the same organization. These companies provide both risk and nonrisk arrangements with providers and traditional indemnity and managed care insurance products. Many of the hybrid models offer several levels of benefits, ranging from the comprehensive HMO-type benefits package to low-option, indemnity-type products. Sometimes referred to as "open-ended" HMOs, these organizations are evolving to compete more effectively with traditional indemnity insurers by offering standard indemnity policies and selling products with large copayments or deductibles and limits on the dollar amount of coverage.

The structure of HMOs is also changing through linkages of HMOs with other organizations by means of joint ventures, networks, management agreements, franchises, syndicating, mergers, and acquisitions. The most common linking arrangement in the HMO industry is the joint venture—an arrangement between two or more organizations, at least one of which is an entity already in operation as a going concern, for the purpose of conducting a new business or providing a new service. On the other hand, management agreements and contracts allow HMOs to purchase administrative and other skills from national health care management firms without merging or franchising with the national firm. Many HMOs, however, have found themselves in weakened positions that force them into a merger with or acquisition by a larger HMO.

References

Arpin, David W. "The 'G' Word." *The Internist,* 28(7):8–9, August 1987.

Boland, Peter. "Joint Venture Relationships Between Preferred Providers and Payers. *Journal of Ambulatory Care Management,* 10(4):1–10, November 1987.

Crane, Mark, and Harry T. Paxton. "Joint Ventures: Which Deals Are the Big Winners?" *Medical Economics,* 64(7):41–45, March 30, 1987.

Egdahl, Richard H. "Foundations for Medical Care." *New England Journal of Medicine,* 288:491–498, March 8, 1973.

Glusman, David H., and John C. S. Kepner. "Strategic Issues in Joint Ventures." *Medical Group Management Journal,* 35(5):18–25, September/October 1988.

Group Health Association of America. *HMO Industry Profile.* Volumes I through IV. Washington, D.C., GHHA, June 1988.

Kirchner, Merian. "Can IPAs Save Small Practices?" *Medical Economics,* 62(15):176–188, July 22, 1985.

Marion Merrell Dow, Inc., *Marion Managed Care Digest. HMO Edition.* Kansas City, Mo., 1988.

_____. *Marion Managed Care Digest. PPO Edition.* Kansas City, Mo., 1988.

Nash, David B. "HMO Practice: Advantages and Disadvantages." *Physician's Management,* 25(5):245–257, May 1985.

Patton, James, and Glenn T. Troyer. "Planning and Implementing the Joint Venture." *Topics in Health Care Financing,* 13(1):86–95, Fall 1986.

Savitz, S. Alan, and Paul R. Roberts. "Some Notes on the Development of an IPA Model HMO." *Journal of Ambulatory Care Management,* 9(2):33–53, May 1986.

Shouldice, Robert G. "HMOs: Four Models Profiled." *Medical Group Management,* 33(3):8–33, May/June 1986.

Troyer, Glenn T. "Joint Venturing." *Topics in Health Care Financing,* 13(1):1–11, Fall 1986.

U.S. Department of Health and Human Services, Health Care Financing Administration, Office of Health Maintenance Organizations. *HMO Governing Board Handbook.* Rockville, Md., DHHS/HCFA/OHMO, April 1981.

Wasserman, Fred W. "For-Profit HMOs and Joint Ventures." *Bulletin of the New York Academy of Medicine,* 63(1):49–60, January/February 1987.

Welch, W. Pete. "IPAs Emerge on the HMO Forefront." *Business and Health,* 5(4):14–16, February 1988.

5

COMPETITIVE MEDICAL PLANS
AND GOVERNMENT CONTRACTING

Another MCO, the competitive medical plan (CMP), is introduced in this chapter. Although a relatively new term, the CMP is not a new concept.

Throughout this chapter and text, organizations that are regulated by the Tax Equity and Fiscal Responsibility Act of 1982 (TEFRA) are described as risk contractors, CMPs, CMPs/HMOs, Medicare risk organizations, or risk organizations.

Historical Development of Risk Contracting

The passage of Medicare in 1965 included opportunities for the federal Health Care Financing Administration (HCFA) to experiment with alternatives to cost-based reimbursement. In fact, the program allowed the government to contract with prepaid group practice plans on a "direct dealing" basis, using a capitation/risk approach, but only for Part B (medical or physician) services; Part A (hospital) payments are made directly to hospitals. Very few groups used this method of payment because of lack of experience, potentially high risks, and the extensive paperwork involved. A notable exception was Group Health Cooperative of Puget Sound (GHC), an HMO prototype that developed a Medicare agreement with the Federal Government effective July 1, 1966. (A risk-sharing contract went into effect in July 1976.) Based on the experiences

---

[1] This chapter is adapted from Robert G. Shouldice and Lynn Peterson-Lowe, *Medicare Risk Contracting with Health Maintenance Organizations and Competitive Medical Plans,* Denver, Colo., Center for Research in Ambulatory Health Care Administration, 1987. Permission by the center to reproduce this material is gratefully acknowledged.

of GHC and other prepaid group practice health plans, it was generally agreed that they were efficient providers of health care.

In 1973, the Health Maintenance Organization Act was passed, providing the legal and financial impetus necessary to develop HMOs on a national scale. Concurrently, the Medicare Act was amended in 1972 to provide incentives for HMOs to enroll Medicare beneficiaries. This legislation allowed the government to develop risk contracts with HMOs for both Part A and B services, contracts that included capitation payments which were paid monthly but based on quarterly estimates of operating costs and enrollment. At year's end, an adjusted average per capita cost (AAPCC) was calculated—an amount that the government would have paid for similar services on a fee-for-service basis. Final payment of up to 100 percent of the AAPCC was then made. If actual costs were less than the AAPCC, the first 20 percent of the "savings" were shared equally by the government and the HMO. Savings beyond 20 percent were to be returned to the government. On the other hand, if actual costs exceeded AAPCC rates, the HMO was solely responsible for the loss. Thus, there were limits on savings but not on the HMO's risks.[2]

Even though they had developed risk-taking programs for enrollees under age 65 and members of commercial concerns, the HMOs preferred not to use the risk approach here. Instead, they continued to provide services to Medicare recipients on a cost-reimbursement basis and made available to this class of enrollee a MediGap or supplemental benefits package, which enhanced the Medicare benefits and created a comprehensive set of benefits for the elderly individual. Group Health Cooperative, however, continued to use its risk contract for Medicare enrollees and was joined by several other health plans; the results were spectacular. Similar to their experiences with under age 65 members, GHC, under its 1966 Medicare agreement and 1976 risk-sharing contract, saw a substantial reduction in hospital days per 1,000 Medicare patients. (Traditional fee-for-service Medicare patients used approximately 4,000 to 4,500 hospital days per 1,000 population, while GHC, under the government risk contract, was experiencing approximately 2,000 to 2,500 days per 1,000 Medicare population.)[3] GHC's experience notwithstanding, the regulatory changes did not result in a major increase in HMO Medicare

---

[2] Laura Himes Iversen and Cynthia Longseth Polich. *The Future of Medicare and HMOs.* Excelsior, Minn., InterStudy, Center For Aging and Long-Term Care, 1985, pp. 7–8.

[3] Karen Wintringham. "Preliminary Results from a Risk-Sharing Health Maintenance Organization." In: *Skills Development for the HMO Managers of the 1980s. Proceedings of the 30th Annual Group Health Institute, Boston, Massachusetts, May 4–7, 1980.* Washington, D.C., Group Health Association of America, 1980, pp. 147–148. At the end of 1977, GHC realized a $1.3 million savings share, with the government's share exceeding $1.7 million. The cooperative's total adjusted costs were 30 percent less than the government's estimated community costs or the AAPCC.

contracts, because the basic payment methods had not changed and HMO "qualification" was now required for an organization to be eligible to contract with the Social Security Administration.

With the enormous growth of the HMO industry, the Federal Government considered expanding its risk-based reimbursement approach to one similar to the GHC experience, where the HMO, in return for payment of a fixed fee per Medicare enrollee per month, would accept the risk for providing all Medicare services. The expectation was that "because the HMO receives a fixed payment from enrollees, regardless of the volume of service provided, there is a financial incentive for the HMO to control costs and to provide the least expensive service appropriate to enrollees' needs."[4] A second expectation was that HMOs would use their expected savings to reduce costs to Medicare beneficiaries and provide more services.[5] Thus, HCFA could finance more Medicare insurance benefits at a lower cost.

DEMONSTRATION PROJECTS

Beginning in 1976, several demonstration projects were conducted to test these assumptions, where HCFA contracted with HMOs on an "at-risk" basis and paid them 100 percent of the AAPCC. The two longest-running demonstration projects, Group Health Cooperative of Puget Sound and the Fallon Community Health Plan in Massachusetts, saved an estimated $2.8 million in 1980 by encouraging fewer hospital admissions, shorter stays, and lower administrative costs.[6] It was estimated by HCFA that, from 1979 to 1984, there was a savings of $50 million, a conservative figure, from 32 risk contracts (covering Medicare Parts A and B). For 1985, HCFA estimated a $34 million savings from all of its ongoing HMO risk contract arrangements.[7] The Bush administration has promoted risk contracts not as cost reduction methods but as methods to reduce paperwork, reporting activities, and other administrative costs to the health plan and, thus, savings in recent years have not been estimated. But, HCFA is

---

[4] U.S. Department of Health and Human Services. "Medicare Program; Payment and Health Maintenance Organizations and Competitive Medical Plans; Final Rules." *Federal Register, 50*(7):1314, January 10, 1985. 42 CFR, Parts 405 and 417.

[5] American Medical Association, Monograph Group on Health Service Policy. *Medicare and Prepaid Health Plans: New Directions for HMOs.* Chicago, Ill., AMA, 1985, p. 9.

[6] "HMOs Expect a Big Influx of Medicare Patients." *Medical World News, 24*(3):102, 107, February 1983.

[7] Group Health Association of America. *HMO Managers Letter, 1*(1):1, September 17, 1984.

finding that the more centralized group and staff model HMOs have realized the largest savings.[8]

TAX EQUITY AND FISCAL RESPONSIBILITY ACT OF 1982

The demonstrated ability of HMOs to contain costs was the impetus for amending Section 1876 of the Social Security Act as part of the Tax Equity and Fiscal Responsibility Act of 1982 (TEFRA), which authorized Medicare to pay, on a prospective rate-setting basis, those organizations that have a cost-based or risk-based contract with the Health Care Financing Administration.[9] This legislation widened the scope of health services organizations (HSOs) that were eligible to contract with Medicare to include not only federally qualified HMOs but also competitive medical plans (CMPs). *A CMP is any organization that meets specific eligibility criteria for Medicare risk contracting but is not necessarily an HMO.* CMPs must be "at risk" and provide physician services primarily through employees of the organization or through contracts with individual physicians or groups of physicians.

Final federal regulations for Medicare risk contracting were implemented on February 1, 1985. As of April 1987, 152 plans had signed Medicare risk contracts, and more than 903,000 beneficiaries were enrolled. HCFA estimates that, in 1990, approximately 1.968 million Medicare beneficiaries received care through HMOs.[10] There is a potential for growth in this market of beneficiaries, whose total number in 1990 approached 33 million nationwide.

Medicare Cost and Risk Contracts

The TEFRA Medicare risk contract is for one year. HSOs, whose eligibility is determined by the Office of Prepaid Health Care, enter into an agreement with the Health Care Financing Administration to provide specific services to Medicare beneficiaries for a predetermined and prepaid capitation sum. There are specific eligibility and contract requirements that must be met,

---

[8] James Bautz Bonanno and Terrie Wetle. "HMO Enrollment of Medicare Recipients: An Analysis, Incentives and Barriers." *Journal of Health Politics, Policy, and Law,* 9(1):41–62, Spring 1984.

[9] Sec. 114(a) of the Tax Equity and Fiscal Responsibility Act, P.L. 97-248, Section 1876; and Title XVIII, Health Insurance for the Aged and Disabled, Section 1876 (42nd U.S. Congress), 1982.

[10] Nancy L. Rucker, *Legislative Issues for Group Practice: 1987,* Alexandria, Va., American Group Practice Association, 1987, p. 8; and U.S. Department of Health and Human Services, Health Care Financing Administration, Office of Prepaid Health Care, Washington, D.C., personal communication, September 19, 1990.

and HSOs that are considering a Medicare risk contract need to review these requirements. Especially important is the capitation methodology used by the government.

COST OR RISK CONTRACTS

Under TEFRA, a "cost" arrangement contract with HCFA may also be developed. Under the cost contract, the HMO/CMP provides services to Medicare recipients and receives interim capitation payments from HCFA. At the end of the year, the payments are adjusted to reflect the Medicare-defined reasonable costs of providing these services. CMPs or HMOs can enter into cost reimbursement contracts if they satisfy all criteria for eligibility as a risk organization; usually these provider organizations choose cost reimbursement if they cannot satisfy HCFA that they can bear the potential losses associated with a risk contract. This arrangement is similar to the traditional cost reimbursement method, where the participating provider bills the Medicare program on a fee-for-service basis and is paid according to Medicare-defined reasonable costs. Cost contracts, however, tie the HMO/CMP more closely to HCFA by identifying in advance the services that are to be provided, by paying an *interim* capitation, and by identifying the number of Medicare recipients that are to be served. Conversely, risk contracts utilize capitation (e.g., prospective) payments similar to other financial arrangements traditionally used by HMOs. Risk contracts are fully discussed in the next section of this chapter. Note, however, that under both arrangements, the Federal Government will not contract for more than 95 percent of the AAPCC for Medicare recipients in the counties served by the CMP/HMO.

ELIGIBILITY REQUIREMENTS

Although federally qualified HMOs and CMPs are eligible to develop risk contracts with HCFA, federal qualification does not guarantee that an HMO/CMP will be approved for a Medicare risk contract. The specific eligibility requirements that must be met are:

1. Organization under state law (a certificate of authority must be obtained)
2. Provision of a minimum range of services, including physicians' services (Part B of Medicare), hospitalization (Part A of Medicare), laboratory and X-ray services, emergency services, preventive services, and out-of-area services
3. Provision of services through physicians and other health care providers who are employees, partners, or contractors of the organization
4. Assumption of full financial risk for provision of services

5. Demonstration of adequate protection for enrollees in the event of insolvency

6. Acceptance of a prospective capitation payment; this payment is fixed regardless of the frequency, extent, or kind of services that are provided to any enrolled Medicare beneficiary

Generally, eligibility requirements for CMPs are more flexible than those for becoming a federally qualified HMO.

The CMP or HMO acts both as an insurer and a health delivery system. It may furnish services directly, arrange to have them furnished, or both. The risk contract places the HMO/CMP at full financial risk for the provision of services, but these risks may be shared with providers or outside insurers.

To become eligible to enter Medicare risk contract negotiations with HCFA, the organization must either enter the federal HMO qualification process or apply to the Office of Prepaid Health Care for CMP qualification. The latter process is generally easier and gives the organization greater flexibility in the development of its benefits package, because only a minimum range of services is required. (See Chapter 2 for an explanation of the HMO qualification process.) TEFRA requirements for Medicare members, however, are identical for HMOs and CMPs.

CMPs and HMOs do differ in several aspects, as noted in Table 5-1. Generally seven major differences are noted.[11]

1. The range of services required of a CMP is minimal in comparison to a federally qualified HMO. The CMP package may exclude coverage for such services as mental health care, substance abuse treatment, and home health care; it is not required to provide for outpatient hospital care except in the case of emergency services. To obtain a risk or cost contract, however, a CMP must make available to its Medicare enrollees the full range of services that are covered by Parts A and B of Medicare, as previously noted.

2. A CMP is not restricted to community rating for non-Medicare members—a feature that many HMOs consider restrictive to their abilities to compete in the marketplace.

3. A CMP may impose deductibles and copayments so long as minimal benefits are provided. The deductible and coinsurance charges to Medicare members are limited.

4. An eligible CMP may permit its members to obtain care from nonplan providers so long as it can demonstrate that members will be treated primarily by the CMP's providers. HMO enrollees are restricted to using providers that are

---

[11] "How Do HMOs and CMPs Differ?" *Outreach, 6*(5):7, September–October 1985.

employed by or under contract to their HMO except in unusual or emergency situations. The CMP must be at risk for members that use nonplan providers and must have utilization controls in place to ensure that the use of nonplan providers will not adversely affect the financial viability of the CMP.

5. HMO regulations require that one-third of the membership of the policy-making body must be members of the organization. CMPs are not required to impose this restriction on their boards.

6. A CMP is not required to demonstrate an enrollment that is broadly representative of the community it serves.

7. A CMP is not required to be a separate legal entity; it may have other lines of business, cost centers, or subsidiary organizations, or it may be a subsidiary of a sponsoring organization, so long as the CMP meets TEFRA requirements. HMOs are prohibited from such arrangements.

The CMP eligibility determination process may take anywhere from 3 to 12 months. Following approval by the Office of Prepaid Health Care, the CMP must begin contract negotiations with HCFA. The time between submission of a contract application and approval of the Medicare risk contract may take from 3 to 6 months. Thus, a year may elapse between the time the decision is made to develop a risk contract until the contract is signed.

CONTRACT REQUIREMENTS

The Final Rules for Medicare risk contracts, published in the January 10, 1985 *Federal Register*,[12] describe a specific set of requirements that an organization must meet for contract approval. Some of the conditions the qualifying organization must be capable of and contract to meet on becoming eligible are:

1. Provide the full range of Medicare services that are presently available in the area
2. Provide an annual open enrollment period of not less than 30 days
3. Use Medicare-qualified providers
4. Provide additional services only if approved by HCFA
5. Follow enrollment rules and regulations
6. Not disenroll because of health status
7. Provide prompt access to services
8. Provide 24-hour, 7-day-per-week emergency services

---

[12] U.S. Department of Health and Human Services. "Medicare Program; Payment of Health Maintenance Organizations and Competitive Medical Plans; Final Rules."

TABLE 5-1 Comparison of Federal Requirements for CMPs and Qualified HMOs

QUALIFIED HMOs (Requirements for commercial members)	COMPETITIVE MEDICAL PLANS (Requirements for commercial members)	HMOs and CMPs (Requirements for Medicare members)*
Provision of Services		
"Provides...services"—no limitations as to time or cost except as prescribed	"Provides...services"—may be limited as to time or cost	Medicare covered services benefits package must be provided if reasonable and necessary
Compensation		
Periodic without regard to date of service	Periodic without regard to date of service†	Same
Fixed, without regard to frequency, extent, and kind of service	Fixed, without regard to frequency, extent, and kind of service†	Same
Community-rated (operational HMOs can phase in)	Not limited to community rating, but compensated on a prepaid capitated basis	Medicare cost calculations are based on adjusted community rate
May be supplemented with nominal copayments as defined in regulation	Copayments and deductibles are allowed—no restrictions†	Copayments and deductibles are limited to the amount actuarially equivalent to those the enrollee would have paid had he or she not enrolled in the plan
Must provide services; often compensation and some state-required automobile insurance policies; other insurance—COB permitted	May be secondary payer to worker's compensation and some state-required automobile insurance policies; other insurance—COB	Medicare is primary payer except in limited circumstances: e.g., automobile no-fault; working aged 65–69
Supplemental payments for supplemental services permitted; must be community-rated if on prepaid basis	No specific provision—payment for supplemental services permitted, but community rating not required	Supplemental payments for supplemental services permitted
No provision re: additional benefits	No provision re: additional benefits	Savings returned to members as additional benefits or as reduction in premium, or both (upon approval of secretary)

Benefits Package

	Physician services provided by doctors of medicine or osteopathy†	Physician services provided by by doctors of medicine or osteopathy‡
Physician services (including consultant and referral services) provided by a licensed physician or other health professional, if permitted under state law	Physician services provided by doctors of medicine or osteopathy†	Physician services provided by by doctors of medicine or osteopathy‡
Inpatient and outpatient hospital	Inpatient hospital†	Inpatient and outpatient hospital‡
Medically necessary emergency services	Emergency services and out-of-area coverage†	In- and out-of-area emergency services and urgently needed services while member is temporarily out of HMO's service area or CMP's geographic area‡
Mental health—20 outpatient visits	No requirement for coverage of mental health care	Limited outpatient mental health
Substance abuse—unlimited detox and referral to ancillary services	No requirement for coverage of substance abuse	Substance abuse covered, with limitations‡
Lab and X-ray	Lab and X-ray†	Lab and X-ray‡
Home health	No requirement for coverage of home health care	Unlimited number of home health visits covered under Medicare
Preventive health services	Preventive health services†	Not covered; Medicare specifically excludes routine physical examinations, eye and ear examinations, and immunizations (with limited exceptions)
Supplementals (optional)	Supplementals (optional)	Savings returned to members as additional benefits or as reduction in premium (upon approval of secretary); other supplementals optional

TABLE 5-1 *Continued*

Providers

Physician services provided *solely* by staff, group, IPA, MDs and other health professionals under contract, any combination of above—excludes unusual and emergency services	Physician services provided *primarily* through the plan's employees or partners, or through contracts with individual physicians or groups (organized on a group practice or individual practice basis)†	See applicable HMO or CMP requirements

Guarantees to Members

Availability, with reasonable promptness	Availability will be evaluated	Availability, promptly as appropriate
Accessibility, with reasonable promptness	Accessibility will be evaluated	Accessibility, promptly as appropriate
Continuity	Continuity will be evaluated	Continuity
Exception re: availability for non-metropolitan area	No provision	Exception re: availability if service not generally available in geographic area and if it is not common practice to refer outside the geographic area
Reimbursement for emergency services	Reimbursement for emergency services	Reimbursement for emergency and urgently needed services not obtainable from HMO or CMP
Ongoing quality assurance	Ongoing quality assurance will be evaluated	Ongoing quality assurance
No requirement for open enrollment	No requirement for open enrollment	Open enrollment at least 30 days
May not refuse to reenroll due to health status	No provision	Medicare member must be reenrolled unless under Section 417.460 HMO or CMP is permitted to disenroll member
Grievance procedures	No specific provision	Grievance and hearing procedures
Protection from HMO liabilities	Protection from CMP liabilities	Protection from HMO/CMP
Confidentiality	No provision	Confidentiality requirements of Medicare program
Offer enrollment to population that is broadly representative of service area	No provision	HMO/CMP not required to accept additional Medicare members if it would make the HMO/CMP population substantially nonrepresentative of the population of the geographic area

No specific provision in Title XIII	Less than one half of the enrollees are Medicare or Medicaid, unless waived by the secretary or an exception is granted (demonstration projects)	Less than one half of the enrollees are Medicare or Medicaid unless waived by the secretary or an exception is granted (demonstration projects)
Full and fair disclosure to prospective members	No provision	Enrollment literature as required by secretary
One-third of policymaking body must be members	No requirement for member representation on board	No requirement for member representation on board
Management and Organizational		
Fiscally sound	Fiscally sound	See applicable HMO or CMP requirement
Adequate provision against insolvency	Adequate provision against insolvency†	Adequate provision against insolvency
Satisfactory administrative and managerial arrangements	Required for HCFA contract	Required for HCFA contract
HMO must assume full financial risk on a prospective basis, but may limit its risk by obtaining reinsurance or sharing risk with providers	CMP must assume full financial risk on a prospective basis, but may limit its risk by obtaining reinsurance or sharing risk with providers	See applicable HMO or CMP requirement
Organization qualified within service area	Organization eligible within approved geographic area	See applicable HMO or CMP requirement
Separate legal entity	Organized under state law	See applicable HMO or CMP requirement
Dual Choice Mandate		
Yes	No	Not Applicable

*TEFRA requirements for Medicare members are identical for HMOs and CMPs.

† Indicates requirements that must be met to be determined an eligible organization by the Office of Health Maintenance Organizations (OHMO). All other provisions pertain to HCFA contract requirements or reimbursement principles.

‡ For Medicare enrollees of both HMOs and CMPs, there are specific limitations in the benefits package (e.g., 60 inpatient days per episode). Refer to Medicare benefits package (Parts A and B) for details.

SOURCE: Beth D. Roy, Director, Division of HMO Qualification, Office of Prepaid Health Care, Health Care Financing Administration, U.S. Department of Health and Human Services. Rockville, Md., DHHS, undated mimeographed paper.

9. Pay for emergency services, urgently needed services, and services ordered by but obtained outside the organization

10. Have a grievance process

11. Maintain an ongoing quality assurance program

12. Enroll any beneficiary who is entitled to Medicare Parts A and B or Part B only, except applicants with end-stage renal disease or in hospice, irrespective of health status

13. Charge no more than actuarial equivalent for deductible/coinsurance amounts

14. Coordinate benefits with other payers

15. Maintain enrollment of Medicare and Medicaid members at not more than 50 percent of plan membership (may be waived if these beneficiaries constitute more than 50 percent of the organization's geographic population)

16. Use any difference between the adjusted community rate (the rate proposed by the HMO/CMP) and HCFA's 95 percent payment to reduce beneficiary charges, provide additional services, return the difference to HCFA, or place a portion in a benefit stabilization fund through HCFA

17. Be able to assume full financial risk

18. Comply with financial disclosure requirements

19. Comply with marketing activity requirements and limitations

20. Have at least 5,000 (nonrural) or 1,500 (rural) under age 65 enrollees prior to initial Medicare enrollment

Although a HMO/CMP may be eligible, contract negotiations with HCFA will determine whether a contract will be awarded.

Contracts are currently negotiated for periods of one year, although HCFA is considering changing this to three-year contract periods.[13] A Medicare beneficiary who joins a CMP or HMO is enrolled for the duration of the contract period.

FINANCING THE CONTRACT

Under risk contracts, HCFA pays the HMO or CMP a premium each month for each Medicare member. Payment is equal to 95 percent of the AAPCC. This amount is an actuarial estimate calculated by the Office of the Actuary of HCFA. First HCFA determines the U.S. per capita cost for all Medicare beneficiaries. This cost is multiplied by the age, sex, and geographic cost indexes that correspond to the counties in which the CMP or HMO operates. The resulting figure represents Medicare's expected per capita cost for beneficiaries in the

---

[13] American Medical Association. *Medicare and Prepaid Health Plans.*

CMP or HMO service area. HCFA then adjusts this rate on the basis of age, sex, institutional status, and welfare status of the Medicare members of the CMP or HMO.[14] Adjustments are developed by using historical cost data from those or similar areas with projections for the contract year. The eligible organization is then provided with a per capita rate of payment for each class of enrollee, published in an AAPCC rate book by HCFA. Rates are updated and published in September of each year.

The HMO/CMP is required to calculate a proposed premium called the adjusted community rate (ACR). This rate is essentially the plan's per capita financing requirement, that is, its "price," including its fixed costs, variable costs, and a profit factor for providing Medicare-covered services; it is adjusted to reflect the higher utilization of services by Medicare beneficiaries. The ACR is the equivalent of the premium that a risk HSO would have charged its Medicare enrollees independently of Medicare payments, using the same rates as charged to non-Medicare enrollees if the benefit is limited to covered medical services. An organization may include in its ACR a reasonable contribution to its contingency reserve fund against the risk of adverse selection or overutilization only if its premium for non-Medicare enrollees includes this element. Note that the CMP must have non-Medicare enrollees (under age 65 commercial members) drawn from commercial employer groups in the service area.

Another way of viewing these costs is to consider the AAPCC as the average *area* cost and the ACR as the average *health plan* cost for the delivery of services to Medicare recipients. If an HSO's proposed ACR is less than 95 percent of the AAPCC, the organization must either provide its Medicare enrollees with additional benefits or accept a reduced monthly payment from HCFA. The additional benefits may be either health benefits beyond the required Part A and B services, a reduction in the HSO's premium rate or in other charges for services furnished to enrollees, or a combination of these. It is important to note that if the calculated ACR is larger than the AAPCC, the organization should not enter into a prospective risk contract with HCFA, because it is doubtful the contract "price" will cover the cost of delivering services.

The HMO/CMP may include copayments, deductibles, and coinsurance in the payment structure so long as the required minimum benefits are provided. The

---

[14] U.S. Department of Health and Human Services, "Medicare Program; Payment of Health Maintenance Organizations and Competitive Medical Plans; Final Rules"; James Lubitz, James Beebe, and Gerald Riley, *Improving the Medicare HMO Payment Formula to Deal with Biased Selection,* Rockville, Md., Office of Research and Demonstrations, Health Care Financing Administration, U.S. Department of Health and Human Services, March 25, 1985, unpublished paper; and M. C. Hornbrook, "Examination of the AAPCC Methodology in an HMO Prospective Demonstration Project," *Group Health Journal,* 5(1):13–21, Spring 1984.

calculated ACR would be decreased by Medicare deductibles and coinsurance. A Medicare beneficiary in a risk contract program may be required to make some payments (supplemental or MediGap coverages—in 1990, the amount was $35.84 for those over age 65) to the HMO/CMP and must continue to pay the Part B premium to the government.

The HMO/CMP must offer a "basic benefits" package, but it may also develop a two-tiered plan, where benefits beyond the basic Medicare-approved benefits package are offered (generally known as a high-option program). Medicare beneficiaries may be required to pass a health status examination to be eligible for a high-option benefits package, although this is strictly prohibited for enrolling beneficiaries in the basic program.

POTENTIAL BENEFITS FOR RISK CONTRACTING ORGANIZATIONS

While the eligibility and contract requirements for the Medicare risk program may seem complex and restrictive, there are several potential benefits for organizations that enter a Medicare risk contract. These include:

1. *Profit factor:* An amount built into the calculation of the premium rate and, if services can be delivered at a cost equal to or less than projected, it is guaranteed. The size of the profit factor may be limited, however, because the ACR calculation is subject to review by HCFA.

2. *Improved budgetary accuracy:* The level of remuneration from HCFA is set prospectively, in contrast to the usual retrospective cost-based reimbursement. This prospective rate information, or known revenue, should increase the organization's ability to budget accurately.

3. *Competitive edge:* Early entry into the Medicare risk contract marketplace will allow the organization the advantage of defining the premium for the regional market. The more cost conscious the initial effort is, the more difficult it will be for subsequent plans to compete with the same premium structure. Also, the first HMO/CMP in the marketplace may likely reach an unbiased patient population, where the incidence of morbidity and mortality are more likely to be representative of the population as a whole.

4. *Improved bargaining position:* The ability of the HMO/CMP to operate several different financing arrangements gives it a better bargaining position when addressing an employer's needs for health insurance, especially if the employee group is aging and a substantial number will soon be covered by Medicare. Moreover, if the Federal Government moves to more capitated programs, especially geographic capitation, the organization that is operating a risk contract will have positioned itself, through its experience in these risk arrangements, to bargain more effectively for these contracts. (Potential

disadvantages of risk contracting are addressed in the following section on operational issues.) The provision that any savings be returned to beneficiaries as increased benefits may also enhance the bargaining position of the HMO/CMP. Services that are likely to be included as increased benefits include those that Medicare does not cover or only partly covers. Some examples are home health services, prescription drugs, eyeglasses, hearing aids, and dental care. If the HMO/CMP seeks to purchase these services for a large number of beneficiaries, it may be able to obtain discounts through competitive bidding.

5. *Decreasing Reimbursement Rates:* This may result from the Gramm-Rudman-Hollings Act where, over time, a decreasing level of payment by the government for Medicare services will occur. It is expected, however, that the extent of the decrease will be lower for risk contracts than for the traditional DRG and reasonable-cost Medicare reimbursement methods, thus rendering risk contracting a potentially more lucrative market.

HMO/CMP Operational Issues

Operational issues concerning the delivery of services to Medicare enrollees by health services organizations will be reviewed in this section. Note that several of the issues presented suggest that CMP contracting has potential disadvantages; these must be considered when an HSO is becoming involved in risk contracting and during the delivery phase.

CONTRACTING DECISION

The first issue to be considered is whether the organization should become involved in risk contracting with the Federal Government and concerns the HSO's current activities and goals. It would be appropriate to become involved if Medicare patients and program payments currently account for a sizable share of the organization's business. This may occur in established HMOs because, over time, members reach the age of 65 and continue their membership, usually on a fee-for-service basis with a MediGap policy. Or, traditional providers such as medical groups or hospitals may find that Medicare recipients comprise a large portion of their activities. A Medicare share of 20 percent or more of the HSO's activities suggests that program involvement is worth the extra effort of contracting with HCFA or contracting as a preferred provider with a local HMO/CMP. It also depends on the organization's future goals and prospects. If the Medicare population is a substantial part of its market, future activities will, in all likelihood, include service to this segment. And as the population ages, this segment will become an increasingly substantial force in the marketplace. Therefore, it might be appropriate to position the HSO to meet this future activity.

All indicators suggest that the Federal Government will continue to press for further risk and capitation contracting for the Medicare population. This is based on the Reagan and Bush administrations' past and current proposals for geographic capitation with or without a voucher system, the expansion of services for the elderly to include catastrophic health insurance coverage, the continuing push for more efficient methods to provide services under the Medicare program and the use of cost containment systems (such as DRGs), and the growth in the current use of risk and cost contracts under the Social Security Act. It may, therefore, be prudent for managers to prepare the HSO for future governmental actions to expand risk arrangements. It also may be useful to become involved at the present time and, thus, to develop contract experience so that future activities will be approached with knowledge gained from the current program.

The HSO may consider the following issues in its contracting decision, including the HSO's efficiency in the delivery of health services, the potential for adverse selection, local assignment rates, supplemental/wrap-around insurance packages, and the local AAPCC. "Other factors to be considered include the capacity for the contract to generate new business; an assessment of the need to provide for additional Medicare services; the impact on management information, financial, and administrative systems; and finally, the need for Medicare-specific marketing plans, Medicare enrollee information, and educational programming."[15] Several of these issues are addressed in the section that follows. But certainly the efficiency and effectiveness of the HSO's current health services delivery system and its relationship to competing providers will affect its ability to be a successful contractor. Relatively more efficient organizations generally have a better chance of success in the HMO/CMP program.

RISKS

Although a cost or risk contract may be developed, generally the cost contract is less risky, because reimbursement is based on traditional fee-for-service payments.

Risks to the HSO under a cost contract arrangement are limited to those the organization currently experiences—that is, risks associated with doing

---

[15] Frederick J. Wenzel. "Medicare Risk Contracts, Success or Failure?" *Medical Group Management, 33*(3):30, May–June 1986.

business in a fee-for-service environment. Cost contracts represent business as usual, but with cost limitations imposed on the HSO at 95 percent of the AAPCC. Risk contracts, on the other hand, allow for "normal" profit, but the contract must still be within the 95 percent AAPCC. With control of inappropriate utilization, the organization could experience an improved net profit from this arrangement.

If the HSO does become involved as a risk contractor, it will assume inherent risks that otherwise would not be taken. First, the contractor may experience adverse selection; Medicare recipients who feel that they will need substantial health services may shop around for the best health insurance program and, thus, will enroll in the HMO/CMP with the expectation that it may provide the most comprehensive coverage at the lowest cost. In fact, the HMO/CMP must have at least 30 days of open enrollment, at which time Medicare recipients can enroll without CMP screening to identify major health problems. If the HSO is the sole provider, it is likely to experience adverse selection.[16] Adverse selection, however, is not a necessary consequence of risk contracting. Many Medicare beneficiaries may elect not to enroll in a HMO/CMP because of a strong, long-standing relationship with an existing provider and because they are currently involved in treatment with that provider.

Second, since the Medicare population, historically, has used services at three to four times the under age 65 population rate, the HMO/CMP may also have difficulty controlling excessive utilization of both physician and hospital services. Without strong physician-initiated controls, budgeted levels of care could easily be exceeded—although only a few risk contractors have experienced this adverse situation.

Third, even though HCFA has created rates that are adjusted for age, sex, county of residence, and institutional and welfare status, there are some inadequacies in the rate-setting methodologies, since rates are not adjusted for major indicators of health status (such as prior hospital or physician utilization). In fact, HCFA's rates reflect the county in which the Medicare patient resides, not where care is received. Research indicates that the factors on which capitation rates are currently based account for less than 1 percent of the variations in per capita costs.[17] By contrast, the DRG methodology accounts for between 30 to 50 percent of the per capita costs. Legislation passed in March 1987 requires that AAPCC rates be adjusted to minimize discrepancies between urban and rural rates; HCFA is currently studying the methodology

---

[16] Ibid, p. 31.

[17] J. W. Thomas et al. "Increasing Medicare Enrollment in HMOs: The Need for Capitation Rates Adjusted for Health Status." *Inquiry,* 20(3):227–239, Fall 1983.

for setting these rates and may improve the rate-setting process.[18] The AAPCC, however, may drop even further than the current 95 percent level. For example, the Gramm-Rudman-Hollings Act mandated a 1 percent reduction in physician payments in 1987, affecting the contracting process. In addition, a reduction in the AAPCC could occur because of (1) the DRG payments to hospitals, which tend to lower the AAPCC for an entire community; (2) the application of the 95 percent of the AAPCC rate in an area where most Medicare recipients are enrolled in one HMO/CMP (e.g., where the capitation for the first year is 95 percent of the AAPCC, for the second year it is 95 percent of 95 percent or 90.25 percent, for the third year it is 95 percent of 90.25 or 85.74 percent, and so on); (3) more tightening of Medicare regulations that would further limit the AAPCC base; and (4) governmental action in changing the rules to make them tougher and less flexible. It is likely that HSOs will continue to use this program until net profits drop to the fee-for-service cost reimbursement levels and then will return to the traditional fee-for-service system, if it is still available.[19]

Stringent limitations on risk reinsurance are another disadvantage of risk contracting that complicate the development of required provisions for such contingencies as insolvency. Not only is risk reinsurance limited, but a major condition for eligibility determination is the assumption of full financial risk by the HMO/CMP. A related disadvantage is that any savings must be shared with HCFA while all losses must be absorbed by the HMO/CMP. Provisions in the legislation have allowed the placement of some money into an HCFA benefit stabilization fund, but this is limited to 15 percent of the difference between the ACR and AAPCC and must be done early in the initial contract period. No interest is earned on funds that are placed in this account.

Thus, when deciding whether to risk contract with HCFA, the potential benefits to the HSO—for example, increased profit potential and competitive edge—must be weighed against the disadvantages or risks. The HMO/CMP is at risk to provide services at a cost equal to or less than the AAPCC. More specifically, the risks that are assumed in risk contracting include biased selection, questionable adequacy of the AAPCC methodology, higher than predicted utilization of services (especially out-of-plan services), stringent limitations on risk reinsurance, and limitations on risk pool contributions.

---

[18] James Beebe, James Lubitz, and Paul Eggers. "Using Prior Utilization to Determine Payments for Medicare Enrollees in Health Maintenance Organizations." *Health Care Financing Review,* 6(3):27–38, Spring 1985.

[19] Robert G. Shouldice. "Are CMPs Right for Your Medical Group?" *Medical Group Management,* 33(6):9–14, November/December 1986.

MARKETING

HMO/CMPs sell their programs to both Medicare recipients and commercial (under age 65) enrollees. The field is experienced in commercial marketing, but has little knowledge and experience in marketing to the over age 65 population. Mathematica Policy Research and the Medical College of Virginia, under contract with HCFA, evaluated the performance of the early demonstration programs and concluded that marketing to a Medicare population requires a very different approach than HMOs/CMPs take with other groups.[20] They suggest that Medicare marketing activities must be directed toward individuals rather than employers/unions.

Unlike commercial marketing activities to employers and unions, which then allow access to employees and union members, CMPs must use different strategies, designed to inform and sell to the Medicare beneficiary directly. Product design should include a package that is financially attractive and can be effectively marketed, given the competing insurance packages that are available to Medicare beneficiaries. Location of provider sites is also a major part of the CMP marketing planning process; new service sites are added in response to the geographic distribution and density of the Medicare population—although this is also a major consideration for under age 65 market planning.

Premiums set by demonstration programs for Medigap or supplemental benefits to Medicare's Part A and B coverages were notably lower than those charged by traditional insurers. "Initial premium differences between demonstration plans and traditional insurers included a plan that offered somewhat expanded benefits and reduced cost sharing for a monthly premium of $26.60, compared with a $46.00 premium charged by the market's major supplemental insurer, and a plan that offered an expanded set of benefits at a premium of $39.00 per month, compared with $70.00 per month for high-option Medicare supplemental policies in the market."[21] Increased benefits at decreased costs, as well as decreased paperwork and predictable monthly fees, are common marketing themes that should be emphasized. Generally, risk-contracting HMOs must operate with a good understanding and awareness of market conditions and competitive pressures; thus, adequate strategic planning is essential for the HSO's success.

---

[20] Kathryn M. Langwell et al. "HMOs in the Medicare Market." *Medical Group Management,* *33*(6):33, November/December 1986.

[21] Ibid, p. 36.

OTHER OPERATIONAL ISSUES

The Mathematica/Medical College of Virginia study of 20 demonstration programs and a terminated demonstration program at the Marshfield Clinic in Marshfield, Wisconsin provides the following list of operational issues for an HMO/CMP when it becomes involved with risk contracting.[22]

1. *Medicare benefits:* The cost to the HMO/CMP for the delivery of these benefits must be well below the AAPCC. A complete analysis of these service units and their costs must be undertaken prior to signing a contract with HCFA.

2. *Minimum inducements:* Only minimum inducements to achieve necessary market projections should be offered. The use of too many added benefits may result in adverse selection, place substantially greater demands for services on the CMP, and place the CMP in a position of greatly increasing the Medigap premium as the AAPCC brings costs down.

3. *Utilization control:* A strong hospital utilization control program must be in place, with the anticipation that there will be a substantial savings in hospital days (usually a drop of 1,500 to 2,000 hospital days per 1,000 Medicare enrollees over traditional fee-for-service hospital use). At the same time, the CMP should anticipate increased utilization of ambulatory services.

4. *Management information system (MIS):* The CMP must have an efficient and effective MIS in place and operational to provide current data on plan operations, including hospital utilization and costs.

5. *Administrative systems:* The CMP's administrative systems should be capable of handling membership accounting, patient transfer functions, one-on-one enrollment procedures, and customer relations. Enrollment of Medicare beneficiaries requires that they be *fully informed* of the implications of their decision to enroll, particularly with respect to "plan use only" requirements.

6. *Marketing plans and capability:* As identified earlier, marketing plans must be well designed and in place, and the CMP must have access to the special marketing techniques and skills that are necessary for Medicare promotion/selling. The plan must protect the program against adverse selection, must allow for a rate of enrollment commensurate with the CMP's ability to deliver services, and should take into account the need for more expensive, one-on-one selling activities.

7. *Delivery system:* Affiliated providers and medical groups must be capable of offering most of the services that are included in their contract with the HMO/CMP or required by HCFA (if the provider or group is the risk

---

[22] Wenzel, "Medicare Risk Contracts, Success or Failure?" p. 31; and Kathryn M. Langwell et al., "HMOs in the Medicare Market, Part 2—Operational Issues," *Medical Group Management,* 34(1):37–44, January/February 1987.

contractor); referral of services outside the group tends to greatly reduce control over utilization and costs. The medical group must be assured that nongroup-provided services can be purchased at rates at or below those paid by Medicare. Because Medicare patients may present more severe and complex health conditions, the medical group should plan on more physician specialists and/or different specialty mixes and more and different types of support staff.

8. *Facilities and sites:* The elderly may require more handicapped parking spaces, wheelchair ramps, an expansion of physical therapy departments, and so on. Also, the geographic location of enrollees should dictate the development of new delivery sites.

9. *Consumer input:* The HSO that is developing a risk contract should work with all local elderly groups in developing the program.

10. *Quality assurance programs:* The nature of risk contracting and the changing nature of provider incentives, as well as the higher frequency-of-service requirement of the elderly, may suggest the need for changes in the frequency and nature of the HSO's quality assurance activities. When an organization applies for HMO qualification or CMP eligibility, the Office of Prepaid Health Care expects the HMO/CMP to develop a comprehensive quality assurance program and commit the necessary resources to implement a broad-based program that will concentrate on the identification and resolution of adverse health outcomes. Under OPHC's guidelines, the ongoing quality assurance program must

- Stress health outcomes to the extent consistent with the state of the art
- Provide review by physicians and other professionals of the process followed in the provision of health services
- Use systematic data collection of performance outcomes and patient results, provide interpretation of these data to plan practitioners, and institute needed changes
- Include written procedures for taking appropriate remedial action whenever, as determined under the quality assurance program, inappropriate or substandard services have been provided or services that should have been furnished have not been provided[23]

11. *Enrollment retention and grievance procedures:* It is necessary to create a member understanding of the "lock-in" provision in enrollment— that most services must be received from plan providers. This provision must be constantly reemphasized with enrollees. Indeed, the greatest number of

---

[23] U.S. Department of Health and Human Services, Health Care Financing Administration, Office of Prepaid Health Care. "Quality Assurance Guidelines for Health Maintenance Organizations and Competitive Medical Plans." Rockville, Md., DHHS/HCFA/OPHC, July 25, 1986, pp. 2–3.

grievances arise because of misrepresentation of this provision. Enrollees also must be made aware that there *is* a grievance procedure that they may use for airing their concerns.

Negotiating the Contract with HCFA

PROGRAM OBJECTIVES

The most obvious reason for federal interest in risk contracting is to effect a reduction in the government's Medicare costs. This objective is accomplished when contracts are signed at the 95 percent AAPCC level; a 5 percent savings is automatically achieved by the government. Thus, the primary goal of this approach is to expand the number of risk contractors and the enrollment of Medicare recipients in these prepaid health care plans. It is hoped that relaxed standards (as compared to the regulations that implemented the HMO Act) for program participation, greater flexibility in benefits packages and delivery options, and the opportunity to earn a reasonable profit will induce more of these plans to develop Medicare contracts.

Data from demonstration programs show a rearrangement in service use.[24] HMOs have experienced reductions in hospital days for over age 65 enrollees similar to those for the under age 65 commercial accounts. Traditional fee-for-service Medicare patients use approximately 4,000 to 4,500 hospital days per 1,000 population annually, while the demonstration HMO programs experienced some 2,000 to 2,500 hospital days per 1,000. These savings translated into financial savings are substantial, and the Federal Government shares 5 percent of them. The remaining savings allow the HMO/CMP to reduce MediGap (supplemental Medicare premiums) costs to Medicare beneficiaries by providing expanded benefits packages and to make a normal profit from this business—a profit margin similar to what the health plan would achieve from its non-Medicare enrollees.

ACHIEVING OBJECTIVES

Current experience suggests that most health plans with risk contracts are able to achieve program objectives. Of the approximately 150 plans with signed Medicare risk contracts in mid-1987, only 13 contracts had been dropped since the risk program began in 1985. The number of risk contracts and applications has continued to increase; as of September 1990 there were 166 contracts in force (97 risk plans, 26 cost plans, and 43 others), and

---

[24] Wintringham. "Preliminary Results from a Risk-Sharing Health Maintenance Organization," pp. 146–147.

the Office of Prepaid Health Care also had 11 applications pending. There have, however, been some notable problems. The Marshfield Clinic had its demonstration contract terminated after it suffered substantial losses because the AAPCC was not sufficient to cover operating costs; Marshfield, in effect, was competing against itself in the AAPCC determination, since it was the only provider in the local area.[25] In May 1987, Blue Cross/Blue Shield of South Carolina dropped its risk contract, noting that the AAPCC payment rate was inadequate, that sudden cost inflation was not built into its 1986 premium, and that HCFA took as long as three to four months to record enrollments and disenrollments.[26] Early in March 1987, Maxicare Health Plans, Inc., based in Los Angeles, California, described significant anomalies in the AAPCC formula methodology, especially the problem with rural/urban county rates, as part of its reason for dropping a Medicare risk contract in Chicago after operating its plan for less than a year.[27] Maxicare reported a $2 million to $4 million second quarter 1986 loss on Medicare revenues of $14 million.[28] But the most problem-plagued Medicare contractor was International Medical Centers, Inc. (IMC), Medicare's largest HMO risk contractor. The HCFA administrator, William Roper, M.D., announced on May 1, 1987 that IMC's contract would terminate as of August 1, 1987 because IMC could not meet the enrollment of less than 50 percent Medicare/Medicaid rule; HCFA also cited a list of consumer complaints about questionable marketing tactics, illegal screening of potential Medicare enrollees, and late bill payments.[29] In last minute negotiations, however, Humana purchased IMC, thereby preserving the Medicare contract and saving HCFA the embarrassment of this potential failure.

The Federal Government is trying to achieve other objectives through risk contracting activities. By consolidating all payments for both Parts A and B of Medicare into a single per capita fee, it is easier for the Federal Government to administer the Medicare program, to control costs, to pass on to the risk contractor the management of the actual delivery of services (and the contractor's piecemeal payment for those services to the providers),

---

[25] Greg R. Nycz and Frederick J. Wenzel, "A View from Under the Microscope, Medicare Prospective Risk Contracting," *Medical Group Management, 30*(3):20–23, May/June 1983; and Wenzel, "Medicare Risk Contracts, Success or Failure?" pp. 30–33.

[26] Maria R. Traska. "SC Blues Plan Drops Medicare Risk Contract." *Hospitals, 61*(9):54, May 5, 1987.

[27] Teri Shahoda. "Unreliable AAPCC Rates Minimize Provider Interest." *Hospitals, 61*(6):34, March 20, 1987.

[28] "Stung by Losses, Maxicare Rethinks Medicare Participation." *Hospitals, 60*(15):14, August 5, 1986.

[29] "Florida Uproar Shakes HMO Movement." *Medicine and Health Perspectives (Supplement), 41*(18):4, May 4, 1987.

and to reduce overall outlays through possible reductions of the AAPCC. The government, however, has noticed that with these risk contracts, there is the potential for a reduction in services and quality of care; it has, therefore, developed regulations to monitor HMO/CMP activities. These oversight activities are included as part of the contract, but significant questions regarding the quality of care in HMOs and CMPs that contract with HCFA (especially the IMC problem) prompted Congress to pass the Medicare Quality Protection Act of 1986, which is described in Chapter 8.

PRECONTRACT ACTIVITIES

TEFRA allows two different kinds of HSOs to develop either risk or cost contracts with HCFA: federally qualified HMOs and organizations certified as eligible CMPs. A qualified HMO has met the regulations prescribed by the HMO Act. This process is not unlike an accreditation activity and includes reviews of health services delivery, marketing, and the financial, legal, and general management of the health plan. After a federal team completes an on-site review, it reports its findings to an HMO case officer, who then reports his/her findings to the administrator of the Office of Prepaid Health Care in Washington, D.C. for final approval or disapproval. The other alternative is to apply to OPHC for certification as a qualified CMP and, concurrently, to negotiate a Medicare contract with HCFA in Baltimore, Maryland. The CMP certification process is similar to the HMO qualification process.

But prior to either of these steps, the HMO or CMP must apply and receive a license to operate in the state. In many states, this process is controlled by HMO-enabling laws and regulations and may take six to eight months or longer. Generally, however, after the state laws are satisfied, federal eligibility for CMPs or qualification for HMOs should be easily met, since most states review the same areas as the Federal Government.

The federal process begins with a CMP Eligibility Application that is submitted to the Office of Prepaid Health Care. The steps in the review process are

1. Receipt of application by OPHC
2. Review of application for completeness
3. Desk review of application by specialist reviewers
4. Site visit
5. Final determination

This process takes approximately four months. Delays in contract negotiations or denial of eligibility generally are caused by one or more of the following seven areas, identified by OPHC from an analysis of 17 CMP applications.

1. Weak quality assurance program or plan
2. Weak utilization controls and risk systems
3. Weak financial position—inadequate capitalization, net income declining, or financial projections not substantiated
4. Inadequate insolvency protection
5. Inadequate management information system
6. Lack of Medicare marketing strategy
7. Lack of written agreements with specialist physicians

KEY ELEMENTS OF CMP ELIGIBILITY

The following key areas are reviewed by OPHC during the preliminary process.

Legal

Organization under state law
Operational status—must have at least 1,000 members at time of application
Insolvency arrangements
Provider agreements
Subscriber agreements

Financial Viability

Performance over the last three years
Budget assumptions
Preliminary ACR
Cost and revenue projections
Capitalization

Health Services Delivery

Availability, accessibility, and continuity of health services
Evidence of physician willingness to serve the Medicare population
Quality assurance management program
Utilization controls/physician risk arrangements
MIS feedback to physicians

Marketing

Enrollment projections and assumptions
Strategy
Marketing materials
5,000 minimum commercial members (1,500 rural)
50/50 rule

When the organization can meet these criteria and become certified, it can then proceed with contract negotiations with HCFA.

CONTRACTING DETAILS

The actual process of implementing a contract with HCFA includes the following steps:

1. *Notification of Interest:* The HSO notifies the Office of Prepaid Health Care of its interest in Medicare contracting. OPHC/HCFA assign a team to conduct an on-site review, send the HMO or CMP background information on Medicare contracts, and request background information on the health plan.

2. *Health Plan Review of Information:* The health plan reviews all the material and sends requested information to OPHC. OPHC then completes its activities, including on-site reviews, to qualify the HMO or certify the CMP. OPHC may provide an orientation on the Medicare HMO/CMP program and will provide assistance for meeting all contract requirements.

3. *HMO's/CMP's Final Decision to Contract:* The HMO or CMP then makes the final decision on whether to contract with HCFA and chooses an effective date. OPHC prepares a report recommending that HCFA enter into a contract with the HMO/CMP.

4. *HMO/CMP Negotiates and Submits Signed Contract:* Although the major issues will have been resolved prior to this step (usually during the review of step 2), the final touches on the agreement are now completed, and the health plan submits three signed copies of the contract to HCFA. They will be countersigned by HCFA, and one copy will be returned to the plan.

5. *CMP/HMO Submits Budget, Enrollment Forecast, and Marketing Material:* Ninety days prior to the contract effective date, the plan submits its budget, enrollment forecasts, and marketing materials. These documents are reviewed by HCFA, capitation rates are set, and low-option premiums and marketing materials are approved.

6. *Enrollment Begins:* The health plan submits initial enrollment data to HCFA by the 15th of the month preceding the contract effective date. HCFA then enters the enrollment data into its records and initiates payments to the HMO/CMP.

ENROLLMENT

All Medicare beneficiaries (those with Parts A and B or Part B only) in the plan's service area are eligible to enroll in the health plan. Enrollment is accomplished through an *open* enrollment period of at least 30 consecutive days during each year. If there is more than one Medicare contracting HMO/CMP in the same service area, the government may require that their open enrollment periods coincide. In addition, the following restrictions apply to the enrollment process:

1. The plan may not enroll more than 50 percent of its membership from Medicare or Medicaid without a waiver from HCFA. Based on the experiences of IMC in Florida, the government is very reticent about approving waivers to this rule.

2. The plan can limit enrollment to maintain a broad range of membership mix by age, sex, and disability level—a membership that is representative of the general population in the plan's service area.

3. Medicare beneficiaries who have end-stage renal disease or have chosen to receive hospice benefits are not eligible for risk contract membership.

4. Conversion is optional for current nonrisk enrollees. An exception is when HCFA determines that, for administrative reasons, all cost enrollees must convert to risk status.

5. Medicare HMO/CMP coverage begins on the first day of the month in which the individual is both eligible for Medicare coverage and enrolled in the HMO/CMP. HMO enrollment commences during the three months following the month in which HCFA receives the completed request to change the beneficiary's Medicare status. HCFA will inform the health plan of the date on which health plan coverage begins for each applicant, and the plan will in turn notify the applicant.

6. The Medicare recipient who enrolls in the HMO/CMP is "locked-in"; for example, the enrollee must use the health plan for all of his/her medical care if the cost is to be covered by Medicare (except for out-of-area, emergency, and urgent services).

7. The ability of an enrollee to leave the health plan and return to regular Medicare coverage is limited by regulation. The enrollee may disenroll at any time by making a dated and signed request; disenrollment would be effective on the first day of the first month after the request for disenrollment is made. Enrollees leaving a service area for a period in excess of 90 days must disenroll; the HMO/CMP is under no obligation to provide benefits to such enrollees.

GENERAL AND SUPPLEMENTAL BENEFITS

Medicare enrollees are entitled to the same full range of Medicare services as their fee-for-service counterparts—both Parts A and B or Part B only—based on their Medicare coverage. These services must be provided directly by the health plan or through preexisting arrangements. Because Medicare limits inpatient coverage to 90 days, with a 60-day lifetime reserve, the Medicare enrollee's coverage may not be as extensive as that of non-Medicare, commercial enrollees. Therefore, the health plan may make available a supplemental, wrap-around, or MediGap package to the Medicare enrollee. These supplemental benefits may include preventive care, reduced coinsurance and deductibles, prescription drugs, and routine eye care, as well as an extension of inpatient hospital stays to 365 days a year. These supplemental benefits fall into three categories: optional, imposed by risk organizations, and required of risk organizations. Optional services may be provided by both risk and cost HMO/CMPs, and enrollees may choose to purchase these supplemental benefits. If approved by HCFA, the health plan may impose or require that all Medicare enrollees purchase a supplemental package. Finally, if the health plan provides the basic Part A and B services for less than the payments that it receives from HCFA, it is required to use these savings to reduce premiums, coinsurance, and deductibles or to provide additional benefits and services. (Note that approximately 70 percent of all contractors have copayments that are the responsibility of the Medicare recipient.)

MARKETING ACTIVITIES

Earlier in this chapter, several marketing issues were reviewed; in addition, TEFRA regulations create specific requirements and prohibitions in the marketing area. HMOs/CMPs that have Medicare contracts must provide interested Medicare beneficaries with "adequate" written descriptions of the rules, procedures, charges, available services, and other information necessary for these individuals to consider health plan membership. Risk organizations must provide written descriptions of any additional benefits or lowered costs that may be available to enrollees and must inform the general public regarding the enrollment period.

The health plan is prohibited from discriminating against particular groups of beneficiaries. It cannot "demarket" low-income areas and place priority on enrollment of Medicare recipients in higher income areas; it cannot mislead or confuse Medicare beneficiaries nor misrepresent the organization, its representatives, or the role of HCFA; it cannot engage in door-to-door solicitation of Medicare beneficiaries; and it cannot offer gifts or payments to entice a beneficiary to enroll.

PRO REVIEW

According to Section 1876 of the Social Security Act, any HMO with a risk contract must submit to PRO review as a condition of that contract. See Chapter 8 for a discussion of PRO review.

Other Alternative Delivery Systems and Managed Care Organizations

The Federal Government, including members of Congress, continues to propose modifications and additions to the growing list of government financing and delivery alternatives that are available in the health services industry. Some of these proposals are reviewed in the sections that follow.

PRIVATE HEALTH PLAN OPTION

First included in the Reagan administration's fiscal year 1988 budget and endorsed by the Bush administration, the private health plan option (PHPO) concept—a euphemism for capitation—would expand the type and number of organizations that could participate in Medicare prepaid arrangements. This concept has also been called "employer-at-risk" capitation—although this "is somewhat misleading since it includes employer-sponsored plans, commercial insurers, unions, combinations of employers and their unions (including Taft-Hartley Health and Welfare Funds), and even broader combinations of employers, unions, their insurers, or others responsible for the medical expenses of health care to groups of Medicare-eligible retirees. Estimates are that as many as six million beneficiaries could be covered by such plans."[30] Thus, the PHPO would expand the Medicare risk contract option to employers and insurers that accept responsibility for their over age 65 retirees' health insurance. HCFA's explanation for this move includes: (1) ensuring that employees who are offered an HMO option are presented a clear choice between health delivery options; (2) a belief that the monetary requirement is an unnecessary intrusion into the marketplace; (3) a belief that the monetary contribution prevents employers from basing their contributions on their population's experience; (4) the possibility of increased employer health benefit costs because of the contribution; and (5) a belief that the Federal Government should no longer have to assess this large industry, given the fact that the original intent of the HMO legislation was to assist in the growth of an infant industry.[31]

Conversely, many in the industry feel that this legislation, known as the Medicare Expanded Choice Act (MECA), would effectively cut Medicare payments, since the employer health plans would be paid by HCFA at 95 percent of what the annuitant group is expected to cost Medicare (95 percent payment rate based on the *group's* experience rather than the AAPCC). Smaller HMOs are uncomfortable with the provision to change the current HMO/CMP lock-in from one year to three years. And the proposal to eliminate the employer contributions may discourage HMO enrollment by offering little or no financial support. Employers, however, may find this eliminated employer contribution of interest.

---

[30] Kevin E. Moley. "Overview of Employer Capitation Activities." *Health Care Financing Review; 1986 Annual Supplement,* 1986, p. 31.

[31] Society for Ambulatory Care Professionals of AHA. "Health Maintenance Organizations/ Competitive Medical Plans." In: *Ambulatory Care Alert,* Chicago, Ill., AHA , May 1987, p. 1.

The draft MECA legislation allows for the establishment of demonstration projects (as of September 1990 only one demonstration project was operating) where employers, county medical societies, physicians, and others can serve Medicare beneficiaries through PPOs and negotiated provider arrangements. It also provides for the following.[32]

1. Employer-based plans could offer "actuarial equivalent" Medicare benefits, rather than specific benefits; offer rebates of up to $500 per year; limit enrollment to their own annuitants (retirees); and be paid by HCFA on the basis of the annuitant group's experience, rather than the AAPCC.

2. Employer-based plans would not have to calculate the ACR, nor would they have to provide physician services completely or primarily under contract. Further, a cost contract option would not be offered.

3. For Medicare risk contract HMOs and CMPs, the legislation would eliminate the ACR for small plans and plans in areas with three or more competing plans; exempt employer plan premiums paid to HMOs/CMPs from Medicare ACR limits; allow HMOs/CMPs to recover revenue that was lost due to legislative action (e.g., Gramm-Rudman-Hollings forced cutbacks); and impose civil monetary penalties for a variety of enrollment and disenrollment violations.

4. Risk-contract HMOs and CMPs also would be allowed to contract for a three-year AAPCC (rather than one year), which would result in a "slightly reduced rate" in the second and third years. The organization would be committed to the preset rates if it selected the three-year option.

SOCIAL HEALTH MAINTENANCE ORGANIZATION

The Social Health Maintenance Organization (S/HMO) is a managed system of health and social services developed exclusively for Medicaid and non-Medicaid Medicare eligibles. As a vertically integrated and capitated system of care, the S/HMO is designed to improve the accessibility and quality of care for the aged, as well as reduce institutional dependency and contain medical costs. In 1980, four demonstration sites were selected by the Department of Health and Human Services Office of Research and Demonstration and were awarded a grant to develop and implement the first S/HMOs. All four sites began marketing in early 1985, and each demonstration ran for a period of 42 months. At the end of the demonstration period, all four sites signed regular contracts with HCFA. The four sites are the Metropolitan Jewish Geriatric Center in Brooklyn, New York; Kaiser Permanente Medical Care Program in Portland,

---

[32] Rucker. *Legislative Issues for Group Practice: 1987*, p. 7.

Oregon; Ebenezer Society in Minneapolis, Minnesota; and Senior Care Action Network in Long Beach, California.

There are many factors that distinguish the S/HMO from the traditional HMO. Unique features of the S/HMO include:

- Providing comprehensive health and long-term care (LTC) benefits
- Providing social and noninstitutional services
- Pooling private and public financing of services
- Providing case-management services
- Providing financial risk for both medical care and LTC benefits for the provider organization
- Permitting participation of both Medicaid and non-Medicaid Medicare eligibles
- Permitting voluntary enrollment of an elderly population that has a broad spectrum of needs

In terms of what services the S/HMO actually provides, the four sites provide all Medicare Part A and B services without the copayments and deductibles associated with these services, as well as acute care benefits such as audiometry, optometry, prescription drugs, and, among other services, preventive visits. All sites also offer unlimited hospital days, and two sites have significantly extended Medicare-type skilled nursing facility (SNF) benefits. The chronic care benefits package at the four sites includes case management, home nursing and therapies, personal care and homemaker services, adult day care, medical transportation, hospice and respite care, and chronic care in an SNF or intermediate care facility. Transportation, escort services, and meals also are provided by the S/HMO.

The S/HMO is financed by pooling public and private dollars, which includes payment from Medicare and Medicaid and self-pay premiums. For non-Medicaid eligibles, the S/HMO receives a capitation payment from Medicare, a monthly premium from the enrollee, and corresponding copayments. For Medicaid eligibles, the S/HMO receives a monthly capitation payment from both Medicare and Medicaid. The capitated Medicare reimbursement is based on the AAPCC, which, in essence, reimburses the S/HMO for 100 percent of what it would have cost Medicare to serve the enrolled population in the fee-for-service sector. The Medicaid reimbursement premium differs in each state and ranges from basing the premium on a rate-book type formula derived from state spending to basing the premium on Medicaid spending data and the site's initial financial estimates. The private premiums are calculated to not exceed the current Medicare supplemental premium.

As mentioned earlier, the target population for the S/HMO consists of both Medicare only and Medicare/Medicaid elderly. Through conventional marketing techniques, the four sites plan to enroll, on a voluntary basis, a balanced population that reflects the local community in terms of health status. In an attempt to achieve this balanced population, the method of "queuing" was adopted by the sites. Queuing, a deviation from health screening, involves putting applicants on a waiting list according to their level of physical impairment. Different from health screening, high-risk applicants are accepted into the program. In effect, the high-risk population is an essential component of the balanced population.

MEDICAID RISK CONTRACTS

The cost to federal and state governments of funding Medicaid, the largest program providing medical assistance to the poor, has grown from a 1965 estimate of $250 million annually to approximately $72 billion in 1990 and an estimated $90 billion in 1991. Lawmakers envisioned that only 2.3 million individuals would be enrolled in the program at any given time, but in 1990, it was esimated that 25.5 million persons qualified for health services assistance and that 27.3 million persons would qualify in 1991. Because states share in these programs, approximately half of the costs are paid by the Federal Government. The escalating cost of the program (average annualized growth, adjusted for inflation, was 14.5 percent), compounded by high health care inflation, led federal policymakers to reevaluate the program and, ultimately, to allow states to explore innovative financing mechanisms as ways to cut Medicaid costs without reducing services covered under the program.

A major financing mechanism that has been explored by states to control costs and utilization involves payments to providers on a capitated basis. Success in the use of capitated systems, including HMO experience in commercial settings and experimental Medicare risk contracting, led Congress to pass legislation in 1976, 1981, and every year since 1985,[33] promoting capitated risk contracting in the Medicaid program. The state agrees to prepay a contracting entity a flat fixed amount per Medicaid recipient for a negotiated period of time—the monthly amount is the capitation rate. In exchange, the organization agrees to provide a negotiated range of services to the Medicaid members. Thus, the contractor/provider is at risk for costs that exceed payments by the state; this gives the contractor a strong incentive to control utilization and costs. Controls include a variety of management techniques that usually combine methods of putting providers at risk for the cost of services with systems that reward them for cost-effective utilization.

---

[33] 1976 HMO Amendments (P.L. 94-460), and the Budget Reconciliation Acts in 1981, 1986, 1987, 1988, 1989, and 1990.

Services required in the contract follow Medicaid (Title XIX) guidelines and are comprehensive in nature, like those of HMO commercial packages and CMPs. States have the option of expanding covered services to include care in intermedicate facilities, dental care, pharmaceutical services, and eyeglasses. Many states prefer a contract with just one regional organization that can provide or arrange for the provision of all covered services; this concept is known as "geographic capitation."

BUDGET RECONCILIATION ACTS AND MEDICAID CONTRACTING

The enabling legislation, especially the 1981 OBRA, has achieved its desired effect. Prior to OBRA, only 17 state Medicaid agencies, including the District of Columbia, had Medicaid risk contracts, covering only 1 percent of the Medicaid population. In June 1989, 28 states had entered into Medicaid risk contracts, covering approximately 2.5 million Medicaid beneficiaries, or an estimated 8 percent of the Medicaid recipients. HCFA estimates that more than 3 percent of the Medicaid population in those 28 states were served by alternative delivery systems.[34] The 1985 OBRA and succeeding budget reconciliation acts provided for large reductions in the federal share of Medicaid program costs and allowed for an expansion of alternative financing approaches, thus providing incentives for the states to develop cost-controlling programs. The legislation stipulates that states may enter into contracts with federally qualified HMOs and other entities provided that they meet the state's definition of an HMO, are organized primarily for the purpose of providing health care, make their services equally accessible to Medicaid and non-Medicaid enrollees, are adequately protected from insolvency, and will not hold members liable for the organization's debts. Medicare and Medicaid membership in these plans can be as high as but cannot exceed 75 percent of total plan membership. States may extend Medicaid eligibility to enrollees for up to six months after an individual's eligibility technically ends—thus resolving many of the administrative difficulties of managing a prepaid system that enrolls members whose eligibility can change monthly. States can also impose a six-month lock-in period on individuals, during which time their membership in a plan is guaranteed, provided that voluntary disenrollment is allowed during the first month of enrollment and disenrollment is allowed

---

[34] Jeffrey Finn, "HHS Pushing for Medicaid HMOs," *Hospitals,* *61*(4):22, February 20, 1987; Janet Firshein, "Medicaid HMO Plans Tackle Quality Questions," *Hospitals,* *60*(6):76, March 20, 1986; and U.S. Department of Health and Human Services, Health Care Financing Administration, Medicaid Bureau, Medicaid Managed Care Office, *Report on Medicaid Enrollment in Capitated Plans as of 6/30/89,* Baltimore, Md., DHHS, June 1990.

thereafter upon showing good cause. Federal "freedom of choice" waivers of these rules also are granted if the state can show such a waiver to be "efficient, cost-effective, and consistent with the objectives of the Medicaid program." For example, the Tax Equity and Fiscal Responsibility Act of 1982 allows for a three-year extension of the 75 percent waiver provided that the plan shows it is attempting to enroll commercial accounts. As of mid-1990, 23 states had freedom of choice waivers, with 32 approved HSO waivers.

ADMINISTRATION OF MEDICAID CONTRACTS

State Medicaid agencies administer the Medicaid program in their respective states and can contract on a risk basis with several types of organizations, including HMOs, prepaid health plans (PHPs) and health insuring organizations (HIOs). All HMO models are now represented with state contracts, with the medical group model exhibiting the lowest enrollment (approximately 6 percent of the total Medicaid population who are enrolled in plans, with enrollment in the other three models equally divided). PHPs do not qualify as HMOs but are (1) organizations that provide health care and have received grants of $100,000 or more (under Section 329(d)(1)(A) or 330(d)(1) of the Public Health Service Act) from the Public Health Service since 1976 or will arrange for the provision of a full range of services under Medicaid, (2) nonprofit primary care entities in rural areas, or (3) organizations that have had contracts with the state to provide services on a prepaid risk basis since 1970. HIOs do not provide services but act as service brokers for the state, meet the state insurance requirements, and are willing to contract for the provision of all or most acute care services to the Medicaid population on an at-risk basis.

The yearly capitation payment to any of the three contracting entities cannot exceed what the Federal Government estimates that the state would pay for the same services in the traditional fee-for-service system. In most cases, states have paid contracting organizations 90 to 95 percent of estimated fee-for-service costs. This approach is generally accepted in capitated medicine because it is felt that inpatient utilization will be dramatically reduced from the high fee-for-service rates (approximately 310 days per 1,000 enrollees—a rate similar to HMO commercial enrollees and half the traditional Medicaid delivery system). Setting the capitation rates, however, has been difficult for the states; the rates must demonstrate a savings over the traditional system and yet be high enough to interest potential contracting entities. Generally, historic "paid claims" data provide the basis for determining what the agencies have paid by county. Then the agency determines the AAPCC, the average cost to the state for providing services to each Medicaid member of the specified population group within a specific geographic area. After additional adjustments by "rate cells," the agency reduces the estimated fee-for-service costs that were developed using the above methodology by a program savings percentage such as 5 percent, creating a final capitation rate that is 95 percent of the fee-for-service cost. States may also deduct a percentage of the capitation rate to cover their administrative expenses.

Not unlike other federal program participation, health services organizations must weigh the benefits of improving Medicaid payments and other advantages against the costs and problems inherent in Medicaid risk contracts. Advantages for HSOs that are already serving Medicaid patients and involved with capitated systems may include improved payment for services, a lock-in on a segment of the market, and greater financial stability for the organization. Conversely, some concerns in developing a state contract are: marketing and enrollment issues, use of appropriate management information systems, and financial issues such as physician reimbursement and adverse risk-taking by the health plan. Marketing is usually handled through or approved by the state Medicaid agency, at least initially, which may create awkward and potentially ineffective activities. Further, little is known about the Medicaid recipient's incentives for enrolling or not enrolling with the plan. Enrollment may be voluntary or mandatory, and questions of extending plan eligibility beyond Medicaid must be considered. Lock-in arrangements add more confusion to the issue. Adequate management information systems and physician compensation questions are common to all HMOs and may or may not pose greater problems in Medicaid risk contracting.

At a time when there has been a phenomenal expansion of capitated medicine through HMOs and CMPs, it appears that most states will expand their efforts to develop Medicaid risk contracts. The slow entry of some states into the HMO market, however, may be the result of abuses in the Medicaid program in the 1970s—especially California's "Medicaid Mills," where HMOs were charged with skimming profits and denying access to health care for the poor. These problems led to significant changes in federal rules governing Medicaid contracts with HMOs; for example, current rules require HMOs to maintain a private enrollment of at least 25 percent and to allow recipients to disenroll if they are dissatisfied. As noted previously, many states are seeking waivers to lock in enrollees so as to guarantee a stable base and to maintain some continuity of care. Some states are making it mandatory for Medicaid recipients to enroll in HMOs, but usually the recipients have several HMOs from which to choose.

These actions by state Medicaid legislators are in response to major concerns and obstacles inherent in the Medicaid program. First, there are difficulties in establishing premium structures that are considered feasible and equitable by both state Medicaid agencies and HMOs—especially since there is the likelihood that Medicaid beneficiaries will require more services than other enrollees and therefore increase costs. Second, Medicaid contracting suggests the lack of a stable population and, because they can become ineligible for public assistance, a high turnover of enrollment among Medicaid beneficiaries. This translates into potentially high rates of disenrollment and higher marketing, administrative, and enrollment costs for the HMO. Third, with high turnover comes higher use of services, since experience suggests that new enrollees use above-average numbers of services.[35] Fourth, the contracting process has included competitive bidding and competitively negotiated prices for hospital and physician services; this suggests that not every provider or HMO is guaranteed or entitled to receive a contract from the Medicaid agency.

Summary

To assist in controlling the increasing costs of Medicare, the Federal Government, from 1965 to the present, has gradually developed legislation that makes Medicare contracting more attractive to prepaid health plans and health services organizations that become eligible competitive medical plans. After HCFA contracted with several HMOs during the last half of the 1970s to demonstrate the Medicare program's effectiveness, the Tax Equity and Fiscal Responsibility Act of 1982 was passed, which included a section that allowed contracts with qualified HMOs and certified CMPs and provided for prospective payments to these organizations for the delivery of Part A and B services to Medicare recipients. Both cost-based and risk-based contracts were allowed. Implemented in February 1985, these risk programs enrolled an estimated two million Medicare recipients in September 1990.

The benefits of contracting with the government include: a potential profit factor that is built into the premium paid by the government, improved budgetary accuracy, a competitive edge over other HSOs, and an improved bargaining position for the health plan when addressing employer needs. Conversely, it is well understood that major problems still remain concerning the development and level of the AAPCC and the control of service delivery through the use of provider incentives. These issues are current topics of study. In addition, the government is interested in further experimentation with risk contracting. For example, under the Medicare Expanded Choice Act program, within the framework of a Medicare Voucher Program—the so-called employer-at-risk capitation concept—or through the use of private health plan options, the fee-for-service medical groups not now under a cost or risk contract may also become participants in these contracting arrangements.

---

[35] Karen Wintringham and Thomas W. Bice. "Effects of Turnover on Use of Services by Medicaid Beneficiaries in a Health Maintenance Organization." *Group Health Journal,* 6(1):13, Spring 1985.

As the authors of *The Future of Medicare and HMOs*[36] suggest, CMP/HMO relationships with Medicare will thrive and have a significant impact on the costs of health services if the following issues are addressed. "First, HMOs must demonstrate that their prepaid capitated systems are cost-effective for Medicare beneficiaries. Second, regulations must encourage rather than hinder HMO participation in the Medicare program, particularly by providing appropriate reimbursement rates. Third, HMOs must develop marketing plans that allow them to successfully compete with fee-for-service physicians and other group health organizations for older clients. And finally, HMOs must maintain a large number of Medicare beneficiaries by providing client-satisfying care that induces members to remain enrolled in the HMO."

These programs provide the precise mechanisms that are needed to serve the elderly—a managed, coordinated, and multidisciplinary approach that ties both short-term and long-term care together. They integrate acute care with preventive and chronic care, and they offer the ability to provide supportive services such as home and hospice care to terminal patients. Together with the ability to control costs, these programs offer great strengths and a hope for better methods of health services delivery to the elderly. With the Federal Government's slow but inevitable push toward what seems to be a totally risk/capitated Medicare system, health services organizations have the opportunity to effectively participate in this new system and to maintain financial success from their operations.

References

Abato, Rozann. "The Role of Managed Care in Meeting the Health Care Needs of the Medicaid Population." In: *Proceedings of the Group Health Association of America, Medicaid Component of Medicare, Medicaid and the HMO Experience, Baltimore Md., August 16-17, 1990.* Washington, D.C., GHAA, 1990.

American Medical Association, Monograph Group on Health Service Policy. *Medicare and Prepaid Health Plans: New Directions for HMOs.* Chicago, Ill., AMA, 1985.

Baldwin, Mark F. "Medicare HMO Option Draws Fire; Critics Call Rate Schedule Flawed." *Modern Healthcare,* 15(22):28, November 22, 1985.

Baldwin, Mark F., and Cynthia Wallace. "Executives of HMOs Are Perplexed by Variations in 1986 Rate Increases." *Modern Healthcare,* 15(23):36, December 6, 1985.

Bonanno, James Bautz, and Terrie Wetle. "HMO Enrollment of Medicare Recipients: An Analysis, Incentives and Barriers." *Journal of Health Politics, Policy, and Law,* 9(1):41–62, Spring 1984.

---

[36] Iversen and Polich. *The Future of Medicare and HMOs,* p. 12.

Christianson, Jon B. "Provider Participation in Competitive Bidding for Indigent Patients." *Inquiry, 21*(2):161–177, Summer 1984.

Diamond, Larry; Leonard Gruenberg; and Robert Morris. "Elder Care for the 1980s: Health and Social Service in One Prepaid Health Maintenance System." *The Gerontologist, 23*(2):148–154, 1983.

Eggers, Paul W., and Ronald Prihoda. "Pre-enrollment Reimbursement Patterns of Medicare Beneficiaries Enrolled in 'At-Risk' HMOs." *Health Care Financing Review, 4*(1):55–73, September 1983.

Firshein, Janet. "HCFA Outlines 1987 Legislative Medicare Agenda." *Hospitals, 61*(4): 50, February 20, 1987.

Fischer, Lee A. "Health Maintenance Organizations and the Medicare Program." *Journal of Florida Medical Association, 72*(9):777–779, September 1985.

Frederick, Larry. "Why Medicare's HMO Express Jumped the Tracks." *Medical Economics, 62*(5):29–35, March 4, 1985.

Greenberg, Jay N.; Walter N. Leutz; and Ruby Abrahams. "The National Social Health Maintenance Organization Demonstration." *Journal of Ambulatory Care Management, 8*(4):32–61, November 1985.

Harrington, Charlene. "Crisis in Long-Term Care: Part 2, Policy Options." *Nursing Economics, 3*(3):109–115, March/April 1985.

Hohlen, Nina M.; Larry Manheim; and Gretchen Fleming. "Access to Office-Based Physicians Under Capitation Reimbursement and Medicaid Case Management." *Medical Care, 28*(1):59–68, January 1990.

Hornbrook, M. C. "Examination of the AAPCC Methodology in an HMO Prospective Demonstration Project." *Group Health Journal, 5*(1):13–21, Spring 1984.

Iglehart, John K. "Medicare Turns to HMOs." *New England Journal of Medicine, 312*(2):132–136, January 10, 1985.

Iversen, Laura Himes, and Cynthia Longseth Polich. *The Future of Medicare and HMOs.* Excelsior, Minn., InterStudy, Center for Aging and Long-term Care, 1985.

Johns, Lucy; Maren D. Anderson; and Robert A. Derzon. "Selective Contracting in California: Experience in the Second Year." *Inquiry, 22*(4):335–347, Winter 1985.

Johns, Lucy; Robert A. Derzon; and Maren D. Anderson. "Selective Contracting in California: Early Effects and Policy Implications." *Inquiry, 22*(1):24–32, Spring 1985.

Krasner, W. "The New Medicare Market for HMOs." *Health Group, 1*(2):7–15, October 1984.

Kuchel, S. A., and K. C. Powell. "The Average Adjusted Per Capita Cost Under Risk Contracts with Providers of Care." *Transactions of the Society of Actuaries,* (23):57–66, 1981.

Langwell, Kathryn M., et al. "Qualification Requirements for CMP Status and Eligibility of Fee-for-Service Medical Groups." Washington, D.C., Mathematica Policy Research, August 1, 1986. Issue paper No. 11 to the Health Care Financing Administration under Contract No. 95-C-98919/3-01

——————. "HMOs in the Medicare Market. Part 2—Operational Issues." *Medical Group Management, 34*(1):37–44, January/February 1987.

Langwell, Kathryn M., and Lyle M. Nelson. "Physician Incentive Arrangements and Use of Hospital Services: A Framework for Analysis." Washington, D.C., Mathematica

Policy Research, June 16, 1987. Prepared for the Health Care Financing Administration under Contract No. 500-83-0047.

Langwell, Kathryn M.; Lyle Nelson; and Shelly Nelson. "Direct Physician Capitation Under the Medicare Program: Evidence and Feasibility." Paper prepared for the Medicare Research Conference, Leonard Davis Institute of Health Economics, University of Pennsylvania, Philadelphia, Pa. October 8–10, 1986.

Lichtenstein, Richard, and William Thomas. "Including a Measure of Health Status in Medicare's Health Maintenance Organization Capitation Formula: Reliability Issues." *Medical Care, 25*(2):100–110, February 1987.

Moley, Kevin E. "Overview of Employer Capitation Activities." *Health Care Financing Review; 1986 Annual Supplement.* 1986, pp. 31–34.

1986 Group Health Proceedings; New Health Care Systems: HMOs and Beyond. Minneapolis, Minn., Group Health Institute, June 1-4, 1986.

Nycz, Greg R., and Frederick J. Wenzel. "A View from Under the Microscope, Medicare Prospective Risk Contracting." *Medical Group Management, 30*(3):20–23, 26–29, May/June 1983.

Shouldice, Robert G. "CMPs: Should We Get Involved?" *Medical Group Management, 33*(5):15–16, 30, September/October 1986.

————. "Are CMPs Right for Your Medical Group?" *Medical Group Management, 33*(6):9–14, November/December 1986.

Stiefel, M., and W. J. Cooper. "The ACR Methodology: Medicare Prospective Capitation in an HMO." *Group Health Journal, 5*(1):8–12, Spring 1984.

U.S. Department of Health and Human Services. "Medicare Program; Payment and Health Maintenance Organizations and Competitive Medical Plans; Final Rules." *Federal Register, 50*(7):1314, January 10, 1985. 42 CFR, Parts 405 and 417.

————, Health Care Financing Administration, Office of Prepaid Health Care. "Quality Assurance Guidelines for Health Maintenance Organizations and Competitive Medical Plans." Rockville, Md., DHHS, July 25, 1986.

————, Office of Health Maintenance Organizations. *CMP Eligibility Review.* Rockville, Md., DHHS, December 9, 1985.

————, Office of the Secretary. *Incentive Arrangements Offered by Health Maintenance Organizations and Competitive Medical Plans to Physicians.* Volume I. Washington, D.C., DHHS, 1990.

Williamson, Helen M. "Social/HMO Serves Aging Population." *Michigan Hospitals, 21*(12):13–17, December 1985.

Wintringham, Karen, and Thomas W. Bice. "Effects of Turnover on Use of Services by Medicaid Beneficiaries in a Health Maintenance Organization." *Group Health Journal, 6*(1):12–18, Spring 1985.

6

THE PROVIDERS

HMOs, PPOs, and CMPs bring together providers and consumers, match health needs with health vendors, and help fulfill the goals of each group. Without consumer demand for health care and providers to supply scarce health resources—manpower, facilities, and equipment—there would be no need for HMOs, PPOs, CMPs, or any other health delivery system. The HMO is one of the best and most efficient ways to match these two components of health delivery systems. PPOs, although perhaps not as efficient as HMOs, allow the purchasers of service—employers—to develop preferred relationships with the providers that they feel will help facilitate their objectives of cost control and, at the same time, provide high-quality medical services to employees and dependents.

Providers—physicians, hospitals, and other components of the delivery element—are discussed in this chapter. Because many HMOs use groups of physicians, a major consideration here will be how these groups are structured and how they are reimbursed for their services. The attitudes of the medical groups, their contractual relationships with health plans, and the control of their activities also will be discussed. Further analyses of physicians who are associated with IPAs will complete the discussion initiated in Chapter 4. Then the relationship of hospitals and HMOs/PPOs will be reviewed. A discussion of the role of the medical director in managed care systems will complete this chapter. The other half of the relationship—consumers—will be considered in Chapter 7: their opinions, attitudes, and viewpoints on the methods used to serve urban and rural populations; and the methods used by HMOs and CMPs to serve consumers in underserved and elderly populations.

Physicians

PHYSICIAN RELATIONSHIPS WITH PREPAID HEALTH PLANS

One of the most discussed issues among physicians and health plans is physician relationships with prepaid health plans, PPOs and other MCOs. Physicians, by training, are generally conservative in approach, using techniques, procedures, and drugs that they learned about in medical school and during their residencies. Changes in practice patterns and payment methods for physicians is slow, difficult, and often unacceptable. From the physician's perspective, developing a relationship with an HMO suggests that the physician's income will change—usually decrease; that the HMO will force controls on the physician's practice behavior; and that the overall quality of the physician's medical services will be diminished. The outcome of these feelings is a very sensitive physician population, concerned about their future, their freedom, and their ability to provide quality service. Conversely, the health plans understand that they cannot market their benefits packages until the physician component of the system is in place and operational; the physicians must be on staff or contracts with individual and/or groups of physicians must be signed. Most importantly, contracts with primary care physicians must be secured, since most care will be rendered and "managed" through referral to specialists by the primary doctors. If problems should arise in physician/health plan relations, such as contract renegotiations, physicians might express negative opinions to HMO patients—a strong message that the HMO's marketing efforts might not be able to remedy. These and other issues must be addressed in the provider agreements and contracts, so as to avoid any problems or misunderstandings.

THE PHYSICIAN PROVIDER AGREEMENT

Provider contracts describe the rights and responsibilities of each of the parties and, like other contracts, must be legally binding, must include an offer and an acceptance, and must provide for a "consideration" or payment. The terms of the contract must be fair and equitable to both parties. From this perspective, because the HMO needs the physician providers, it most likely will negotiate "in good faith" and, initially at least, will be very fair with the physicians. The physicians may also need the relationship—to meet competition from physicians who also have joined the HMO, to use the HMO as a marketing device to develop larger practices, to ensure that current patients will not be drawn to other HMO "participating" physicians, and to prevent being "locked-out" of a substantial group of enrollees who have joined the HMO or PPO.

Contract provisions should address as completely as possible all the concerns that might arise during the contract period, which normally is a year. These provisions should include the items listed in Table 6-1. Although each provision in this list is important, several have become critical to successful health plan/physician relationships. These are discussed under the general headings that follow.[1]

Financial Arrangement: As discussed in Chapter 4, physicians may be paid via salary, fee-for-service, capitation, or a combination of these methods. For physicians serving HMO members, two questions should be considered when developing contract arrangements: (1) Should risk be accepted through withholds and capitation payments? and (2) If capitation is accepted, how close do those payments approximate earnings under the traditional fee-for-service system? Most physicians will try to resist the HMO's efforts to share some level of risk with them. Depending on the physicians' ability to avoid assuming HMO risks, several financial arrangements can be used.

Physicians' first preference is a contract for full charges (described as usual and customary), based on current scheduled fees-for-services. This allows the physicians to cover both their fixed and variable costs as well as their mark-up or profit margin.

A somewhat less-acceptable arrangement includes discounted charges. If the HMO can provide strong guarantees that the contract will provide a substantial increase in new patients, the medical group and IPA physicians may be willing to negotiate a discount. Small discounts would lower fees and reduce profit margins but would at least cover fixed and variable costs, while substantial discounts might wipe out the physicians' profits and not cover all variable costs. In the latter situation, physicians may be willing to provide sizable discounts because the HMO volume would allow them to at least cover their fixed costs and remain operational. This concept is known as "contribution margin," and it would be used by physicians in serious need of additional business or those who fear they might lose business to competing physicians who do sign with the HMO.

The third method, capitation, places the physicians at risk that premiums collected will not cover all costs of inpatient and physician services. The physicians may accept capitation because (1) it is the only way that the HMO will agree to do business; (2) the HMO will give the medical group or IPA physicians an exclusive contract, similar to a franchise, under which the HMO agrees not to contract with other area physicians; (3) the HMO provides guarantees of substantial increases in the physicians' business; (4) a long-term arrangement

---

[1] This discussion is adapted from Robert G. Shouldice, "Negotiating with Alternative Delivery Systems," *Medical Group Management,* 34(1):9–11, January/February 1987.

TABLE 6-1 Physician Provider Contract Provisions

1. The relationship of the parties to one another; specify whether the contract creates an agency relationship

2. A definition of terms used in the contract

3. The method of payment, timing of payments, and methodology used in determining the payment rate

4. Incentives that will be used to control utilization; specify the level or percentage of the withhold, how losses and profits will be apportioned, and the overall level of risk that is assumed by the physician

5. A prohibition against member surcharges being levied and collected by the physician

6. Limitations on the number of enrollees to be served by the participating physician or medical group practice

7. An exclusivity clause limiting the physician's participation in provider contracts with other HMOs and PPOs

8. Limitations on fee-for-service practice

9. Quality assurance (QA) and utilization review (UR) responsibilities, and mandatory participation in established programs

10. Record keeping requirements on and provisions for the HMO's access to plan members' medical records for the purpose of QA and UR review

11. Privacy and confidentiality of members' records

12. Credentialing of participating physicians

13. A dispute resolution, which may include mandatory arbitration

14. A requirement of prior health plan approval of provider subcontracts

15. A procedure for prior approval of hospital admissions, concurrent reviews of hospital stays, and approval for referrals to specialists

16. Procedures for emergency cases

17. A clause regarding an updating of the provider listing to whom the participating physician can refer members; in IPA model HMOs, the contract provision should require that the IPA periodically provide to the HMO an updated list of contract physicians

18. A detailed list of services to be provided, including a list of exclusions, limitations, and copayments

19. A description of marketing responsibilities and the physician's role in marketing

20. The state law governing the contract

21. The term of the contract, causes for termination, and termination procedures

22. Member's rights upon termination, for example, the member's right to select another provider in the network or IPA

23. Automatic contract renewal or renewal procedures

24. Procedures for amending, a requirement that amendments be in writing, and notification for amendments

25. The required liability insurance, including workers compensation and medical malpractice insurance

26. The limitation of liability for the debts of the other party beyond what is agreed upon in the contract

27. A hold harmless clause, or an agreement by each party to indemnify and hold the other party harmless for its own negligence

28. A statement that enforceability of the contract is not affected by unenforceability of any single contract term or provision

29. A statement that the contract is the entire agreement between the parties

30. A statement that the contract does not create any rights in third parties, that is, limit assignment without written consent

31. A nonwaiver of defaults; for example, lack of strict compliance with any term or condition of the contract is not a waiver of any term or condition of the contract

between the HMO and the physicians is anticipated; (5) the medical group or IPA receives assurances that its cost and profit margin will be covered by the capitation; (6) there will be controls on inpatient care costs; and (7) reinsurance will be available in the contract to cover substantial losses that the physicians may experience.

Utilization of Physician Services: An actuarial study is the best method for understanding the relationship between the utilization of services by members and the capitation paid to physicians. Some groups want the capitation based on what they would receive from fee-for-service equivalent services; this can only be accomplished by knowing the level of services that will be needed by the HMO enrollees. Actuaries and other financial/insurance experts provide these data based on experience of like populations, or on the actual experience of the HMO's members. Negotiations can then proceed in earnest. A rule-of-thumb formula is that physician capitation should range between 35 to 45 percent of the total premium—based, of course, on the kinds and levels of services to be provided by the physicians.

Hospital Utilization: Total payments to the group may also be tied to the hospital risk pool and hospital use by members. If physicians are able to control utilization at negotiated levels, then they will share in the savings. Again, actuaries can help the physicians determine the appropriate levels of hospital use for the local area, and the group can then negotiate the sharing arrangement with some confidence. Based on 1990 data, hospital days per 1,000 commercial enrollees were 339.4, and for Medicare enrollees, 1,628.0. The plan and group could set these figures as optimum levels of use, with the savings below or the costs above these figures to be shared 50/50 with the health plan, with certain limitations in effect.

Gatekeepers: Some HMOs, especially IPA models, will establish primary care providers as gatekeepers for most or all of the services available to enrollees. The primary physicians are paid a capitation for *all* services and are then responsible for arranging referrals to specialists. This system could create some animosity toward the gatekeepers. Again, the HMO and its providers should critically analyze the political, professional, and financial ramifications of having the physicians act as primary and specialty gatekeepers.

Copayments: The agreement should describe the copayments that enrollees will be required to pay when receiving physician services. Copayments should be made at the time the services are delivered and should be collected and retained by the group. These copayments should *not* be used to reduce capitation payments, but their level may be taken into consideration when capitation rates are negotiated. The providers may argue that copayments are used more as a method of controlling enrollee behavior than of raising revenue; indeed, the collection of copayments for the physicians may cost more administratively than the amounts collected.

Physician Management Fee: If the HMO uses a gatekeeper or case-manager approach, it might be appropriate for the physicians to negotiate a management fee for handling patient activities. Justification for this fee is the extra burden that is imposed on primary physicians to coordinate and control enrollee care. Payment of this fee may be based on a flat amount per member per month and included in the capitation.

Ancillary Services: If physicians provide ancillary services—pharmacy, lab, radiology, physical therapy—they may want to include the use of these services in the HMO contract; conversely, the health plan will attempt to limit the use of these services through payments or utilization review. Because of the substantial profit in these areas, the physicians will want to negotiate vigorously.

Management Information: Most of the current and future negotiations will depend on the plan members' use of services, as will the control of day-to-day utilization. The agreement should specify that this information will be provided to the physicians in a timely fashion, including a list of current members, specialty providers, hospital and physician utilization, actuarial data, and so on.

Utilization and Quality Reviews: All HMOs are involved with utilization and quality reviews. Usually under the direction of the HMO's medical director, the reviews are used to deny claims, change practice patterns, and generally control some of the physicians' long-established activities. The physicians will want a strong role in the review process by having their representatives sit on the health plan's committees, with veto power on nominations for the plan's medical director. Physician representatives take an active role in medical practice issues and provide a balance in decisions by the HMO's medical director that may be potentially detrimental to the physicians.

Timing of Capitation Payments: By definition, capitation is a prospective payment made to the provider per member per month. The HMO will attempt to make payment on or about the 15th of each month, after some services have been provided. Physicians will want to negotiate that payments be made on a timely basis, as close to the beginning of the month as possible. Conversely, the health plan will argue that the use of the premiums for the first 15 days of the month creates income for the HMO to help hold premiums competitive and to operate the plan effectively. Generally, the HMO will offer a lower capitation if the payment date is set earlier in the month so as to take advantage of the time value of money.

Caveats: Contracts with restrictive clauses may work to the advantage of only one of the parties and may unfairly limit the activities of the other. For instance, HMOs may attempt to include a restrictive covenant that limits the physician's private practice. Prior to the 1988 amendments to Title XIII, federally qualified HMOs were required by law to maintain a provider panel that was dedicated to delivering services to the health plan's enrollees. Thus, provider contracts were developed with a clause that required the physician to limit fee-for-service patients to no more than 50 percent of his/her practice. With the passage of the 1988 amendments, however, these practice limitations should no longer be necessary.

Similarly, restrictions on competition may be found in provider contracts; a clause that creates an "exclusive" service relationship between the HMO and the physician is sometimes used by the HMO to limit the ability of other health plans to develop an appropriate provider panel and the physician's ability to develop a larger practice by serving more than one HMO.

A third issue is the potential conversion of the physician's current private patients to HMO membership. Conversion clauses may work to the advantage of both parties; the HMO will increase enrollment, and the physician will retain current patients and increase his/her practice. Conversely, these individuals become health plan enrollees. If the HMO and the physician terminate their relationship, the provider usually loses the former patients. Finally, if problems develop between the plan and the physician, a clause that cancels the contract within a stated period, such as 30 days, is helpful; however, a 60- or 90-day equal rights clause that defines and states the rights of each party at the time of separation might be more useful.

Physicians and plans should develop agreements with the objective of a long-standing relationship, but the understanding that contracts can be terminated will put the relationship in better perspective. With this in mind, the health plan should develop sufficient provider agreements to allow for coverage should some of their provider groups decide to cancel their contracts. Similarly, the physicians should not become overly dependent on HMO patients, but, if possible, should continue to build their private practices. As plan providers, the physicians must respect the HMO's procedures, including preauthorizations for hospital admissions or referrals, utilization control and peer review, and so on. To ignore the HMO's rules could mean loss of payment to the physician. And expectations of full fee-for-service equivalent reimbursement from the HMO could lead to provider problems; working with a managed care system ordinarily means discounts from traditional fee schedules because of volume. Finally, a good faith commitment to the contract by both parties is customarily expected. If the providers do not commit to the concept, by verbally abusing the health plan system in the presence of enrollees or by treating plan patients differently than FFS patients, the relationship will rapidly disintegrate.

SUMMARY OF CONTRACT AND RELATED PHYSICIAN CONCERNS

Frequently, physicians will be faced with the proposition of joining more than one MCO and will be approached by representatives from other HMOs or PPOs. In determining which offer of participation is most appropriate or whether to join with any plan, physicians need to evaluate the following issues.

1. The ethical question of being offered a monetary incentive to possibly restrict the use of health care services
2. The level and method of payment for services
3. The likely delays in receiving payments
4. The amount of any withhold and the likelihood of recovering all or part of the withhold from the health plan
5. The conflicting obligations to the health plan, usually a corporation, and the patient
6. The corporation's conflicting obligations to patients, policyholders, and investors
7. The financial soundness of the health plan
8. The up-front costs of joining the health plan
9. The number of enrollees in the plan and an estimate of the number who will use the physician's services
10. The role of the primary physician as gatekeeper, or as the referring physician receiving patients from a participating primary physician acting as gatekeeper
11. The manner in which the physician's compensation differs from the compensation of other physicians participating in the health plan
12. The risk that the health plan may be unable, in future periods, to compensate the physician for service delivery
13. The level and scope of added administrative burdens, that is, utilization reporting, business and medical audits, patient-management activities as a gatekeeper, and so on
14. The past history of the health plan's executive director and medical director as health services administrators
15. The potential for intrusion and interference by the health plan in the physician's standard operating procedures and office practice patterns

THE PHYSICIANS' GROUP AND PRACTICE SHARING

The medical group practice arrangement utilized by group and staff model HMOs began in the 1880s with the formation of the Mayo Clinic in Rochester, Minnesota. With the increasing number of specialty boards in the 1930s

TABLE 6-2 Number of Medical Group Practices and Physicians Practicing in Groups in the United States—1926 to 1988

Year	Number of Medical Groups	Percent Change	Number of Physicians in Groups	Percent Change	Average All Group Sizes	Average Multispecialty
1926	125	–	–	–	–	–
1932	220	76.0	–	–	–	–
1959	1,546	602.7	13,009	–	8.4	–
1965	4,289	177.4	28,381	118.2	6.6	–
1969	6,371	48.5	40,093	41.4	6.3	10.1
1975	8,483	33.2	66,842	66.7	7.9	13.2
1980	10,762	26.9	88,290	32.1	8.2	15.2
1984	15,485	43.9	140,392*	59.0	9.1	26.6
1988	16,579	7.1	155,628	10.8	9.6	24.2

*These figures represent physician positions; physicians may practice in more than one group, which may tend to overstate this figure.

SOURCE: B. E. Balfe and Mary E. MacNamara, *Survey of Medical Groups in the U.S., 1965*, Special Statistical Series, Chicago, Ill., American Medical Association, 1968, p. 2; American Medical Association, *Medical Groups in the U.S., 1984*, Chicago, Ill., AMA, 1985, pp. 4–9; and Penny L. Havlick, *Medical Groups in the U.S.: A Survey of Practice Characteristics*, Chicago, Ill., American Medical Association, 1990, pp. 33–34.

and a concurrent increase in the number of physicians who continued their education to qualify for board certification, physicians sought an environment in which they could practice in their limited specialities and a situation where other disciplines of medicine, as well as specialized equipment and diagnostic facilities, would be readily available in the same location. "Other factors which contributed to the rapid growth of medical groups include the surge of definite surgery, with its concomitant need for technical coworkers and team work; the early popularity of spas and sanatoria, with their need for specialized staff; the development of large individual practices, with the consequent need for professional associates; and the gradual development of group patterns in clinical teaching."[2]

The number of medical groups has increased dramatically since the 1880s, as shown in Table 6-2. In 1926, there were 125 groups; the American Medical Association estimated that there were 15,485 medical groups in 1984 and approximately 20,000 in 1990; this last figure represents an annual growth rate

[2] American Association of Medical Clinics, American Medical Association, and Medical Group Management Association. *Group Practice, Guidelines to Joining or Forming a Medical Group*. Chicago, Ill., American Medical Association, 1970, pp. 1–2.

of more than 20 percent.[3] In 1990, of the approximately 587,700 physicians in the United States, some 165,000 were practicing in groups.[4] Because HMOs utilize multispecialty groups, however, it is useful to understand the growth in the size of these groups. The average size of a multispecialty group in 1969 was 10.1 physicians; by 1988, the size of these groups more than doubled to approximately 24 physicians per group. In 1965, more than 10 percent of the nation's nonfederal physicians were practicing in groups, compared to approximately 17.6 percent in 1969 and 28 percent in 1988. These trends toward more multispecialty groups, larger groups, and more of the total physician work force involved in multispecialty group practice will continue through the 1990s.

PREPAYMENT AND CAPITATION

In 1969, an AMA survey indicated that approximately 6 percent of medical groups, representing 6,540 physicians, were involved with a varying proportion of prepayments and fee-for-service payments. In a Louis Harris and Associates survey, the number of physicians considering affiliation with an HMO increased to 46 percent of the sample in 1984, as compared to 27 percent in their 1981 survey.[5] Some 60 percent of non-HMO-affiliated physicians included in the Harris survey said they believed prepaid plans would affect their practices over the next 10 years, and almost 26 percent expected to be substantially affected. Officials of the Medical Group Management Association suggest that in mid 1991, 30 to 40 percent of its 5,000 member group practices will be involved with managed care.

DEFINITION OF GROUP PRACTICE

The most commonly accepted definition of group practice is that provided by AMA: "Group medical practice is the application of medical services by three or more physicians formally organized to provide medical care, consultation,

---

[3] American Medical Association, Division of Survey and Data Resources, Group Practice Data Base, 1988 Group Practice Census. Personal communication. March 31, 1989.

[4] American Medical Association, personal communication, March 31, 1989; Health Insurance Association of America, *1986–1987 Source Book of Health Insurance Data*, Washington, D.C., HIAA, p. 73; and _____, *HIAA Source Book of Health Insurance Data 1990*, Washington, D.C., HIAA, 1991, pp. 76 and 85.

[5] "HMOs Win Physician Support, but Quality Questions Remain." *Medical Staff News, 14*(8):3, July 1985.

diagnosis, or treatment, through the joint use of equipment and personnel . . . and with methods previously determined by members of the group."[6]

Title XIII of the Public Health Service Act (P.L. 93-222, the HMO Act and its amendments) further describes the requirements for medical groups and individual practice associations that were met by federally qualified HMOs. These requirements are provided in Chapter 5. The definitions of AMA and the federal regulation requirements both emphasize the organization of physicians within a formalized, coordinated setting that has become a legal entity—either a partnership, corporation, association, or some other arrangement. Even the individual practice association, as defined by the HMO law, requires a formalized joint effort by individual participating physicians. There are advantages and disadvantages to group practice, as described in these definitions.

ADVANTAGES AND DISADVANTAGES OF GROUP PRACTICE

Dr. William A. MacColl, for 20 years associated with the Group Health Cooperative of Puget Sound, identifies 12 advantages of group practice to physicians:[7]

1. Sharing of knowledge and responsibility, which allows the physician to concentrate on that part of the practice of medicine for which he/she is best trained.

2. Utilizing the best skills of the specialist as well as those of the general primary care practitioner. The specialist in a group is not required to function as a generalist, and, conversely, the generalist can act in the capacity of "manager" of the patient's care by controlling the overall care of the patient.

3. Keeping up with all the developments in medicine more easily than in solo practice because of the free exchange among the specialists and primary care physicians in the group.

4. High standards resulting from this interchange of ideas. Since no one in a group wishes to be associated with a second-rater, the net standard tends to be the sum of the high standards of the individuals. Each physician's practice is open to other group members through the use of unit medical records— one record for each member, which follows the member throughout his/her enrollment in the HMO.

---

[6] American Association of Medical Clinics et al. *Group Practice*, p. 3.

[7] William A. MacColl. *Group Practice and Prepayment of Medical Care*. Washington, D.C., Public Affairs Press, 1966, pp. 89–91.

5. Money and time for study and training, which are usually considered a part of the group physician's remuneration. In fact, group practice physicians normally spend less of their time seeing patients than do doctors in fee-for-service—five hours a week less. This time becomes available for hospital obligations, study, and continuing education and training.

6. Regular rotation of hours and a sharing of after-clinic emergencies. Thus, most of the staff is relatively free in the evenings, on weekends, and on holidays. Scheduling of vacations with the knowledge that several of one's associates are available to care for patients provides for greater continuity of care.

7. The availability of immediate income to the physician who has just completed the long and costly training period, plus a ready-made practice that can be built upon as the young physician's reputation and skills increase. Starting incomes in group practice are comparable to those in the local community and continue to parallel communitywide incomes as the physician's practice increases.

8. Additional benefits, including malpractice insurance, time-loss and medical coverage, life insurance, occasionally an automobile, social security and retirement programs, and incentive payments.

9. Relief from the business aspects of the practice of medicine, for which most doctors are not trained. The physician does not have to be directly concerned with the billing and collection of fees, the employment of personnel, purchase of supplies and equipment, payment of rent, and so on. He/she usually is not required to make a large capital contribution to join the group and has a reasonable assurance of a stable income.

10. The ability to present his/her views concerning policy and programming within the group within a very short period after joining. Most groups are autonomous and self-governing, and the young physician may be granted voting privileges after a short probationary period, usually one to three years.

11. Availability of ancillary services, personnel, and facilities.

12. Cooperative spirit engendered in the "family of doctors for the family of patients." The group practice physicians share in the professional care of the group as the patients share in the total services the group has to offer. The sense of professionalism is enhanced; group practice is said to offer a check on the possibility of error and a friendly support in adversity.

There are several disadvantages to physician participation in group practice.[8]

---

[8] American Association of Medical Clinics et al., *Group Practice*, p. 11; see also, _____, "Advantages and Disadvantages of Group Practice," *Illinois Medical Journal*, *135*(4):512–513, April 1969.

1. Physicians may experience some loss of freedom to practice as they wish and some loss of individuality. Because group practice requires a coordinated effort, individual physicians must conform to group patterns, guidelines, and behavior. Work schedules, sharing of patient loads, and questioning by one's peers of treatments provided are a part of group practice.

2. Two aspects of physician income may present a problem—level and method of sharing. Most group practice salaries are based on several factors that are not relevant to solo practice. First, the level of compensation usually follows the median income per specialty earned by solo practitioners in the community, with a few group practitioners receiving either lower- or higher-than-average salaries. The opportunity for huge solo practice incomes does not occur in group practice. Second, the group physicians must arrive at a suitable income-sharing arrangement, usually on a yearly basis. Acceptable arrangements, especially when HMO capitation payments are a part of the group's revenue, are sometimes difficult to achieve, with the potential for disputes ever present.

3. Physicians have to conform to established formularies, levels of practice, quality of care, and operating procedures. Physicians not familiar with such organizational constraints may find these limitations unacceptable.

4. Patients are plan patients, not a single physician's patients. As such, the control of the patient's care may reside with several rather than with one practitioner, and patients may not always see the same physician each time they come in for medical care. Some health plans assign a managing physician who is responsible for the total coordination of the enrollee's medical care. Nevertheless, each of the group's physicians shares and suffers to some degree from the errors of his/her associates. Sharing the liability of the group may be unacceptable to some physicians.

5. Finally, because of the division and departmentalization of effort in group practice, an undesirable degree of overspecialization may result.

THE MEDICAL DIRECTOR

Essential to the medical management of managed care models is a physician in the role of medical manager or director. The complicated business aspects of health maintenance organizations and medical group practices have brought many nonphysician administrators into these organizations, but because the primary objective of the HMO remains the delivery of high-quality medical services, there is a particular role and affiliated responsibilities that only a physician manager can fulfill. Thus, the role and position of medical director has been created in both the health plan and in affiliated medical group practices.

Medical directors are physician leaders and managers. They are physicians who have "consciously made a commitment to spend at least part of his or her time as a health care manager. These individuals occupy a variety of positions, both part-time and full-time, in numerous and varied organizations."[9] They hold a variety of titles and carry out administrative responsibilities that relate to the professional actions of physicians and other providers. Generally, these individuals continue to pursue their chosen clinical activities and are recognized for these clinical skills by others in the profession or by members of their medical group practice. Their managerial role requires frequent decisions requiring professional medical expertise and, therefore, is quite distinct from that of the health plan CEO and the group practice administrator.[10] The role of medical director varies, depending on the type, size, and organizational structure of the HMO, but, generally, two distinct functions have surfaced: first, that of medical executive and, second, that of medical group leader.[11]

As the medical executive, the medical director is involved in the administrative medicine aspects associated with the HMO, with responsibilities in the following areas: medical input into HMO planning and operations, utilization review, quality assurance, hospital/medical staff affairs, and enrollee relations. As such, the medical director plays a key role in the design of the benefits package and associated financial planning and budgeting for medical services. This may include the establishment of contract patterns for providing primary and specialty care, selection of clinic sites, and decisions on how to market the medical services of the HMO. Table 6-3 is based on studies completed in 1979 and again in 1985 by Witt Associates, Inc. of Oak Brook, Illinois and Carol Betson for the American Academy of Medical Directors. These data suggest that medical directors are primarily involved with the management of the medical staff—utilization review, quality assurance, physician recruitment, credentialing, disciplinary action, and the development and implementation of policies and procedures related to medical services. To a lesser extent, they are involved with medical manpower planning and the recruitment of other personnel.

A primary responsibility of the medical director is monitoring and controlling the HMO's use of medical and hospital services. Thus, the HMO must have an effective method of monitoring the quality of care; the medical director

---

[9] American Academy of Medical Directors. *The Physician Manager in HMO/Pre-Paid Health Plans.* Tampa, Fla., AAMD, 1984, p. 6.

[10] John M. Harris, Jr. *The Role of the Medical Director in the Fee-for-Service/Prepaid Medical Group.* Denver, Colo., Center for Research in Ambulatory Health Care Administration, 1983, p. 2.

[11] Gordon Mosser, M.D. *The Provider as Medical Manager.* Minneapolis-St. Paul, Minn., Aspen Medical Group, 1986, pp. 1–11.

TABLE 6-3   Functions of Medical Directors: Results of Two Studies

Function	Percent of Sample Involved in Function	
	Witt Study*	Betson Study†
	%	%
Utilization review/data management	93.7	100.0
Quality assurance review	91.6	94.6
Medical staff affairs	80.0	94.4
Physician recruitment	73.7	94.4
Credentialing	64.2	100.0
Disciplinary action	63.2	88.9
Medical manpower planning	52.6	94.4
Recruitment of other personnel	47.4	61.1
Risk management	41.1	33.3
Medical education	38.9	55.6
Salary negotiation	37.9	77.8
Nursing service	27.4	—
Institutional liaison work	27.4	77.8

*Based on a 25.2 percent response (99 HMOs) to a questionnaire sent to the 393 existing HMOs in 1985, excluding those HMOs in operation less than one year.

†Based on a sample of 18 HMOs and enrollment of from 10,000 to 50,000.

SOURCE: D. Garry Belton and Carol Richards Baron, "Profile of the HMO Medical Director," *Medical Group Management, 34*(2):18, March/April 1987; and American Academy of Medical Directors, *The Physician Manager in HMO/Pre-paid Health Plans,* Tampa, Fla., AAMD, 1984, pp. 21–24.

sets the approach to quality control when he/she decides the acceptability of hospitals, physicians, specialists, and others as contractors to the HMO. The medical director establishes medical standards for quality care, designs a method for monitoring compliance, and acts as a liaison between HMO management and the providers—physicians and hospitals. He/she participates in negotiating contracts, in establishing risk arrangements, and in evaluating contract compliance. As final arbiter of member complaints about the medical services that are being provided or are lacking, the medical director interprets the provisions of the benefits package to both physicians and disgruntled members. With these wide-ranging and significant responsibilities, the medical executive/director functions as a member of top management of the health plan. Along with the chief executive officer, the medical director usually reports directly to the board of the health plan.

Medical Directors in Group Practices

The second role of the medical director is that of medical group leader. The terminology for this position may be center medical director in staff model

HMOs, or chairman of the board, managing partner, CEO, or medical director in a medical group serving an HMO. The chairman of a group practice board or managing partner of a smaller medical group carries both the administrative and medical management functions as the CEO of the medical group practice. In this situation, the CEO is both the medical group leader/medical director and the operations manager. The primary responsibilities of the medical director as CEO of the medical group are to lead the medical group in all its activities, many of which are separate from the HMO. In larger groups, these responsibilities may be shared with a business or clinic manager who is hired by the group of physicians to carry out the business functions of the company. Other medical groups separate the business and medical administrative functions, and the medical director has only medical administrative responsibilities. These responsibilities are similar to those described for the medical executive, but at a somewhat different level, and may include medical group planning and operations, medical staff affairs, utilization review and quality assurance, and representation of the group to patients and outside organizations.

Specifically, the medical group leader as medical director undertakes the functions listed in Table 6-3. He or she establishes or rearranges the organizational structure, performs planning activities, arranges both physician and nonphysician staffing, implements compensation systems, and participates in budgeting. In a group with a significant prepaid component, the medical director establishes mechanisms to monitor and control utilization, especially in the areas of ancillary services and hospitalization. He/she may even act as the authorizing agent for such services for colleagues in the medical group and referral specialists outside the group. This responsibility includes establishing an effective management information system or using an MIS provided by the health plan. Data derived from such a system are utilized by the medical director in internal quality assurance and peer review programs.

As the representative of the group to patients and outside provider organizations, the medical director deals with patient complaints and problems that patients and physicians face with the HMO. This task, therefore, includes interacting with the HMO on initial and continuing contracts, on HMO marketing efforts, and with employers who offer the HMO products. Obviously, the medical directors of the physician group and HMO must work closely together, with each representing the primary interests of their own organization.

Medical Director in Staff and IPA Model HMOs

In staff model HMOs, the medical executive, medical director, and group manager are often the same person. The medical staff and the medical director are employees of the HMO, and the goals and operations of the medical group are the same as those of the HMO. The medical director is the line supervisor for medical services delivery, is usually a full-time employee, and is in the difficult and unique position of representing both the needs of the HMO and the medical staff under his/her control.

Medical executives in IPA HMOs interact with the medical group managers of many medical groups and individual physicians under contract with the health plan. In this model, both the HMO and the physicians have greater autonomy and, therefore, less control over the operations of one another. The medical directors of the medical groups and the IPA model HMO are often part-time employees, except in the case of very large HMOs (perhaps over 30,000 enrollees). Their roles and responsibilities are similar to those of medical directors in other model HMOs, but because of the independence of the medical groups, there tends to be a lack of coordination, cooperation, and overall effectiveness in the IPA HMO's operations in comparison with other HMO models.

Medical Director Qualifications

Medical managers in groups must be respected colleagues, possessing leadership abilities and strong reputations as physicians. They must understand what it is to be a clinician and how to deal with a clinician's problems—to have empathy with fellow physicians. They must understand the immediate goals of the physicians for their individual patients and, at the same time, comprehend the broader goals of the group practice and the HMO and how these goals relate to the needs of the community.[12] As good managers, they must have skills in the functions of management—planning, leading, organizing, directing, controlling, decision making, coordinating, communicating, and so on. Since most physicians are not trained in these skills, most medical directors learn on the job and through executive training programs and seminars sponsored by national associations. Recently, graduate schools in management have established programs that are specifically designed for physicians who need to study and develop managerial skills in preparation for medical management positions.

Some important qualifications for medical directors include being personally well organized, productive, able to delegate, and astute at solving problems. Other useful attributes of good managers and leaders are good communication

---

[12] Ernest W. Saward, "The Role of the Medical Director in a Group Practice HMO," In: *Proceedings of the Medical Directors Conference, Los Angeles, Calif., June 19–20, 1977*, Vol. 2, No. 1, Washington, D.C., Group Health Association of America, 1981, p. 248; and J. G. Smillie, "Skills Required for Physician Management," In: *HMO Physician Manager: Managing HMO Physicians, Proceedings of the Medical Directors Conference, Denver, Colo., February 13–14, 1981*, Vol. 5, No. 3, Washington, D.C., Group Health Association of America, 1981, pp. 3–4.

skills, an understanding of group dynamics, and the ability to deal with interpersonal relationships, especially in an organization where consensus within a group of highly trained professionals is always an issue. This is especially important in a practice committed to the principles of income pooling, where income is derived from both fee-for-service and capitation.

It is essential that the medical director and the group's chief corporate officer or managing partner, the clinic manager, and the health plan's executive director and medical director have a relationship of mutual respect and trust. This relationship can only be created if the medical director understands the HMO's business affairs—actuarial, underwriting, and budgeting affairs of the plan; marketing; using demographic, epidemiological, and socioeconomic data to plan and staff effectively; and enrolling and other nonmedical and nontraditional health services delivery functions. To this end, it is expected by experts that in the near future, a management specialty may be created within medicine where physicians will be trained beyond their clinical specialties. Studies would include epidemiology, strategic planning, organizational development, finance, computer science, and marketing, leading to physician certification by the American College of Management in Medicine.[13]

While many of these functions can also describe the role of a medical director in a totally fee-for-service group practice, a prepaid practice requires that the time and talents of the medical director be directed to controlling resources and monitoring quality, activities that are essential to the success of a prepaid group. In many respects, the medical director polices the activities of the group's physicians, based on utilization and quality standards established by the group and HMO. In the long term, the medical director plays a key role in educating the group's physicians on the need to control health services costs and providing them with feedback to assess their practice patterns. This control-with-feedback loop may be a passive system of merely supplying data for use by individual physicians in gauging their activities against preset goals or against other colleagues. It also may be a more active system, with the feedback used for corrections—more evaluation and judgment on behalf of the medical director—or to reinforce appropriate physician behavior through formal recognition, bonuses, praise, and so on. The medical director must lead the group in establishing utilization and quality standards that will ensure high-quality care but will not equate quality with excessive use of physician time or ancillary services.[14]

---

[13] Harris. *The Role of the Medical Director*, p. 6.

[14] Ibid., p. 8.

Physician Personnel Administration and Human Relations

The physician evaluation process begins when a physician is hired by the group or the HMO, or when the HMO contracts with a medical group or with individual physicians. Similar to hospital credentialing processes, the initial evaluation of the physician's qualifications provides a thorough review of his/her character and record of adequate performance. HMOs have often relied on the credentialing process of their affiliated hospitals as a proxy for their own credentialing processes. This has several distinct disadvantages. First, some physicians that the plan may require so as to maintain a smooth, on-going operation may not have admitting privileges and, thus, may not have gone through the hospital's credentialing process; this is especially true for primary care physicians who may limit their services to ambulatory care only and refer their patients to specialists when they need hospitalization. Second, because of the unique nature of the HMO's benefits package and services offered, the hospital's processes may not fully evaluate the physician's qualifications to deliver the benefits offered to members. Third, and most important, the 1986 Health Care Quality Improvement Act (P.L. 99-660) specifically mentions HMOs as organizations in which a formalized due process in the physician sanctioning procedure is appropriate; if the HMO does not follow these procedures in evaluating and taking action against one of its physicians, the HMO loses its legal protection from antitrust action, at least for sanctions involving quality of care.[15] Finally, within the medical group, different physicians may have a variety of clinical and administrative responsibilities, which are the basis of their initial evaluation for the job, and for evaluations of performance over time.

Initial credentialing of physicians entails the collection and analysis of documentation regarding the physician's licensure, education and training, board certification, reference checks (perhaps through the clearinghouse that is mandated by the Health Care Quality Improvement Act), standing in the medical community, staff privileges at hospitals, and the like. The HMO may also require that the physician obtain malpractice insurance and disclose whether there are any previous malpractice claims against the physician, either settled or outstanding. If the health plan and/or medical group provides malpractice insurance for its physicians, it may need to obtain a tail-coverage policy to protect the group from previous suits against the physician that may affect current coverage. Finally, if the physician has not practiced in the area, application for hospital staff privileges and membership in the local medical societies may be requested prior to completing the credentialing process.

---

[15] Peter R. Kongstvedt. *The Managed Health Care Handbook.* Gaithersburg, Md., Aspen Publishers, Inc., 1989, p. 82.

Ongoing Physician Evaluation

To be effective, ongoing physician evaluation by the HMO and/or medical group must:[16]

- Be conducted regularly, usually yearly
- Cover the total sphere of influence of the physician within the group
- Be conducted by a person with knowledge of the physician's performance, often a clinical department chairman
- Be tied to a feedback mechanism, typically an incentive or bonus program

Evaluations should be structured to consider the physician's unique individual clinical and administrative responsibilities. They should be based on written descriptions of his/her role in the organization; in many instances, such a job specification is created during the physician recruitment process and modified as the physician's responsibilities change. Some medical groups may utilize a physician rating process in the income distribution formula that may also be applied to overall physician evaluations. Important areas that may be included in the evaluation are the physician's clinical knowledge and skills, rapport with patients, ability and willingness to work with other staff and on committees, and productivity. A multidimensional evaluation system may consider the physician's ability to control utilization and cost, but only in relation to other attributes that may be equally important to the group. Obviously, this system should be tied to physician income, bonuses, sanctions, advancement within the group, and other actions similar to personnel programs for nonphysician employees. The evaluation process also gives the medical director another tool for educating physicians about the goals of managed care systems. His/her most challenging task may be motivating and managing physicians who are in the business of providing primary health services within a setting that curtails their independence, where the enrollees may be particularly demanding, and where the provider might make less income than in a comparable fee-for-service practice.

PHYSICIAN ATTITUDES CONCERNING GROUP MEDICAL PRACTICE AND HMOs

Ever since the start of the prepaid group practice movement, organized medicine has posed a threat for, and has resisted, the closed-panel concept.

---

[16]Robert Match. "The Keystone of the HMO—Its Medical Director." In: *Proceedings of the Medical Directors Conference, Denver, Colo., April 1973*. Edited by Michael A. Newman, M.D. Washington, D.C., Group Health Association of America, 1973, pp. 17–18.

A closed panel is an arrangement where membership in a physician group is restricted by the present membership to selected individuals. Local medical societies objected to this concept because they felt that prepaid group practice would severely limit the solo practitioner's ability to compete for patients, that prepaid plans and group practice represented a step toward socialized medicine, that there would be corporate control and lay interference in the doctor-patient relationship, and that the use of advertising by the plan and the potential corporate practice of medicine were unethical. Strong resistance from these local medical societies took the form of "professional isolationism," with plan physicians ostracized, denied hospital privileges, and refused membership in the medical society. Recruitment of physicians by health plans became difficult, and final resolution of the early plans' grievances was achieved only after long legal actions in which the prepaid group practice concepts were upheld. The most important case resolving such a situation involved staff physicians at Group Health Association (GHA) in Washington D.C. and the District of Columbia Medical Society. In January 1943, the Supreme Court of the United States held that the American Medical Association and the District of Columbia Medical Society had violated the antitrust laws and the rights of GHA by conspiracy in restraint of trade.

Today, however, most local medical societies do not openly confront existing or newly developing HMOs. There continues to be some resistance, but usually only on the part of a few members; generally, the local medical societies have reluctantly accepted HMOs and other managed care systems as competitors. This reflects an important change in the attitudes of individual physicians toward managed care systems, as mirrored in the results of studies indicating that approximately half of all physicians prefer some type of prepaid capitation practice over fee-for-service practice.

In a 1975 study conducted by David Mechanic,[17] the orientations and attitudes of a group of prepaid physicians were compared to those of a group of nonprepaid physicians. He found that doctors have a concept of how much time they should devote to their practice relative to payment received. Physicians receiving a capitation felt no financial incentive to deal with increased patient demand by increasing their work hours, while nonprepaid physicians were more likely to increase their hours to meet high patient demand. Moreover, the study showed that the fee-for-service doctors spent more time in direct patient activity than prepaid doctors, with "patients seen" as the best indicator of income for fee-for-service physicians. Prepaid doctors were more likely to deal with increased patient demand by delaying patient care, using the queue

---

[17] David Mechanic. "The Organization of Medical Practice and Practice Orientations Among Physicians in Prepaid and Nonprepaid Primary Care Settings." *Medical Care, XIII*(3):189, March 1975.

as a rationing device, or allowing patients to see a specially available, urgent care physician.

This practice could result in an assembly-line practice and consequent consumer dissatisfaction with the patient-physician relationship. Thus, there is the tendency in HMOs to limit not only inpatient hospital care but also the resources available for ambulatory medical care relative to demand. This can be resolved by adding more ambulatory care resources, developing better patterns of manpower utilization, and using physician surrogates and other paraprofessionals—in other words, by becoming more efficient.

In 1984, the results of a nationwide Harris survey of HMO activities found that approximately half of the responding physicians held a very favorable or somewhat favorable attitude toward HMOs, compared to 36 percent in a 1981 Harris survey. Harris found only a small decrease, however, from 71 percent to 64 percent, in the number of physicians who believed that HMOs offer lower quality care than traditional systems. Most responding physicians, 78 percent, felt that HMOs were very or somewhat effective in containing health care costs; however, 65 percent thought that the cost containment incentives of HMOs reduced the quality of services to an unacceptable level. For example, physicians surveyed noted that HMOs perform fewer tests than necessary, employ fewer well-qualified doctors, and do not provide opportunities for the development of adequate physician-patient relationships.[18] Conversely, surveyed physicians in fee-for-service practices and in HMOs showed similar levels of personal satisfaction, with HMO physicians indicating greater satisfaction with peer support, affiliation with a major medical center, and time available to devote to nonprofessional interests.[19] Harris concluded, however, that "there is no evidence in this survey. . .that HMOs employ physicians of lower caliber than the physician community as a whole (as measured by board certification and length of practice). Moreover, HMO members are satisfied with the quality of their doctors."[20]

Plan administrators and medical directors should recognize that physicians are concerned with these issues, address the issues in physician recruitment efforts, and develop methods for ensuring that the problems are adequately solved. Informal progress reports should be included in the executive and medical director's conversations with plan physicians to help pinpoint any issues that have not been resolved or to allay any continuing fear or skepticism on the part of the physicians.

---

[18] Louis Harris and Associates, Inc. *Summary Report, A Report Card on HMOs: 1980–1984.* Menlo Park, Calif., Henry J. Kaiser Family Foundation, 1985, pp. 12–13, 28–29.

[19] Ibid.

[20] Ibid., p. 28.

Another indicator of physician attitudes toward HMOs is turnover rate—the number of physicians who decide to terminate their provider relationship with an HMO within a year. In general, turnover rates for physcans who have been with a plan for more than two or three years appear to be very low—from 2 to 3 percent per year. For the Kaiser Foundation Health Plan, Northern California Region, the rates generally have been close to 6 percent. The reason proffered for the higher than average turnover rate is the lure of higher outside incomes. In three other HMO prototypes, the turnover rate is less than 2 percent— Group Health Cooperative of Puget Sound (Seattle), Group Health Plan of St. Paul, Minnesota, and Health Insurance Plan of Greater New York. Rates are somewhat higher during the two-to three-year physician probationary period most plans maintain.[21] It appears that after the physicians are in the program for more than three years, their feelings toward the HMO become more positive.

Characteristics of HMO Physicians

Several studies, including a 1982 study by Goodman and Wolinsky[22] on physician choice of practice modality, have analyzed the major differences between physicians in solo versus group practice and in traditional fee-for-service versus prepaid medical practice. The findings of this study indicated that the choice of practice modes was more a function of professional autonomy and individual preferences than expected income among the potential alternatives of solo and group practice. Physicians who joined groups tended to be board-certified and younger and practiced in high bed-to-population communities, as compared with those in solo practice. Luft[23] found that physicians in prepaid group practices (PGP) worked relatively shorter work weeks than physicians in traditional settings, and that PGP physicians spent more time in the office and less time in the hospital than their FFS counterparts. Held and Reinhardt,[24] in an analysis of the effect of economic incentives on physician productivity, concluded that physicians in PGPs were generally

---

[21] U.S. Department of Health, Education, and Welfare, Health Maintenance Organization Service, *Questions Physicians Are Asking About HMOs and the Answers,* Rockville, Md., DHEW, 1972, pp. 3–4; and Wallace Cook, "Profile of the Performance of the Permanente Physician," In: *The Kaiser-Permanente Medical Care Program,* Edited by Anne Somers, New York, Commonwealth Fund, 1971, p. 104.

[22] L. J. Goodman and F. D. Wolinsky. "Conditional Logit Analysis of Physicians' Practice Mode Choices." *Inquiry, 19*(3):262–270, Fall 1982.

[23] Harold S. Luft. "Assessing the Evidence on HMO Performance." *Milbank Memorial Fund Quarterly, Health and Society, 58*(4):501–536, 1980.

[24] Phillip J. Held and Uwe E. Reinhardt. "Analysis of Economic Performance in Medical Group Practices." Princeton, N.J., Mathematica Policy Research, July 1979, p. 295. Final Report Under Contract HRA-106-74-0119

younger and more likely to be female, spent an average of 10 to 15 percent less time per year on patient care, and earned approximately $4,000 to $6,000 less per year than physicians in traditional medicine. These findings are supported by the data provided in Table 6-4, which suggest that, on average, HMO physicians practiced approximately one to two hours less per week than fee-for-service physicians and, except for staff model HMOs, HMO physicians provided more office visits per week than their FFS counterparts while providing an average of four hospital visits fewer than FFS physicians (HMO physicians averaged 24.9 hospital visits while FFS physicians averaged 28.9). Held and Reinhardt attributed these findings to differences in style of practice and the allocation of time between the office and hospital. Mechanic[25] assessed the effects of payment scheme and practice mode. He found that, on average, PGP physicians had lower incomes, worked fewer hours, had longer waiting times for appointments, and tended to practice in larger communities located on the West Coast. Conversely, FFS physicians had shorter waits for appointments, worked more hours, earned higher incomes, and tended to optimize the personal aspects of their independent practices.

Goodman and Swartwout[26] evaluated the effects of financial arrangements and the organizational setting on the socioeconomic aspects of four delivery systems, including solo and group practice and independent versus prepaid practice. In their study, Goodman and Swartwout found that solo FFS physicians tended to be older, were nonboard certified, preferred autonomy over earnings, and had more patient visits, longer hours, and shorter waits for appointments. Prepaid group physicians tended to be younger, preferred a specific practice location and predictable schedule, and had lower incomes and expenses, coupled with fewer patient visits, shorter work weeks, and longer patient waiting times. Their studies clearly indicate that income maximization is not one of the major goals of prepaid group physicians, a finding supported by the studies referred to previously. Moreover, Goodman and Swartwout's study, along with that of Luft and the 1984 Harris survey, found that physicians in fee-for-service and prepaid group practice showed comparable levels of personal satisfaction—they were equally satisfied with the internal arrangements of the practice.[27] Given the tendency for physicians to provide services in both the fee-for-service and prepaid modes, these differences may disappear; however, if

---

[25] Mechanic. "The Organization of Medical Practice and Practice Orientations," p. 189.

[26] Louis J. Goodman and James E. Swartwout. "Comparative Aspects of Medical Practice." *Medical Care*, 22(3):255, March 1984.

[27] Louis Harris and Associates, Inc., *Summary Report, A Report Card on HMOs: 1980–1984*, p. 19; Harold S. Luft, *Health Maintenance Organizations: Dimensions of Performance*, New York, John Wiley and Sons, 1981, pp. 52–57; and Goodman and Swartwout, "Comparative Aspects of Medical Practice," p. 261.

TABLE 6-4 Average Weekly Workload and Amount of Time Spent with Patients

Practice Setting	Total Hours Worked	Patient Care Hours	Number of Office Visits	Number of Hospital Visits	Office Visits (minutes)	Hospital Visits (minutes)
Kaiser model HMO	48.7	45.1	120.0	23.6	17.6	26.3
Other group model	48.0	43.3	105.7	18.9	19.3	35.1
Staff model HMO	48.6	43.3	85.2	26.9	21.8	41.5
IPA model HMO	50.2	45.3	100.5	30.3	21.1	30.9
Group fee-for-service	50.5	45.6	97.8	31.4	21.7	30.5
Solo fee-for-service	50.5	45.5	94.8	26.3	22.6	36.8

SOURCE: Robert Carlson. "Study Shows No HMO Stereotypes." *Medical World News*, 27(5):129–130, March 10, 1986.

the number of capitated and managed care systems and medical group practices continue to grow, medical practice in the United States may well take on more of the characteristics of the prepaid group practitioners described in these studies.

WHY PHYSICIANS JOIN STAFF AND GROUP MODEL HMOs

The advantages for physicians joining an HMO have been discussed, but what are the reasons why physicians who are organized like a medical group practice join an HMO? Based on Kaiser-Permanente experience and that of other HMO prototypes, the following list recounts some of the reasons:

1. The growing national reputation for quality prepaid multispecialty HMO practice

2. The presence of personal friends and professional associates who practice in the group

3. The ability to practice medicine without immediate financial consideration

4. Time off, colleague availability for consultation, good coverage for calls, and time for nonprofessional interests

5. Excellent retirement plans and malpractice coverage

6. A preference for capitated rather than fee-for-service practice

7. Security, convenience, and stability of practice within the group, and the affiliation with a major medical center

8. Incomes comparable with those of colleagues in fee-for-service practice

The Structure of Physician Groups and Panels

Like the administrative unit of the health plan, the HMO medical panel must be organized so that medical care can be provided in a coordinated, efficient, and effective manner. The group must maintain an adequate level of professional and paraprofessional staff, as well as adequate facilities for their practices.

STAFFING

Earlier in this chapter, AMA's definition of what constituted a medical group—three or more physicians formally organized—was discussed. From studies by AMA and others, it appears that groups of five or fewer physicians are not as successful as groups of between 5 and 8 physicians, with the average around 20 to 25 physicians. This does not suggest that there is an optimal size for HMO medical groups; it only suggests that most staff and group HMOs must have a small, five-primary-physician group in place before marketing and enrollment can proceed. Second, many mature staff and group HMOs function effectively with panels of 20 to 25 physicians—replicated as often as necessary to accomplish requisite staffing ratios for the HMO's enrollment levels. Staffing levels depend on several factors, paramount of which is number of enrollees; the higher the number of enrollees, the larger the physician panel(s).

Two methods can be used to plan for staff. First, staffing guidelines for the total full-time equivalent (FTE) physicians, including both primary and specialty physicians, may assist in overall yearly planning for medical staff. The second approach is the development of staffing levels for primary service physicians only, since much of the care delivered to HMO members (probably 70 to 80 percent) will be primary in nature.

Using the first method, the staffing of HMOs usually is developed around a staffing ratio of 1 full-time equivalent physician for each 1,000 to 1,100 enrollees (see Table 6-5). This ratio is much lower than the national norm (1:420 in 1989) because of the unified efficiency, competition, and effectiveness of HMO operation. Moreover, the ratio varies with the age of the HMO, the demographic characteristics of the population served, and the expectations of the membership population concerning the availability of medical care. Plans just beginning operations show fairly high ratios of 1 physician per 500 or 600 enrollees because of the normally low number of enrollees at an HMO's onset, while highly competitive, mature IPA plans might show a ratio of 1 physician per 1,200 enrollees or lower.

The second approach is to develop primary physician staffing using the ratio of 1 primary care physician for 1,600 members, but again this ratio may

TABLE 6-5　Staffing Levels in Seven Staff and Group Model HMOs; Members Per Physician

Physician Occupation	*HMO Examples*						
	A	*B*	*C*	*D*	*E*	*F*	*G*
Internal medicine, family practice, general practice. . .	2,400	2,700	2,300	2,700	3,080	2,115	2,700
Pediatrics	6,000	4,500	6,000	5,200	5,710	10,100	4,545
OB/GYN	10,000	9,000	10,000	10,000	11,100	11,760	9,090
Surgery	10,000	17,000	10,000	10,000	11,100	2,050	1,670
Urology	50,000	100,000	50,000	75,000	66,600	47,600	100,000
Orthopedics	35,000	25,000	35,000	35,000	25,000	47,600	25,000
Ophthalmology	50,000	33,000	50,000	37,000	33,000	47,600	–
Otolaryngology	45,000	50,000	45,000	45,000	33,300	71,400	50,000
Dermatology	40,000	–	40,000	29,000	33,300	35,700	100,000
Radiology	35,000	25,000	35,000	38,000	25,000	35,700	25,000
Pathology	80,000	–	–	85,000	66,600	71,400	–
Psychiatry	100,000	–	–	42,000	66,600	35,700	–
Anesthesiology	80,000	–	–	–	40,000	35,700	–
Neurosurgery	150,000	–	150,000	–	100,000	71,400	–
Allergies	100,000	50,000	–	52,000	66,600	–	50,000
Neuropsychiatry	–	50,000	–	–	–	–	–
Neurology	60,000	–	–	91,000	200,000	142,800	–
Overall ratio of members to physicians:	1,015	1,053	1,044	1,000	1,053	1,075	1,100

SOURCE: U.S. Department of Health and Human Services, Office of Health Maintenance Organizations, "Medical Care Data from HMOs," *National Trend Data Issuance No. 2, May 13, 1980*, Rockville, Md., DHHS, 1980; and *Proceedings of the Medical Directors Educational Conference, New Orleans, Louisiana, February 4–5, 1977*, Washington, D.C., Group Health Foundation, 1977, pp. 1 and 3.

vary, based on the characteristics of the health plan and its membership.[28] In this situation, primary care providers cover internal medicine, family practice, general practice, pediatrics, OB/GYN, and general surgery; it should also be understood that approximately 60 percent of the care provided by OB/GYN physicians and general surgeons is primary in nature, with the remainder described as specialty services. Obviously, if OB/GYN physicians and surgeons practice as specialists only, the primary care physician ratio will need to be adjusted accordingly—that is, fewer members per physician. Leaner ratios suggest that the primary physician who carries most of the service delivery load will be working at close to full capacity over extended periods of time. Under these stressful conditions, there will be higher physician turnover, resistance to accepting committee assignments and other nonpatient duties, loss of morale, decline in the quality of services, and so on. The impact on members may

---

[28] Kongstvedt. *The Managed Health Care Handbook*, p. 27.

be even greater than on staff, with extensive waits to obtain appointments, high consumer dissatisfaction with the plan, and increased disenrollment during open season. Ratios lower than 1:1,600 may mean that the plan cannot effectively compete in the open market with leaner health plans. To assist in setting staffing ratios, Table 6-5 provides some ranges of selected physician specialists; these data are provided only as examples, and staffing should be based on the actual needs of the HMO's population.

In staff and group model HMOs, physicians are added to the staff on a full-time basis when it has been determined that it is costing the plan or group practice more for fees, retainers, or part-time salaries than it would for an equivalent full-time physician. Figure 6-1 provides a guide for determining at what enrollment level full-time physicians should be added to the staff. This guide is based on the premise that staff is added on a full-time, incremental, and straight-time basis.

The computation of required full-time equivalent physician (FTEP) complements shown in Figure 6-1 can be performed as follows: assuming the initial enrollment will range between N_{min} and N_{max} and the range of full-time equivalent physicians needed is between 1:600 FTEP/enrollees and 1:1,200 FTEP/enrollees, then the maximum physician complement ($FTEP_{max}$) is

$$FTEP_{max} = N_{min} \frac{(1)}{600}$$

Example: For a minimum initial enrollment of 10,000,

$$FTEP_{max} = 10,000 \frac{(1)}{600} = 17.0 \text{ full-time equivalent physicians}$$

The minimum physician equivalent requirement ($FTEP_{min}$) is

$$FTEP_{min} = N_{max} \frac{(1)}{1,200}$$

Example: For a maximum initial enrollment of 20,000 enrollees

$$FTEP_{min} = N_{max} \frac{(1)}{1,200} = 20,000 \frac{(1)}{1,200} = 16.7 \text{ full-time equivalent physicians}$$

The plan needs 16.7 to 17.0 full-time equivalent physicians of all varieties to provide adequate health services to its enrollment of 20,000 members. During the feasibility, planning, and developmental stages, the physician complement should be based on revised enrollment expectations using the

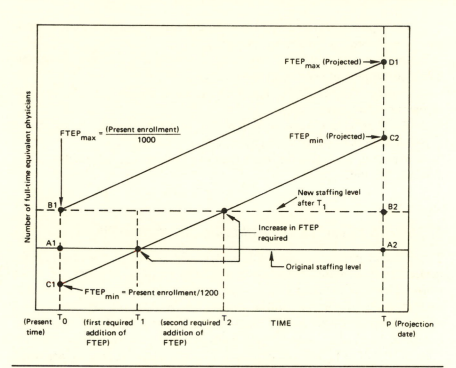

FIGURE 6-1 Full-time equivalent physicians over time.

above method. During plan operation, when enrollment growth stabilizes, physician complements can be more easily assesed. The ratio of all FTE physicians to enrollees will range between 1:1,000 and 1:1,200 and should be based on close monitoring of utilization, cost, and need. Enrollment growth, then, will be a major input. Analysis during the operational stages can be done by substituting the values of 1:1,100, for example, for 1:600 and using present enrollment for N_{min} and projected enrollment for N_{max}, and primary care physician needs can be obtained by using the ratio of 1:1,600. Note that these ratios for all physicians and primary physicians are planning assumptions agreed to by the health plan's board, management, and physicians as appropriate levels of physician service delivery. Extrapolating the data over time provides the timing for adding physicians to the staff.

The following steps can be used to project the FTEP needs using Figure 6-1:

1. Draw the present FTEP line A_1A_2 for the present number of full-time equivalent physicians.

2. Draw points B_1 and C_1, representing the maximum and minimum FTEP, based on the present enrollment level at T_0.

3. Draw points D_1 and C_2, indicating the maximum and minimum FTEP, based on the present enrollment level at T_0.

4. Connect C_1C_2 and B_1D_1, based on expected growth (i.e., the example assumes a linear growth rate).

5. The time T_1 at the intersection of A_1A_2 and B_1B_2 indicates the time (T_2) at which additional physicians must be added to the HMO.

6. Line C_1C_2 represents the upper limit of physician equivalents that can be added to the staff.

FULL-TIME EQUIVALENT PHYSICIANS BY SPECIALTY

Three further points are important. First, as the size of the membership and medical staff increases, the need for specialist services increases. Table 6-6 provides some guidelines for appropriate staffing levels of medical specialists. Second, specialty coverage will be needed by the HMO on a full-time basis at the 20,000 to 30,000 enrollment level—the level that is widely accepted as the breakeven point for an HMO.[29] Third, plans that anticipate an initial enrollment level of 10,000 to 15,000 should include full-time equivalent physicians in the following specialties: gynecology, pediatrics, and surgery. These generalists and specialists should provide 70 to 80 percent of all health services needed by enrollees.

Another method for assessing the number of physicians by specialty can be accomplished by using the maximum and minimum full-time equivalent physicians formula developed in Figure 6-1. Three steps should be followed.

1. Compute the expected maximum and minimum full-time equivalent physician complement expected for the projected enrollment level.

2. Compute the maximum and minimum full-time equivalent physicians for each specialty, using the percentage distribution of physicians by specialty (the specialty distribution value provided in Table 6-6).

3. Adjust the value for variations in plan benefits, operating policy, specific needs, and so on.

---

[29] Dustin L. Mackie and Douglas K. Decker, *Group and IPA HMOs,* Gaithersburg, Md., Aspen Publishers, Inc., 1981, p. 139; U.S. Department of Health, Education, and Welfare, *Questions Physicians Are Asking About HMOs,* p. 1; and Norbert Goldfield and Seth B. Goldsmith, *Alternative Delivery Systems,* Gaithersburg, Md., Aspen Publishers, Inc., 1987, p. 136.

TABLE 6-6 Specialty Distribution × Full-time Equivalent Physician Needs

a.	General Practitioners and Internal Medicine	= 0.500 ×	FTEP
b.	Dermatology	= 0.036 ×	FTEP
c.	Urology	= 0.016 ×	FTEP
d.	Obstetrics and Gynecology	= 0.093 ×	FTEP
e.	Allergy	= 0.007 ×	FTEP
f.	Pediatrics	= 0.160 ×	FTEP
g.	Orthopedist	= 0.028 ×	FTEP
h.	General Surgery	= 0.056 ×	FTEP
i.	Otolaryngology	= 0.028 ×	FTEP
j.	Ophthalmology	= 0.027 ×	FTEP
k.	Psychiatry	= 0.009 ×	FTEP
l.	Radiology	= 0.015 ×	FTEP
m.	Other	= 0.025 ×	FTEP

SOURCE: Texas Instruments, Inc. *Development of an Implementation Plan for the Establishment of a Health Maintenance Organization.* Rockville, Md., Health Maintenance Organization Service, U.S. Department of Health, Education, and Welfare, 1971, p. 118.

Example: Where $\text{FTEP}_{max} = 17.0$ and $\text{FTEP}_{min} = 15.4$

    a. General Practitioners and Internal Medicine = 0.5 × FTEP, maximum = 8.5; minimum = 7.7

    b. Dermatology = 0.036 × FTEP, maximum = 0.612; minimum = 0.554

NONPHYSICIAN STAFFING

Nonphysician staffing includes personnel involved in both the delivery of services and the operation of the health plan. For staff model HMOs, both categories of personnel are recruited and hired by, and work directly for, the health plan, while in all other HMO models, health services delivery personnel work either for a group practice or directly with individual physicians; only nondelivery personnel, for example, marketing, finance, claims processing, and the like are employed by the health plan. The staffing levels of a group practice with nonphysician personnel depend on several factors, the most important of which are the physicians' practice patterns. It has been found that the ratio of prepaid group practice staff to physicians is from four to five direct paramedical personnel per physician, with the average usually on the lower side.[30] Table 6-7 provides the results of the 1989 Medical Group Management

---

[30] Medical Group Management Association. *The 1989 Cost and Production Survey Report.* Denver, Colo., MGMA, 1989, p. 24.

TABLE 6-7   Nonphysician Staffing: Mean Number of FTE Employees per FTE Physician by Percent Prepaid Income for Multispecialty Groups, 1988 Data

Employee Category	Percent Prepaid Income				
	No. Prepaid	1% to 10%	11% to 20%	21% to 50%	over 50%
Total group employees per FTE physician	4.22	4.00	4.19	5.03	5.31
Executive staff	.19	.14	.16	.12	.17
Business office	.70	.59	.62	.72	.63
Data processing	.21	.16	.17	.18	.18
Other administrative	.20	.15	.15	.26	.29
Registered nurses	.54	.46	.55	.60	.50
Licensed practical nurses, aides	.78	.70	.79	.82	.98
Medical receptionists	.58	.55	.56	.64	.91
Medical secretaries/transcribers	.29	.32	.28	.29	.20
Medical records	.32	.30	.30	.41	.50
Nonphysician providers	.18	.12	.14	.21	.24
Laboratory	.37	.38	.32	.37	.38
Radiology	.24	.22	.21	.23	.26
Physical therapy	.27	.10	.10	.11	.11
Optical	.10	.07	.04	.06	.11
Housekeeping/maintenance/security	.19	.14	.19	.18	.17
Certified registered anesthetists	.16	.12	*	*	*
Other support	.34	.31	.30	.52	.53

NOTES: An asterisk indicates that data are suppressed when the number of responding groups is less than 6. Data for university and government-affiliated medical groups are excluded from this table.

SOURCE: Medical Group Management Association. *The 1989 Cost and Production Survey Report.* Denver, Colo., MGMA, 1989, p. 24. Reprinted with permission of the Medical Group Management Association. See also John R. Colman and Frank C. Kaminsky, *Ambulatory Care Systems, Volume IV: Designing Medical Services for Health Maintenance Organizations.* Lexington, Mass., Lexington Books, 1977, pp. 101–111.

Association's *Cost and Production Survey Report* regarding 1988 medical group staffing levels in both prepaid and nonprepaid groups. Interestingly, the groups with limited prepayment (1 percent to 10 percent) had the lowest nonphysician staffing levels at 4.00 FTE employees per physician, while those groups with more than 50 percent of their business with HMO patients reported the highest staffing levels at 5.31 FTE employees per physician. It is evident that as medical groups serve more HMO patients as a percent of their total clientele, they increase their staff in two major areas. First, administrative and other support employees increase from approximately 0.50 FTE per physician in nonprepaid groups to 0.83 FTE in groups of 50 percent or more prepaid. Second, paramedical personnel, excluding radiology and laboratory, increase from 1.86 to 2.63 FTE in the same group categories; however, the use of medical receptionists and physical therapists decreased in these same categories.

TABLE 6-8 An Example of Nonphysician, Nonhealth Services Delivery Health Plan Personnel Staffing at Two Enrollment Levels

Category	Staffing by Level of Health Plan Enrollment	
	< 25,000	> 25,000
Executive Offices:		
Executive Director	1	1
Assistant Executive Director	1	1
Staff Associate	1	2
Secretaries/Receptionists	2	2
Finance:		
Finance Director	1	1
Assistant Finance Director	0	1
Accountant	1	1
Claims Administrator	1	1
Accounts Payable/Claims Processing	1	2
Accounts Receivable/COB	1	2
Actuary	0	1
Other Financial Functions	1	1
Marketing:		
Marketing Director	1	1
Plan Representatives	4	4
Marketing Secretary/Receptionist	1	1
Enrollment Clerk	1	1
HMO Medical Director's Activities:		
Patient Ombudsman	1	1
Utilization Coordinator	1	1
Secretary/Receptionist	1	1
Health Educator	0	1
Data Processing:		
Director of Management Information Systems	1	1
Processors	1	2
Other Personnel:		
Personnel Director	0	1
Research	0	1
Housekeeping and Maintenance	1	1
Total Health Plan Personnel	24	33

Nonphysician, nonhealth services delivery personnel employed by the health plan may include the categories of nonphysician personnel listed in Table 6-8. Note that staffing of the administrative unit is provided for two levels of enrollment—fewer than 25,000 and more than 25,000 members. Table 6-8 is only an example of HMO staffing; actual health plan employee arrangements are based on the individual characteristics of the HMO's operation. Generally, most of these personnel categories remain relatively constant, regardless of enrollment level. The exceptions are in the finance department and data processing; as enrollment increases so does the level of staffing in these areas.

For example, Colman and Kaminsky[31] found that "on average the finance and business department (of 20 HMOs) employed 4.79 full-time equivalent employees per ten thousand members. This staffing pattern represents one full-time employee per 2,097 members." They go on to point out that as enrollees increase, the business staff increases proportionately. "When the HMO begins operation it will need to have 2.75 full-time employees working in the finance and business department. When plan size approaches twenty thousand enrollees this staff should consist of 9.16 full-time equivalents. This increased size in staffing is obtained by adding one staff member to the department for every 3,125 new members enrolled in the plan."[32]

The size of the data processing staff depends on several factors, especially the level of enrollment; the type of management information system being used, including the variety of data collected, organized, and reported; and the level of computerization of the data system. In some plans, data processing is provided under contract with an external data processing company, although most health plans now have developed significant internal data handling capabilities. Based on Colman and Kaminsky's studies,[33] the data processing function will initially require 2 persons and then will increase at the rate of 1 staff person for every 10,000 enrollees until HMO membership reaches 50,000 members.

Group Practice Organization and Physician Payment

What is the organizational relationship of a group practice to the HMO? Again, the answer differs with each HMO model, because physician groups organize themselves most frequently as profit-making enterprises and many health plans are not-for-profit. Moreover, to avoid possible antitrust actions, the group practice must be "at arm's length" from the health plan in matters concerning control of the HMO's operation and physician compensation. In all HMOs—both not-for-profit and investor-owned—it is advisable that the medical group be autonomous and free to make decisions concerning medical matters and compensation for physicians. The medical groups should be self-governing, although they may rely on the health plan's executive or medical director for counsel and advice or even for administration of the group.

---

[31] John R. Colman and Frank C. Kaminsky. *Ambulatory Care Systems, Volume V, Financial Design and Administration of Health Maintenance Organizations.* Lexington, Mass., Lexington Books, 1977, p. 38.

[32] Ibid., p. 39.

[33] Ibid., p. 43.

FORMS OF ORGANIZATION

Group practices have four general forms of organization available to them—solo proprietorship, partnership, unincorporated association, or corporation. In the last case, several options are available: regular corporations with stockholders, Subchapter S corporations, foundations, and professional corporations or professional associations. Obviously, the form chosen depends on many factors, although, based on a 1969 AMA survey, the partnership form was chosen by almost 70 percent of the groups. By 1984, however, the majority of medical groups had gone through reorganization, with more than 70 percent choosing the professional corporation legal form of organization.

Generally, one method is chosen over others because of tax advantages, personal liability of the group members, size of the group, control of operations, capital acquisition, and programs for retirement funds.[34] Health plan/medical staff organizational relationships can be categorized according to the method of physician compensation. Three methods are prevalent—physician ownership of the HMO, contract, and salary.

For-profit HMOs developed, owned, and operated by the medical group, described in Chapter 4 as the integrated group model HMO, control all aspects of the health plan, including the method of physician compensation, usually based on salary and bonus. More frequently, medical groups may be under contract with the HMO, as described earlier in this chapter. The proprietary medical group may take any of the aforementioned forms but must follow the arm's length rule with the health plan. The medical group negotiates with the HMO concerning capitation rates, number of enrollees to be served, and acceptable utilization ranges. It controls physician membership selection, vacation scheduling, night coverage, and professional standards and establishes its own internal payment formula and bonus program. Problem areas that the health plan may encounter in its relationships with contract medical groups may be standards of quality; utilization levels; use of the health plan's facilities, equipment, and personnel; mix of fee-for-service and health plan patients served; and financial remuneration for enrollees served.

In staff model HMOs employing a salaried medical staff, a separate contract is prepared for each physician by the health plan. Payment to physicians can be based on a per capita arrangement, hourly pay or salary, straight retainer, or fee-for-service, although the last method is rare. In some instances, the issue of corporate practice of medicine has been raised with regard to the salaried method of physician payment. Even though a direct individual payment is made

---

[34] For a discussion of these organizational forms and issues, see American Association of Medical Clinics et al., *Group Practice*, pp. 23–28.

to each physician, the medical staff is still organized as a group practice; it is autonomous concerning medical matters and is self-governing.

PHYSICIAN COMPENSATION AND PAYMENT FORMULAS[35]

Most group practices associated with HMOs pool their income. Compensation plans developed by the medical group are used to reward individual physicians for their level of training and productivity while simultaneously encouraging appropriate use of medical services. There is no ideal compensation formula. In essence, the efficacy of a specific formula depends on such variables as group size, geographic location, physician goals, and, among other factors, specialty representation. A compensation formula deemed good today may not promote group interests tomorrow.

In the following discussion of compensation formulas used by group practices, various methods of physician compensation developed by capitated groups are reviewed, and the factors that should be considered in the development of any compensation plan are described.

Traditional Fee-for-Service Formula

Some groups choose not to change their existing compensation formula and continue rewarding physicians strictly on the basis of productivity. These groups do not separate fee-for-service from prepay revenue, but treat all dollars as if they were derived from fee-for-service. Physicians, in turn, are compensated according to a formula that is based on billed charges and their collection ratio. Because this formula is predicated on the economics of the fee-for-service system, more volume (more physician charges) ostensibly yields more profit. This theory does not apply in a capitation arrangement, where a group's revenue does not rise in direct proportion with the volume of services rendered. Instead, profit is realized prior to the delivery of services, therefore, essentially less volume yields more profit. But, even with this major flaw, studies of medical groups suggest that compensation plans based on productivity are most prevalent in groups receiving less than 40 percent prepay revenue.

In this system, after expenses are drawn, the net income is distributed on a yearly basis in accordance with a prearranged schedule developed by the

---

[35] This discussion is adapted from Robert G. Shouldice and Lana Bornstein. "How Capitation Payments Are Included in Your Income Sharing Formula." *Medical Group Management Journal,* *34*(6):11–13, November/December 1987.

physicians themselves. One method of dividing income is for each partner to share equally in the net income, based on the principle that as a member of the medical team, each is considered to be of equal value to the group. More frequently, the schedule is not an even distribution but is based on a point-rating formula that considers a physician's total bookings (i.e., the total number of patients served), total collections, length of service, formal training, research efforts, experience, board specialty, standing in the medical community, and other subjective factors.

Modified Fee-for-Service Formula

A modified fee-for-service formula involves separating fee-for-service from prepay revenue and compensating physicians using a formula with two components: (1) billed fee-for-service charges, and (2) a percentage of the capitated physician fund. Billed charges are handled by following the group's traditional fee-for-service income-sharing formula. Capitated funds received by the medical group are placed in the physician fund—the monetary pool established by the capitation payment to the group practice and maintained for all of the group's physicians.

The pool may be divided into primary and specialty care pools. Based on the experience of the group or other providers, a percentage of the total fund would be allocated for primary care (e.g., 80 percent) or specialty care (e.g., 20 percent). Payments to the group's physicians, as well as to outside referral physicians, would then be drawn from the appropriate pool, with the understanding that limits on physician incomes are established by the limits of funds available in each pool.

A portion of the physicians' fund may also be restricted for the payment of the group's operating expenses. For example, 70 percent of the fund (or 70 percent of the physician's fee) would be distributed to the physicians based on the group's current fee schedule. The remaining 30 percent of the service fee would be held in the pool until the end of the year or other accounting period. In the event that general service use and referrals outside the group are within the capitated target for the year as established jointly by the HMO and the group's physicians, the excess would be distributed either equally, according to specialty, or based on productivity. In this way physicians are guaranteed a minimum percentage of their service fee (in this example, 70 percent), even if referrals or other service utilization exceed the target. Additionally, many groups choose to award primary care physicians a greater percentage of the excess pool than specialty physicians in an attempt to adequately compensate the primary care physicians for managing patients and other administrative work involved with their HMO patient practice.

Fixed Compensation Plans

Fixed compensation plans reward physicians through either a negotiated salary or equal distribution. Basically, a negotiated salary entails compensating a physician as an employee with a yearly salary from the physician fund. (Negotiated salaries may be used even though the owner-physician is not an employee of the group.) Under this system, physicians usually elect a board for performance review so as to regulate and develop the physician's salary/income. This form of compensation is most prevalent in large group practices, many of which are nonprofit. Conversely, compensation through equal distribution is most prevalent in small, less-diverse groups.

Cost Accounting Plans

Another alternative is to account for the individual physician's cost of operation, which may be applied on a physician-by-physician basis, whereby the physician's gross income is reduced by the cost of personnel, space, equipment, malpractice insurance, and other costs directly attributed to the physician. In effect, the direct cost of nursing personnel, receptionists, examination rooms, office space, special-purpose equipment, and other items that vary significantly from physician to physician are deducted from the physician's income. These direct costs may be charged in full or on a percentage basis (e.g., 50 percent) to the responsible physician.

Relative Value Approach

A fifth type of compensation plan is based on the relative value of the services provided by the physician. This method attempts to address the level of complexity and activity in the individual physician's practice. Under this system, the medical group develops relative values for all physician services.[36] Using a management information system that identifies services provided to the group's patients (those served on either a capitation or noncapitation arrangement) the physician's gross income is created by the application of the relative values of the services provided minus the costs associated with the delivery of service.

---

[36] A source of these values might be Christopher J. Woodthorpe, ed., *Relative Values for Physicians,* 2nd Edition, Princeton, N.J., McGraw Hill, 1984.

The Hospital Pool

As part of their capitation agreement with an HMO, many physicians have agreed to share risks for overutilization of hospital care, but have also agreed to share in the savings from their control of hospital admissions. In this relationship, the health plan establishes a hospital fund for hospitalization expenses. Savings from this pool, for example, may be shared 50/50 by the physicians and the HMO. Losses would likewise be shared with the physicians— the physicians' share is limited to available funds in the pool (and a possible assessment against their share of future hospital-pool savings). Assuming that there are savings, the physicians may distribute this income according to one of the previously described methods or may create a separate distribution system, such as one based on documented days saved by individual physicians, the level of the individual physician's hospital activity—expressed in days—as a percentage of all hospital days generated by group physicians, and so on.

COMPENSATION/CAPITATION RELATED ISSUES

Because of the distinct nature of the capitation arrangement, many issues have surfaced concerning the efficacy of a compensation formula that is developed by a group accepting HMO payments. The physicians' goals may become unattainable owing to some internal incentives inherent in a particular compensation plan. Topical issues that are related to groups accepting prepaid patients include group solvency, excess service use, productivity slowdown, group harmony, quality of care, and patient satisfaction.

The issue of group solvency is associated with excess service use and rewarding physicians strictly on the basis of productivity. Groups receiving more than 40 percent prepay revenue and using the traditional fee-for-service compensation formula may, in fact, jeopardize the group's solvency. As mentioned earlier, under a capitated arrangement, a group's revenue does not rise directly with the volume of services provided, rather, profit is realized prior to the distribution of services. Under a capitated system, a group's income rises as

- The number of HMO patients choosing the group as their provider increases
- The HMO premium and the group's capitation increases
- The efficiency of the physicians increases
- The day-to-day management of patient care improves

Capitation arrangements conflict with the inherent incentive characteristic of the traditional fee-for-service compensation formula—more volume yields more profit. In the event that service distribution exceeds the capitation target for the year, the group will experience a financial loss. Some groups have managed this issue by providing risk-sharing arrangements, stop-loss insurance, and the use of a gatekeeper to prevent excess service use.

Groups using fixed compensation plans, such as equal distribution or straight salary, may experience a problem in group harmony and physician productivity. A group that compensates physicians on the basis of equal distribution does so on the premise that all physicians and their services to the group are of equal value. With the additional administrative responsibilities imposed on the primary care physician to regulate service use, the issue of fairness may disrupt the internal esprit de corps of a group. In effect, primary care physicians may resent the specialist who is not burdened with extensive administrative duties, yet receives the same percentage of the group's profit. Further, in a multispecialty group, due to the differences in professional training and risk associated with given procedures, some physicians may become resentful of those who deliver less-complicated services but receive the same percentage of the group's profit. Similarly, resentment may build because some group physicians refer capitation patients to outside-the-group specialists more frequently than others, thus significantly depleting the capitation by fee-for-service payments to outside providers. Another problem associated with equal distribution and straight salary compensation plans may be productivity slowdown. In essence, equal distribution and salary plans afford no extra incentives for greater effort to promote patient satisfaction, and a reduction in service distribution may result in a lower quality of care. Bonuses or mechanisms by which salaries are revised tend to alter this trend and promote greater productivity and efficiency.

Quality of care is an issue of major concern in capitation arrangements. As previously mentioned, under a system where "less is more," there is an inherent incentive for physicians to reduce the amount of services provided. In effect, this reduction in service delivery may take the form of fewer follow-up visits, procedures, and inoculations, which, in turn, may negatively affect the quality of medicine. Further, groups accepting both fee-for-service and prepay patients may be inclined to treat prepay patients as second-class citizens in a two-tier system, whereby the number and type of services distributed to the prepay patient differ from those distributed to the fee-for-service patient. This quality of care problem may be resolved by rewarding physicians according to a fee-for-service/prepay productivity ratio or by instituting strict measures of utilization/quality control.

Agreeing on an acceptable payment formula may be the most troublesome area for group members. Recognizing this fact, the group practice administrator should build a strategy for the group around the following set of principles:[37]

1. Each member of the medical group is considered equal.

2. Incomes must be competitive with private practice and high enough to attract and hold well-trained and competent doctors.

3. Length of training should be recognized only when it increases competency.

4. Although special competencies should be considered, length of service with the group should be a major factor for increasing income.

5. Admission to the partnership, where applicable, should bring increased income.

6. Because the physician is concerned with keeping the enrollee well and increasing his/her productive years, rather than with sporadic episodes of illness, the physician receives compensation regardless of fluctuations in load (just as the patient pays a monthly premium whether ill or well).

7. Because of the limited supply of certain specialists, somewhat higher income may be necessary for these physicians.

8. Physicians considered for partnership or for purchasing a share of the business, where applicable, should serve a probationary period of from two to three years.

Most HMO and CMP models share the risk of overuse of services by members during a specific period with the providers of care. *Risk sharing, at risk,* and *risk assumption* are terms that refer to the financial risk of ensuring and providing health services by the plan. *Risk* in this sense is defined as the possibility that revenues will not be sufficient to cover expenditures incurred in the delivery of contracted-for services. *Risk sharing* means that physicians and hospitals have agreed to a financial stake in the health plan's operation; their compensation is based, to some degree, on their ability to hold the use of services at an appropriate level and to decrease the use of the more expensive sources of care. One of the key philosophical issues concerning HMOs is that of risk sharing through provider incentives. The fee-for-service system can be said to encourage inefficient use of medical resources because of the financial incentives for overutilization of the most expensive health services. In the HMO, physicians may increase their compensation if they can control utilization at appropriate levels, with the outcome that risk sharing encourages efficient use

---

[37] MacColl. *Group Practice and Prepayment of Medical Care*, p. 109.

of facilities and resources. Since hospitalization is the most expensive part of medical service delivery and in many instances the most abused service, HMOs and CMPs emphasize methods to control unnecessary hospital use through incentive arrangements. Operationally, risks that do not affect incentives in the system but are truly unforeseen hazards that cannot be controlled by prudent patient or administrative management should be covered by insurance. Inappropriate hospital use can be controlled by physicians; therefore, they should be given financial and other incentives to control it.

In group model HMOs, physicians are placed *at risk* when the agreement with the health plan provides for a compensation process that distributes to the physicians as a group the surplus (savings) or loss from the group's operation over a specified period of time. Several risk-sharing models are currently being used; some are described in the discussions that follow. For the group practice manager, it is important to realize that physician risk-sharing models are a desirable means by which to influence the management of medical care resources: they must be compatible with the various elements of the group's operation, they are seldom permanent, and the more risk that is reinsured by a private carrier, the lower the capitation to the group.

Before discussing the various methods by which prepaid plans share risks with providers, it will be useful, for comparison purposes, to review the incentives and levels of risk taking by providers in traditional fee-for-service practice. Providers in nonprepaid systems do take risks—the outcome of doing business, such as bad debts and uncollectables, uninsured losses, bad business decisions, and questioned clinical practice, usually called malpractice. *Risk assumption*, that is, insurance risks accepted by HMOs and capitated providers, where premiums and capitation rates might not cover medical care expenses, are clearly not a part of the traditional fee-for-service environment. With regard to incentives, the traditional fee-for-service system creates financial incentives to provide more rather than less—through the fee-for-service payment mechanism, the design of benefits packages that emphasize the use of expensive hospital care, and the practice of protective medicine so as to avoid malpractice suits. Obviously, the need to attract and maintain patients and the physician's professional ethics and moral obligation to society help govern his/her practice patterns as much as the financial incentives. But, since these nonfinancial issues are a part of all provider practices, it must be the opportunity for financial gain that motivates the traditional fee-for-service providers to give more than appropriate levels of medical services.

PHYSICIAN AND HOSPITAL RISK-SHARING MODELS

Like the fee-for-service providers, prepaid providers are also motivated by the need to avoid malpractice situations, by their professional ethics and moral

TABLE 6-9 Methods of Compensating Primary and Specialty Care Physicians by Model Type in 173 HMOs

| | Model | | | | |
| | (Percent of total using method) | | | | |
Method of Compensation	Staff N=22	Group N=29	IPA N=59	Network N=19	Mixed Models N=44
Primary Care Physicians:					
Any use of salary	100.0	13.7	0.0	5.3	34.2
Any use of capitation	18.2	88.8	78.0	100.0	81.8
Primary Care Physicians:					
Salary exclusively	72.7	17.2	0.0	0.0	6.8
Capitation exclusively	0.0	62.1	50.8	73.7	50.0
Salary and capitation	18.2	10.3	—	5.3	18.2
Salary and other methods	9.1	—	—	—	2.3
Capitation, salary, and FFS	—	3.4	—	—	2.3
Capitation and FFS	—	—	18.6	5.3	—
Capitation and discounted FFS	—	3.4	3.4	15.8	4.5
Capitation, discounted FFS, and other methods	—	3.4	5.1	—	6.9
Discounted FFS	—	—	10.2	—	4.5
FFS exclusively	—	—	8.5	—	—
Other	—	—	3.4	—	4.6
Total	100.0	99.8	100.0	100.1	100.1
Specialty Care Physicians:		*Number of Plans**			
Salary	13	0	0	0	0
Capitation	13	26	7	4	20
Charges	0	0	14	—	15
Discounted charges	15	19	18	11	30
Other	—	—	8	—	—

*HMOs may report using more than one method.

NOTE: Dashes represent items that were not reported in the study for the particular HMO model.

SOURCE: Adapted from Marsha Gold and Ingrid Reeves. "Preliminary Results of the GHAA-BC/BS Survey of Physician Incentives in Health Maintenance Organizations." In: *Research Briefs.* Monograph of the Group Health Association of America. Washington, D.C., GHAA, November 1987, pp. 7–10.

obligations to patients and society and even by their desire to maintain a stable practice and retain satisfied patients. In addition to these incentives, prepaid providers are usually placed at risk and agree to financial incentive arrangements that usually involve a capitation arrangement, in all but a staff model HMO. For example, recent data regarding compensation methods for primary care physicians in 173 HMOs, representing approximately half of the enrollment in HMOs in early 1987, are presented in Table 6-9; all HMO models used capitation as the dominant method of physician compensation, with the exception of staff models, which used this payment mechanism the least (only 18.2 percent reported any use of capitation).

Capitation payments vary by type of physician specialty; most primary physicians will be compensated on a capitation basis (except in staff models), while most specialists will be compensated on a discounted fee-for-service or other method. Even specialists are compensated by HMOs through capitation payments in many instances, especially in staff, group, and mixed models. IPA and network models usually pay specialists using fee-for-service or discounted fees. Given these data, the implication is that primary care physicians in all but staff model HMOs are compensated by capitation payments, a structure that tends to reduce unnecessary and expensive treatments and service modalities, while primary care physicians in staff model HMOs, who are rarely compensated through capitation, have little incentive to control utilization. But, most staff models provide primary physicians with the opportunity to earn bonuses if utilization is controlled appropriately. Moreover, even specialists in many HMOs are placed on capitation, ostensibly with the same conservation incentives as their primary care counterparts.

Health plans use a variety of motivators to supplement capitation and bonuses, including withholds from capitation and fee-for-service payments. Withhold incentives are usually associated with the use of specific services or risk pools: as services are used, a stated percentage of the capitation or fee for the service is withheld from the group's or individual provider's payment— usually 10 to 25 percent of the fee. After a specified period of time, usually a year, the health plan accounts for service use by risk pools and, if utilization is within budgeted levels, the entire withhold is paid to the provider. Conversely, if services are above budgeted limits, the withhold is used to make up deficits— usually shared by the health plan. According to the Group Health Association of America, withholds are more likely to be used for primary care pools than for specialty pools and least likely for inpatient pools; they occur more frequently in network and IPA model HMOs than in group and staff model plans.[38]

It is also important to realize that the capitation, in many instances, is paid to a medical group or IPA under contract with the HMO and not necessarily to the individual physicians. As discussed earlier in this chapter, compensation to individual group practice physicians is based on internal-to-the-group income-sharing formulas. Thus, the group as a whole may have incentives to control utilization, but individual physicians may not personally feel much direct

---

[38] Marsha Gold and Ingrid Reeves. "Preliminary Results of the GHAA-BC/BS Survey of Physician Incentives in Health Maintenance Organizations." In: *Research Briefs*. Monograph of the Group Health Association of America. Washington, D.C., GHAA, November 1987, p. 4.

pressure to conform to the group's objectives. Physicians may be motivated not only by group norms that include the financial well-being of their company, but also by those other nonfinancial incentives previously mentioned. Again, according to the the GHAA survey,[39] in plans that use the financial incentives discussed above, "40 percent use only group performance measures for initial distribution, 11 percent use only individual measures, and 49 percent use combinations of group and individual measures of performance." The study also found that individual performance is more likely to be used in the distribution of incentive payments for primary care pools, rather than for inpatient or specialty referral services. But, overall, it is more likely that funds will be distributed on a combination of individual and group performance measures. This helps to maintain a certain level of morale and esprit de corps, as well as group philosophy in medical group practices.

Another study, by Lewin/ICF, Inc.,[40] a health management consulting firm under contract with the Federal Government examined the incentive payment plans in 215 federally qualified HMOs and CMPs to determine the nature of the risk that physicians were accepting, the extent of that risk, and the distribution of the risk (either aggregate health plan or group performance, or individual physician activities). Their conclusions were somewhat similar to the GHAA analysis, in that more than two-thirds of the plans had arrangements that were based on aggregate distribution factors, with only 15 percent of the arrangements based on individual performance relative to utilization targets. GHAA researchers,[41] however, feel that their data suggest that substantially more than 15 percent of the plans use individual factors because "some distribution based on individual performance was used also in some plans where initial distribution was based on group measures (30 percent of the sample)."

It is reasonable to assume that physicians in HMOs and CMPs are under considerable financial and managerial pressure to limit unnecessary care. But, by limiting services, especially hospital services, do these plans affect the quality of care or patient outcome? Although these two studies do not address this question, the topic of quality in managed care systems is reviewed in Chapter 8 of this text. In the following sections, a categorization of incentive/risk-sharing models is provided, based on the Lewin/ICF, Inc. study.[42]

---

[39] Ibid., p. 4.

[40] Lewin/ICF, Inc. *Incentive Agreements Offered by HMOs and CMPs to Physicians. Executive Summary*. Washington, D.C., Office of Assistant Secretary for Planning and Evaluation, U.S. Department of Health and Human Services, October 27, 1987, p. 3.

[41] Gold and Reeves. "Preliminary Results of the GHAA-BC/BS Survey," p. 5.

[42] Lewin/ICF, Inc. *Incentive Agreements Offered by HMOs*, pp. 15–16.

Type 1. Shared Surplus: Physicians share only in the amount (of revenues) in excess of budget over costs. Two subcategories of this method are commonly used.

    a. DISTRIBUTION BASED ON INDIVIDUAL FACTORS: The surplus is distributed to individual physicians based on their own performance.
    b. DISTRIBUTION BASED ON AGGREGATE FACTORS: The surplus is distributed to the individual physicians based on factors of performance of the health plan and/or the larger group of physicians as a whole.

Type 2. Risks for Deficits Only: Physicians are at risk for a percentage of their compensation if deficits occur. This usually involves a withhold, through which the health plan accumulates funds to cover any future deficits. After deficits are settled, the remainder of the withhold is distributed to the physicians. Again, this might be on an individual or aggregate factor arrangement.

    a. DISTRIBUTION BASED ON INDIVIDUAL FACTORS: The withholds are used to cover deficits; residuals are then distributed among physicians on the basis of relative individual performances measured against utilization targets. For instance, the HMO may withhold 20 percent from its capitation payments to individual physicians and apply these funds to negative balances in the individual physician's hospital and specialist pools. The physician is responsible for the deficit up to the amount of the withhold and cannot share in any net surplus that the HMO may experience. Note that the physicians' risks are limited to some percentage of their compensation from the HMO.
    b. DISTRIBUTION BASED ON AGGREGATE FACTORS: The physicians are at risk for deficits, but their risk is limited to some percentage of their compensation from the plan. A withhold may be used to accumulate funds to cover deficits. After deficits are resolved, the remaining withheld funds are distributed among the physicians on the basis of aggregate performance factors. The group then determines how to distribute the withheld funds to individual physicians.

Type 3. Surplus and Deficits Shared: Physicians share in both the excess and shortage of budgeted funds (or revenue) as compared to costs, and the surplus and deficits are distributed among individual physicians.

    a. DISTRIBUTION BASED ON INDIVIDUAL FACTORS: Surplus or deficit is shared on the basis of individual factors. For example, a portion of physician fees might be withheld, with the physicians then responsible for deficits in certain risk pools up to the amount withheld. If a surplus occurs, the physicians receive their total withheld funds and share in the surplus, based on their individual, relative performance in the group.

    b. DISTRIBUTION BASED ON AGGREGATE FACTORS: Similar to Type 3.a., surpluses and deficits are shared, but the sharing is based on aggregate rather than individual factors.

Type 4. Full Risk for Deficits: Physicians are at full risk for deficits. The responsibility for deficits is distributed to individual physicians based on the performance of the whole group, even though the apportionment among physicians may be based on their relative individual positions in the group.

Type 5. Acceptance of Surplus and Full Risk for Deficits: Physicians not only are at full risk for deficits, but if surpluses occur, they are the recipients of those profits. The sharing of deficits and surpluses is at the discretion of the group; usually the arrangement is described in the income-sharing formula. This model may occur in HMOs that are owned and operated by the medical group practice itself.

Another issue relating to incentive arrangements concerns the level of services for which the physician is at risk. In some situations, the primary physician is responsible for primary services only; primary and specialty services; or primary and specialty physician services and institutional services such as acute hospital care and skilled nursing home care. The physician is at lowest risk when primary care is the only service at risk and at greatest risk when institutional services, which are the most costly of all services, are included in the capitation. Placing the primary physician at risk for more than primary services may also increase the possibility that the physician will be more reluctant to refer patients to specialists or to use inpatient care, and thus affect the quality of care, although there are no studies to support this claim.

    Finally, many plans agree to stop-loss provisions for their physicians and may, indeed, obtain stop-loss coverage for the HMO itself. In these situations, the losses of the health plan, medical group, or individual physician are limited after a predetermined level of service has been provided to an individual or group of members. Arranged with an independent insurer, the HMO and physicians bear the cost of providing services until health care expenditures for any enrollee reach a certain dollar figure or the cost to the plan for their population as a whole reaches a certain dollar amount. The insurer pays the losses above this point. For example, all costs over $35,000 per enrollee per year are paid by the third-party insurer. GHAA[43] reports that two-thirds of the

---

[43] Gold and Reeves. "Preliminary Results of the GHAA-BC/BS Survey," p. 5.

health plans studied having financial incentives for physicians also have some provision for stop-loss coverage, especially for inpatient services and specialty referral services. They suggest that there is a relationship between the use of stop-loss protection and the risk-sharing model used, although, again, this topic needs further study to come to any firm conclusions.

Two Risk Sharing Examples

BAND MODEL: A modification of the Type 3 incentive/risk-sharing model, Surplus and Deficits Shared, is the "band model," which calls for "bands" or parameters to be placed around anticipated use rates for hospitalization and/or medical services. The health plan assumes all the risk of use falling within the band. The health plan, physician group, or other third party—such as an indemnity carrier—assumes the risk of overuse (or gain, in the event of underuse) if the utilization level falls outside the preestablished bands. The health plan otherwise would assume small losses or gains if use was contained within the bands. Note that the health plan and physicians must develop expected levels of use and must also reach an agreement (including an outside insurer, if used) concerning the bands and the loss- and surplus-sharing formula. Table 6-10 shows an HMO that shares its gains and losses equally with its physician group and the outside indemnity carrier. In other cases, a reinsurance carrier may underwrite a portion of the gains or losses outside the bands, with or without health plan or physician-sharing arrangements. Deficits, as in other Type 3 models, would be covered up to the amount of the withhold.

TABLE 6-10 Band Model

Actual Use	Percentage of Anticipated Use	Cost Associated with Various Use Levels	Effects
140	140	$140	Insurer assumes loss of $20 and physician loses $20
120	120	120	Plan loses $20
100 Expected level	100	100	—
80	80	80	Plan gains $20
60	60	60	Insurer assumes gain of $20 and physician gains $20

INCENTIVE MODEL: Incentive payments can be tied directly to hospital use and can take many forms. The following example illustrates a simple method of determining a physician's bonus or incentive:

Anticipated hospital days per 1,000 enrollees = 450
Utilized hospital days per 1,000 enrollees = 360
Incentive rate = $800 per day saved
Total incentive payment = $72,000
(450 − 360) × $800 = $72,000

In another example, the incentive model couples the physicians' share of any surplus to the hospital utilization rate. As the rate decreases, the physicians' share increases to some maximum level (e.g., 50 percent). To illustrate, the physicians' share of the surplus created from lower-than-expected hospital use would be computed as follows:

Percentage Rate	if	Number of Hospital Days per 1,000 Enrollees Is Achieved
30		500
35		475
40		450
45		425
50		300

The medical group's share of the incentive fund is not allowed to exceed 20 percent of the total yearly capitation.

HOSPITALS

There are several approaches to providing for inpatient services to health plan members. The health plan can own and operate the hospital facilities, contract or have an agreement with one or more hospitals for services, or basically, rely on the hospital staff admitting privileges of the HMO physicians. Few HMOs own and operate hospitals; some of the well-established plans that do are the Group Health Cooperative of Puget Sound, the Kaiser Health Foundation, and the Health Insurance Plan of Greater New York. Most HMOs use one of the other methods to ensure that hospital services are available to enrollees, although some, like Group Health Association of Washington, D.C., provide in their contracts with policyholders that the health plan will make only its best efforts to provide hospital services. They do not guarantee that hospital services will be available, although it is very infrequent that health plans will have problems finding hospital beds—especially with the low occupancy rates most hospitals are now experiencing.

The least effective approach is providing for hospital services through the use of HMO physician staff privileges only; usually, this approach provides no assurance that hospitals will willingly participate with the HMO in its utilization and quality control activities, and hospitals certainly will not provide discounts to the HMO. More frequently, the HMO is able to develop agreements and contracts with hospitals, either directly or indirectly, which include some assurance that services will be available at discounted rates. Many approaches are used in these agreements, including the following:[44]

1. The HMO negotiates directly with the hospital, the output of which is an agreement or formal contract that defines the relationship between the two institutions, including methods and levels of payment for services. Payments are made directly to the hospital by the HMO.

2. The HMO contracts with one or more medical groups and/or IPAs; the contract specifies that the HMO will include in its capitation rate to the medical groups and IPAs monies for inpatient services. In turn, the groups or IPAs will pay for hospital services used by health plan members; in effect the groups and IPAs are placed at risk for hospital as well as physician services under this approach. There is no direct contract between the HMO and the hospital.

3. The HMO enters into a contract with a fiscal agent such as Blue Cross or an indemnity insurer, which then acts as a third-party administrator (TPA) to reimburse hospitals and, perhaps, other institutions for member services.

4. Finally, the HMO contracts with a fiscal intermediary for specific services, usually a nationally known insurer such as Blue Cross, which then acts as a TPA paying both in-area and out-of-area emergency claims. In many instances, the name and logo of the TPA appear on the HMO member's identification card, with a statement indicating that the insurer is responsible for reimbursement. In this way, providers outside the HMO's immediate service area are more willing to accept the HMO member's card for payment assurances—a substantial, advantageous marketing strategy for the HMO.

Financial arrangements between HMOs and/or their TPAs and hospitals vary, depending on the ability of each party to effectively negotiate for its position. Arrangements agreed to will be one of the following:

---

[44] U.S. Department of Health and Human Services, Health Care Financing Administration, Office of Health Maintenance Organizations. *Guide to Development of Health Maintenance Organizations*. Rockville, Md., DHHS, 1982, pp. III-25–III-26. DHHS Publication No. (PHS) 82-50178

1. *Full fee-for-service charges:* Under this arrangement, the HMO and its participating physicians are treated like any other purchaser, that is, beds are made available on a first-come, first-served basis, and the hospital bills the HMO or TPA at full fee-for-service rates. This is the rate that a self-responsible, private patient without insurance coverage would be required to pay. In some instances, the hospital will agree to ensure bed availability to HMO patients and to provide admitting privileges to qualified HMO physicians meeting hospital credentialing processes.

2. *Discounted fee-for-service charges:* This method is similar to the first except that the HMO agrees to pay billed hospital charges minus a fixed percentage, which is based on the efficiencies of guaranteed payments, usage protocols utilized by the HMO, and so on.

3. *Billed charges with maximum:* The hospital and HMO agree that the HMO will pay billed charges, but a cap or maximum is placed on charges, with the HMO responsible for all charges up to the maximum.

4. *Reimbursable costs:* Allowable costs are determined according to a formula negotiated by the hospital and HMO. The HMO then reimburses the hospital retrospectively, based on the costs incurred according to the agreed upon formula.

5. *Prospective per diem:* An average per diem rate is set in advance—a set rate per patient per day. The HMO is then charged that rate for each day its members are hospitalized. Multiple per diems may also be used if different rates are established for type of service or minimum usage for each type of service.

6. *Prospective rate per group:* In this situation, the hospital charges the HMO on the basis of the federally recognized diagnostic-related grouping (DRG) classification system, which is widely used to reimburse hospitals for services to Medicare patients.

7. *Prospective rate per case:* The hospital sets rates based on an assumed average length of stay per admission, and the HMO is charged this rate for each member admitted. This method may or may not have unique rates differentiated by diagnosis.

8. *Flat rate per bed:* The HMO guarantees payment at a set rate for a predetermined number of beds—a leased-bed arrangement. The hospital provides services to HMO patients on the condition that the HMO does not exceed the number of beds for which payment has been made. The predetermined rate can vary for different types of beds (service).

9. *Capitation rate:* The hospital and HMO negotiate a per enrollee, per time period (usually monthly) rate. The hospital provides all contracted for services to members for a prospective payment without retroactive adjustments, so the hospital is at risk that the capitation rate will not be sufficient to cover all of the costs of providing inpatient services to HMO members.

TABLE 6-11   HMO Payment Methods Used in Hospital Contracts, by Ownership: 1985

Payment type	Related Hospital Owns HMO %	Related HMO Owns Hospital %	Independent Formal Contract %	Independent No Formal Contract* %
Fee-for-service	5.4	50.0	22.0	59.3
Discounted FFS	28.4	10.0	26.7	14.4
Billed charges, up to a maximum level	5.4	10.0	2.9	1.7
Reimbursable cost	1.3	–	2.5	2.1
Prospective per diem:				
A. Single rate	21.6	30.0	18.0	5.3
B. Multiple rates	13.5	–	15.0	8.4
Prospective rate per Case or Group	17.4	–	7.4	7.7
Flat rate per bed	2.7	–	0.8	–
Capitation rate	4.0	–	4.5	1.0
Total†	99.7	100.0	99.8	99.9

*Includes those with and without letters of understanding, verbal agreements, or other formal or informal agreements.

†May not add to 100 percent due to rounding.

SOURCE: Adapted from Gary J. Rohn and M. R. Traska. "Riskier HMO Payment for HMO-related Hospitals." *Hospitals, 61*:(16)42, August 20, 1987.

Generally, hospitals prefer to use full-charge or discounted-charge methods, while HMOs attempt to negotiate capitation contracts; however, accommodations are usually reached somewhere between these two points as shown in Table 6-11. Note, however, that hospitals related by ownership to HMOs are more likely to give the HMO a discount or to use a per diem or DRG approach, while hospitals independent of HMO ownership may agree to full or discounted charges approximately 74 percent of the time. Independent hospitals with formal contracts use either single or multiple per diem payment approaches 33 percent of the time.

Many factors are considered by hospitals when deciding whether to become involved with HMOs. These include the number of competing hospitals in the HMO's service area, the supply of beds and ancillary services and the occupancy rates for those beds, the hospital's share of the market, its ability to control financial risks under an HMO capitation contract, the hospital's level of security in its current market share, the ability to obtain stop-loss or excess-loss insurance, the probability that HMO patients will require an increased intensity of services, the ability of the HMO to improve the hospital's cash flow, a heightened or diminished image because of the HMO affiliation, medical staff relations, especially if the HMO contract calls for staff privileges to HMO providers not presently on the hospital staff, and so on. A hospital that is operating at 50 percent occupancy, for instance, will probably agree to an HMO contract if it means additional patients and compensation at or near billed charges; improved occupancy, however, will only occur if the HMO expands the already existing hospital service area, since HMOs tend to reduce hospital days per 1,000 population and would diminish even further the hospital's occupancy rate if only existing hospital markets were enrolled in the health plan. Complicating the hospital's analysis would be the effect of competing hospitals, as well as many of the issues noted above. Obviously, HMO affiliation is not an easy decision for hospitals. Indeed, in areas where HMO and other managed care programs hold more than 50 percent of the health insurance market, hospitals have been forced to participate to survive and, in some cases, have been forced to close because of dramatically lowered occupancy and cutthroat competition among competing hospitals for HMO business.

One last comment regarding HMO hospital services is important. The concerns of hospitals about the impact of HMOs on the economic viability of community hospitals are well founded. Based on the number of hospital beds nationwide, the United States has approximately 4.5 inpatient hospital beds per 1,000 population; however, the well-established HMOs that own and operate their own hospitals maintain a ratio of only 1.5 to 2.0 beds per 1,000 enrollees. As the number of HMOs and other managed care groups grows, hospital bed use will continue to drop. This fact raises serious public policy questions regarding the availability of hospital services in an increasingly difficult financial and economic period for the inpatient sector of the health services industry.

OTHER PROVIDERS

Benefits packages may require the services of other providers, including all levels of long-term care facilities; pharmacy, dental, and optical services; home health care; and so on. Plans may wish to own the facilities and directly control the delivery of these services or they may find it more advantageous to contract with outside organizations, especially for services that are infrequently used.

Summary

This chapter deals with providers of care—physicians, nonphysician staff, and hospitals. The medical director's role in both the health plan and in medical groups and IPAs is presented. Emphasis is placed on physicians in group practice because of their major role in the provision of services to HMO subscribers.

The American Medical Association defines a medical group as three or more physicians formally organized and providing care through the joint use of facilities and personnel, with income distributed according to a prearranged formula. The aforementioned statistics use the "three or more physicians" definition as the basis for growth trend analyses. Most important, however, is the fact that the average size of all medical groups was 9.6 physicians in 1989, and multispecialy groups averaged 22.9 physicians in the same year.

The major advantages to physicians in groups are the sharing of knowledge, talent, responsibility, and ideas; regular rotation of hours and coverage for evenings, weekends, and vacations; immediate practice and income for young physicians; salaries comparable to fee-for-service practice; and relief from the business aspects of practice. Disadvantages include loss of freedom and some loss of individuality; problems with the level of individual physicians' incomes and the establishment of an equitable income-sharing arrangement; conformity to the group's standards of practice, conduct, and operating procedures; sharing in the group's liability; and the loss of the physicians' patients to the plan.

The attitude of physicians toward medical group practice HMOs and their participation in HMO activities can be traced from the initial outright, vocal, and legal resistance on the part of organized medicine to the present resigned acceptance on the part of most individual physicians. Physicians are becoming participants in HMOs because of their desire to maintain or increase their current practices. Where HMOs present a competitive threat, some medical societies or physician groups have developed IPA model HMOs in an attempt to retain the fee-for-service, solo practice concept for members. Other individual physicians have joined with HMOs on a full-time or part-time basis. Research suggests that physicians now have a more positive attitude toward practicing in a prepaid group practice setting, although they still have doubts concerning such associations. Paramount among these are the fear that they will lose status in the eyes of medical colleagues and patients, lack of time to do a good job, a breakdown in the patient-physician relationship, possible loss of income, unpredictable growth of HMOs, loss of freedom to practice and set fees, and advancing the physician turnover rate. Turnover rates of from 2 to 3 percent per year are normal in HMOs, suggesting that physicians like to practice in the HMO setting once they complete the initial probationary period.

Physicians and HMOs negotiate agreements and contracts that address the concerns that might arise during the contract period, normally a year, including a description of the services to be provided to enrollees, methods and timing of payments, incentives and risk sharing, quality assurance and utilization review, credentialing, prior approval for referrals to specialists and hospital stays, gatekeeping, collection of copayments, and information and record keeping requirements. Issues such as exclusive contracts, the ability to terminate the relationship, and the ethical and professional question of participating in financial incentives that may lower the quality of care are other concerns that physicians and health plans address in their contracts.

The size of the medical staff of the health plan is based on some generalized guidelines; a staffing ratio of 1 physician for 1,000 to 1,200 subscribers for fully operational plans is the national level. The ratio, however, varies with the membership's medical expectations. Generally, there will be a higher ratio of physicians to subscribers during the early months of operation, even as high as 1 physician to 500 enrollees, and a lower ratio (as low as 1:1,200) for mature plans.

Physicians are added to the staff on a full-time basis when it has been determined that it is costing the plan more for fees, retainers, or part-time salaries than it would for a full-time equivalent physician. The full-time equivalent physician groups should include the following specialties: general medicine, general practice or internal medicine, obstetrics and gynecology, pediatrics, and surgery. Nonphysician staffing also depends on several factors, most important of which are the physician's practice patterns and the use of physician extenders. Experience shows that HMOs staff at a ratio of four to five direct paramedical personnel per physician.

Group practices follow several forms of organization—solo proprietorship, partnership, unincorporated association, or corporation. A 1969 AMA survey reported that approximately 70 percent of all medical groups were formed as partnerships. By 1984, the majority of groups had gone through reorganizations, with more than 70 percent choosing the professional corporation as a legal form of organization. The relationship of physicians can take several forms, including physician ownership of the health plan, a contract with the plan, or full-time salaried employment in the plan. These arrangements affect the method by which physicians are compensated for their services. Compensation formulas in medical groups normally are developed by the physician group on a yearly basis. Expenses are paid first; net income is then distributed according to a prearranged formula. Groups have a more difficult time arriving at an income-sharing formula when capitation income is included. Since capitation payments create incentives to contain the use of service, the traditional productivity factors that groups customarily use to rate physician activities no longer apply to all sources of group income and distribution.

Most physicians associated with HMOs are placed at risk for service use and are given financial and other incentives to control plan costs. Incentive systems are based on the principle that physicians will be more productive and more satisfied with their lot if their superior service both individually and as a group is tied to additional income. Likewise, inferior service and/or inability to manage the group's time effectively at an acceptable level results in sharing losses sustained by the plan and by the medical group. Thus, many incentive systems and risk-sharing models have been developed.

Risk sharing through provider incentives is a key philosophical issue of HMOs, because the physician decides whether to use HMO funds and the form of health care services to be administered. To share in the risk that these funds will not be sufficient to cover all health care services places the provider in a position to hold use at an appropriate level and to appropriately decrease utilization of expensive hospitalization. This philosophy is the opposite of the fee-for-service system, in which the physician, because of the enticement of larger income not regulated by a fixed monthly payment, increases the units of services provided.

Although most services are provided by the group practice, other, more expensive services are provided by hospitals. HMOs seldom own, control, or operate their own hospitals. Inpatient hospital services are arranged through several mechanisms—ownership of hospital, staff admitting privileges of plan physicians at a nonplan hospital, contracts between the hospital and plan for beds, or informal working arrangements with staff-admitting privileges. HMOs are in the most favorable position with regard to controlling use and inpatient costs if they have their own hospitals. The least favorable position is the granting of staff-admitting privileges without the advantage of an informal or formal working arrangement. Services other than outpatient and inpatient hospital beds may be provided by the HMO through ownership of facilities, contractual arrangements, or informal working arrangements with outside providers.

References

Abrahamsen, Maria B. "Hospital/HMO Contracts Need Careful Evaluation." *Michigan Hospitals, 21*(6):21–25, June 1985.

Anderson, Odin, et al. *HMO Development: Patterns and Prospects,* Chicago, Ill., Pluribus Press, Inc., 1985, Chapters 3, 4, and 5.

Colman, John R. and Frank C. Kaminsky. *Ambulatory Care Systems. Volume V, Financial Design and Administration of Health Maintenance Organizations.* Lexington, Mass., Lexington Books, 1977.

Girard, Robert D. "Legal Issues in Contracting with HMOs." Parts 1 and 2. *Hospital Progress, 55*:45–62, August 1974, and *55*:66, September 1974.

Gold, Marsha and Ingrid Reeves. "Preliminary Results of the GHAA-BC/BS Survey of Physician Incentives in Health Maintenance Organizations." In: *Research Briefs.* Monograph of the Group Health Association of America. Washington, D.C., GHAA, November 1987.

Goodman, Louis J. and James E. Swartwout. "Comparative Aspects of Medical Practice." *Medical Care,* 22(3):255–267, March 1984.

Harris, John M., Jr., *The Role of the Medical Director in the Fee-for-Service/Prepaid Medical Group.* Denver, Colo., Center for Research in Ambulatory Health Care Administration, 1983.

Kongstvedt, Peter R. *The Managed Health Care Handbook.* Gaithersburg, Md., Aspen Publishers, Inc.,1989.

Kralewski, John E.; Dennis D. Countryman; and Laura Pitt. "Hospital and Health Maintenance Organization Financial Agreements for Inpatient Services: A Case Study of the Minneapolis/St. Paul Area." *Health Care Financing Review,* 4(4):79–84, Summer 1983.

Kralewski, John E.; David S. Doth; Robert G. Rosenberg; and Daniel G. Burnes. "HMO-Hospital Relationships: An Exploratory Study." *Health Care Management Review,* 8(2):27–35, Spring 1983.

Krasner, Wendy. "Multi-Hospital Sponsored HMOs." *Health Span,* 2(10):16–20, November/December 1985.

Louis Harris and Associates, Inc. *A Report Card on HMOs: 1980–1984.* Menlo Park, Calif., Henry J. Kaiser Family Foundation, 1984. Study No. 844003

Luft, Harold S. *Health Maintenance Organizations: Dimensions of Performance.* New York, John Wiley and Sons, 1981, Chapters 2 and 12.

Morrisey, Michael A. "The Nature of Hospital-HMO Affiliations." *Health Care Management Review,* 9(2):51–60, Spring 1984.

Morrisey, Michael; Geoffrey Gibson; and Cynthia Ashby. "Hospitals and Health Maintenance Organizations: An Analysis of the Minneapolis-St. Paul Experience." *Health Care Financing Review,* 4(3):59–69, March 1983.

Mosser, Gordon, M.D. *The Provider as Medical Manager.* Minneapolis-St. Paul, Minn., Aspen Medical Group, 1986.

Scitovsky, Anne A.; Lee Benham; and Nelda McCall. "The Use of Physician Services Under Two Prepaid Plans." *Medical Care,* 17(5):441, May 1979.

Sims, Phyllis D.; David Cabral; William Daley; and Louis Alfano. "The Incentive Plan: An Approach for Modification of Physician Behavior." *American Journal of Public Health,* 74(2):150, February 1984.

U.S. General Accounting Office. "Physician Incentive Payments by Prepaid Health Plans Could Lower Quality of Care." Report to the Chairman of the Subcommittee on Health, House Committee on Ways and Means, House of Representatives, U.S. Congress, Washington, D.C., U.S. Government Printing Office, 1988.

7

CONSUMERS AND PURCHASERS
OF MANAGED CARE

The consumer is the third segment of the HMO triumvirate—health plan, providers, and enrollee groups. In this chapter, consumer opinions, attitudes, roles, and levels of satisfaction are appraised. The issues of access, continuity of care, members' viewpoints, and a profile of members are presented. Because members are, in effect, beneficiaries under contracts that the health plan maintains with employers, unions, associations, and governmental agencies, these purchasers of MCOs are also discussed. Together, this information will set the stage for the discussions of marketing prepaid health plans in Chapter 10. This chapter concludes with a discussion of the one major aspect of HMOs and CMPs that concerns all members of the triumvirate – the members' perception of the quality of medical care in the HMO setting. In Chapter 8, quality assurance and utilization review are more fully reviewed from the perspective of providers and health plan managers, including a discussion of methods of measurement and methods of maintaining quality in prepaid health plans.

Title XIII of the Public Health Service Act—the HMO Act (P.L. 93-222) and its guidelines—defines the HMO consumer as an individual who has entered into a contractual arrangement with an HMO for specified health services for the individual or his/her family, or one for whom such a contractual arrangement has been made who does not work for the HMO.[1] This definition of a consumer is used here as a synonym for *enrollee, subscriber,* or *member* of the HMO.

---

[1] U.S. Department of Health, Education, and Welfare, Health Services and Mental Health Administration, Health Maintenance Organization Service. *Proceedings: National HMO Consumer Program Development Workshop.* Rockville, Md., 1973, p. 5.

The Consumer Voice and Public Expectations

Consumers are demanding an opportunity to participate in matters that concern them—an opportunity to speak out, to generate their own representation, to expand their economic influence, and to keep current with new developments and services. In the health services field, consumer demands include expressions of attitudes and opinions concerning the health care organizations and their providers and the evaluation of health services. They feel the latter can be adequately performed not only by professionals but also by the recipients of the service. This point of view is partly due to the increasing number of individuals with health insurance coverage; care through the health insurance mechanism is purchased by the consumer who is not sick but well—not dependent but resourceful, and generally not locked into only one health plan but provided with several choices of plans in which to enroll.

The consumer's interest and influence are based not only on his/her purchasing power but on a number of other factors, including higher education levels, improved communication, higher disposable incomes and higher standards of living, and the frustrations that develop when the limited supply of health care services does not match the growing demand for, and quality of, the services desired. Consumers are becoming more capable of making choices between the alternatives available to them. And employers, business coalitions, unions, associations, and others who represent the consuming public, who have a vested interest in maintaining efficient work forces, and who pay most of the health plan premiums on behalf of their employees are establishing a new economic relationship with medicine.

The new consumer influence is being felt in the areas of cost and the methods of financing care, the adequacy of manpower, and the quality and organization of health services. Previously, such considerations have been solely professional decisions. Although consumers have had to accept much of what traditional fee-for-service and prepaid medical care have offered, they are beginning to exercise independent judgment. In the decade of the 1980s, consumers, purchasers, and payers have exerted a decisive influence on medical policy, a process that will continue to sharpen as the number of HMOs and PPOs and enrollment in such managed care plans increase.

Consumer Participation

In a free-market economy, the consumer participates by deciding what product or service shall be used and for whom it will be available; this is a distinctive feature of our society. In health care, such participation has not always held true; only in recent years has there been a general consumer awakening, because health services organizations, especially HMOs, have used marketing techniques previously reserved for commerce. Through the market analysis process, consumer participation is being sought to help decide what health plan benefits packages and covered medical care should be included and what they should accomplish. In fact, most health care observers agree that more consumer involvement is needed in decision making to overcome deficiencies in the health system. Consumer participation also is seen as a motivation mechanism; people are more likely to accept decisions that they helped to make. For the health planner, although consumer participation is now common in policy formulation, such participation is less common in the more specific operational aspects of facility management. Because consumer participation of necessity redistributes responsibility, power, and control, its use in both planning and health care operations is viewed by some as the first step to a more socialized and consumer-controlled health care system.

What is the level of consumer involvement or interest? In the classic study conducted by Jerome L. Schwartz[2] of six consumer-cooperative HMOs and six private physician HMOs, 11 aspects of the evaluated programs were compared, including the policymaking processes, the value of consumer participation to the members, the degree of consumer participation, and the amount of influence exerted by consumers, physicians, and administrators in setting health plan policy. Schwartz found that participation changes with the age of the plan. Newly developing plans have general member participation; most of the initial work is voluntary, and decisions are shared by the entire group. As the organization grows, a staff is hired and functions are delegated. The membership's influence begins to decline when professional or technical services are required or when specific knowledge, training, or education are needed for making decisions. Thus, three indicators of membership participation are customary. First, early tradition embodied in the cooperative effort can set the mode for participation. Second, membership size affects participation: the larger the organizaton, the lesser the activity by total membership, because members lose interest as the professionals exert more influence. Third, the complex decisions of large organizations require the input of expert opinion; therefore, the enrollees' influence is diminished.

Schwartz made the following generalizations regarding consumer participation:

1. Individual participation in member organizations, in political as well as community life, is low.

---

[2] Jerome L. Schwartz. *Medical Plans and Health Care.* Springfield, Ill., Charles C Thomas, Publisher, 1968, p. 219.

2. Most organizations have an oligarchical structure with an active minority and an inactive apathetic majority.

3. The few members who are active are likely to be from the higher socioeconomic level and to have more education and higher income.

4. Policy is rarely made at the membership level—it is usually set and controlled by boards of officials.[3]

When consumers are elected to the governing body, they participate in policymaking. Their level of activity is related directly to their personalities and the management style exhibited by the president of the board and the plan's administrator—strong authoritative styles tend to restrict consumer participation. Administrators, physicians, and key staff members often have a more significant voice and influence in deciding policy. Conversely, consumer plans that encourage consumer board participation generally have better programs in the following four areas: individual enrollment practices, eligibility policies, complaint procedures, and medical benefits. This may be due to pressures from large, organized purchasers, such as unions or employers, to add extra benefits. The policies of consumer plans that Schwartz studied were more favorable to enrollees than were the policies of physician plans.[4]

Other major findings of the Schwartz study are:

1. Consumer sponsorship of the HMOs had no more impact than physician sponsorship on basic and preventive coverages offered by the plans. This generalization also can be extended to group enrollment procedures, health education and information programs, evaluation of the quality of care practiced in the clinic, and assessment of consumer satisfaction.

2. Since some of the consumer-sponsored plans had difficulty attracting specialists (a problem not shared by physician-sponsored plans), consumer sponsorship may have been a deterrent in obtaining specialists.

3. Both consumer and physician governing boards devoted approximately the same amount of attention to various subjects at board meetings.

4. Doctors were the most influential group in policymaking decisions in physician-sponsored plans.

5. General member participation in consumer medical cooperatives was low in terms of attendance at meetings, voting, and other activities.

6. In general, administrators and physicians were more influential in deciding policy in consumer-sponsored plans than were the lay board of trustees.

7. Administrators generally had the most important role in cooperative plans and physicians had the second most important role. In plans with professional or executive trustees, however, the board had a major voice in policymaking.[5]

---

[3] Ibid., p. 58.

[4] Ibid., p. 221.

[5] Ibid., pp. 223–225.

Most importantly, Schwartz concluded from the study that consumer sponsorship of HMOs and consumer participation in the plans can have a favorable influence on health plan programs. It is discouraging to note that there are fewer consumer-sponsored prepaid health plans as other sponsors enter the field. Chapter 4 provides a review of sponsorship and health plan models.

Profile of Prepaid Health Plan Members

There is also some discussion in Chapter 4 about the growth of HMOs and the number of members. Who are these HMO members, why do they choose to enroll, and what are their characteristics? In the discussion that follows, data regarding HMO versus non-HMO members are provided.

The most complete description of HMO membership comes from the Louis Harris and Associates, Inc.[6] study of attitudes and experiences with HMOs. The following discussion draws on the data and conclusions of this study. The study found that 62 percent of the HMO members were below 40 years of age, 55 percent had household incomes exceeding $25,000, 63 percent were married, 66 percent were employed in organizations with 500 or fewer employees, and 52 percent did not have children under 18 years of age. Between 1980 and 1984, Harris noted substantial shifts in the demographic makeup of HMO enrollees. In 1984, a significantly larger proportion of members were below the age of 40 and a smaller proportion were age 50 and above. It appears that enrollment in HMOs is occurring more frequently among younger, under age 40 individuals than among those who are over age 40. Although data are not available to support this conclusion, enrollment in HMOs by individuals over age 65 may be increasing because of the federal emphasis on risk contracting with qualified HMOs and eligible CMPs. Thus, enrollment since 1984 shows an increase in both the under age 40 and the over age 65 categories. Additionally, although all income levels among HMO members were evenly represented in 1980, by 1984 a majority earned more than $25,000, with a significantly smaller proportion earning $15,000 or less. More members were white collar workers than skilled laborers, a finding that did not change between the 1980 and 1984 surveys, and there were fewer union members enrolled in HMOs in 1984 than earlier. Single or previously married adults represented a larger minority of HMO members in 1984 than in 1980, although the family size and sex profile of HMO members remained the same between the two study periods. Finally, 40 percent of HMO

---

[6] Louis Harris and Associates, Inc. *A Report Card on HMOs: 1980–1984*. Menlo Park, Calif., Henry J. Kaiser Family Foundation, 1984. Study No. 844003

enrollees had been members for two years or less, while 22 percent had been members for more than seven years.[7]

HMO members were questioned about their level of satisfaction with prepaid plans. An overwhelming 91 percent responded that they were at least "somewhat satisfied" with the services provided by HMOs. This was similar to Schwartz's finding 16 years earlier—there was a small group in all organizations, perhaps 6 to 8 percent of the membership, that were dissatisfied with the system in which they were enrolled. Members of group or staff model HMOs expressed greater satisfaction with HMOs than did IPA members, but, by and large, 92 percent of all HMO members felt that their prepaid plan met or surpassed their expectations. Only 5 percent indicated that HMO services were worse than their initial expectations.[8]

Most HMO members were more satisfied with their health care services, plan coverage, and costs than comparable non-HMO members. But, the greatest difference between HMO members and nonmembers was in satisfaction with the cost of health services; with regard to out-of-pocket costs for health care, 59 percent of the HMO members were very satisfied, while only 21 percent of eligible nonmembers expressed the same satisfaction level. A greater percentage of HMO members than nonmembers were satisfied with the availability of doctors and medical services, the ability to see a doctor whenever needed, and the quality of hospital care. Insignificant differences were found between members and nonmembers regarding the quality of doctors and their ability to see a specialist when needed. The area of greatest dissatisfaction expressed by HMO members (32 percent) was waiting time, but even in this area, nonmembers (40 percent) were more likely to be dissatisfied than HMO members. As one might expect, group and staff model members were more likely to be highly satisfied with the 24-hour availability of physicians and services and with their low out-of-pocket costs. Conversely, IPA model members were more satisfied with their ability to see a specialist when needed than were members in the other models. As the use of gatekeepers by IPA HMOs increases, this difference should disappear. When the responses of HMO members to questions of satisfaction were compared to those of nonmembers, satisfaction with HMOs by members remained high, while satisfaction with the traditional forms of health care slipped between 1980 and 1984, especially with respect to the ability to see a doctor whenever needed, the quality of doctors, and the time that elapsed between calling for an appointment and actually seeing the doctor.[9]

---

[7] Ibid., p. 20–23.

[8] Ibid., p. 42.

[9] Ibid., pp. 58–59.

The Harris survey compared HMO member satisfaction with eligible non-members and the public. By a margin of 9 to 39 percentage points, HMO members were found to be especially satisfied with how much their health plan paid for their major medical expenses, their lab tests, treatment for minor illnesses, and visits to their doctors. Fewer than 10 percent were dissatisfied with these expenses. Additionally, in areas where HMO members were particularly satisfied—treatment of minor illnesses, lab tests, and doctor's visits—eligible nonmembers expressed dissatisfaction; nonmembers expressed much lower levels of satisfaction with major medical expenses and how much they had to pay over what their insurance or plan paid. Overall, HMO members felt that prepaid care was better than the traditional system. The opinion of the general public (45 percent) and eligible nonmembers (53 percent) was that HMOs were better, although 25 percent of the general public and 23 percent of nonmembers felt that there was no difference between traditional and HMO systems.[10]

In general, then, HMO members might be characterized as under age 40, predominantly white collar, upper middle class, and married, with approximately half of the enrollees having children under the age of 18. Most are well satisfied with the cost, benefits, and quality of physicians and services offered by the prepaid plans. Dissatisfaction with HMOs occurs in certain elements, including the length of waiting times and the ability to see a specialist. The question of consumer satisfaction is continued in a later section of this chapter.

Unions and Business: The Purchasers

For a variety of reasons, unions have been compelled to seek health care primarily through collective bargaining and then to press for it in the political arena. Employers, competing for the best workers, bowed to the demands of the unions for more comprehensive health services in health insurance benefits packages. Progress by unions for health services increased during World War II, when, due to wartime control over wages, employee fringe benefits—including health and welfare—were expanded through collective bargaining. It was during the late 1940s that the first effort toward national health insurance was made by unions and socially oriented and concerned groups such as cooperatives and consumer organizations. Resistance from health providers, especially physicians organized as the American Medical Association, defeated this early effort; but unions intensified their bargaining for health services, primarily the financing and level of benefits. It was this

---

[10] Ibid., pp. 63–64, 70, and 73.

collective bargaining that promoted the rapid growth of the Blue Cross/Blue Shield plans as mechanisms for prepaying hospital and surgical fees, as well as the growth of several major prepaid group practice plans.

Year after year, collective bargaining brought forth more monies to pay for spiraling costs. Many times unions had to accept losses in the middle of a contract or had to go to the members for contributions to continue the benefits. Because there were frequent discussions concerning benefits at union meetings, union members were well educated regarding benefits packages and the bargaining process. This transformed the consumer from a passive recipient to an articulate "demander" of all kinds of medical services. As the consuming public became more sophisticated and the mystery surrounding the practice of medicine continued to be dispelled, greater interest was directed toward the quality of care. Today, most people feel that access to high-quality medical care is a right, not a privilege.

With millions of members and their families supporting them, unions were a considerable force in the development of comprehensive health services programs and dual- or multiple-choice agreements with HMOs. Dr. I. S. Falk of Yale University summarized the union's influence:

The unions' increasing interest in health and their goals in matters of medical care are important not only to their own members but for society as a whole. Many union activities are conducted in the framework of communitywide services. Union policies and practices for their own members tend to set patterns for others as well.[11]

Except for the Federal Government, business employers are the largest purchasers or payers of health services through employer-sponsored health insurance benefits.[12] As union and worker demands for more benefits heightened during the 1950s through the 1970s, employers acquiesced, but not without paying dearly for these added fringe benefits; unionized companies spent an average of $2,364 per employee per year for health benefits in 1987.[13] Employer contributions for employee health insurance rose from $1.8 billion in 1955 to $101 billion in 1985—a 5,511 percent increase in 30 years.[14] By 1990, the average cost of employer medical plans had increased 21.6 percent over 1989,

---

[11] Douglas M. Haynes, ed. *Louisville Area Conference on the Delivery of Health Care.* Louisville, Ky., University of Louisville, 1971, p. 17.

[12] Chapter 5 includes a discussion of governmental involvement as a purchaser and governmental contracting with competitive medical plans and qualified health maintenance organizations.

[13] A. Foster Higgins and Company, Inc. "Foster Higgins Health Care Benefits Survey." *Medical Benefits,* 5(4):1–2, February 29, 1988.

[14] Suzanne V. Klett. "Corporate America Opens the Door to Managed Care." *Medical World News,* 27(1):60, January 13, 1986.

from $2,600 per employee in 1989 to $3,161 per employee in 1990.[15] Employers and unions, therefore, have become deeply involved in measures to reduce their costs, including reviews of current health benefits and the companies writing their own coverage, becoming self-insured for health benefits, and evaluating alternatives to the traditional Blues and indemnity coverages, including PPOs and HMOs. These actions can be categorized into five areas:

1. Using administrative and insurance funding more efficiently
2. Shifting costs to employees
3. Redesigning benefits packages
4. Using a self-insurance approach to fund care
5. Changing patterns of delivery and buying medical care[16]

All five areas have been used by employers, but only the fifth category will effectively reduce costs for both the employer and the employee.

Many employers and unions have joined with other area employers to form business or health coalitions. Such coalitions have actively studied the rising costs of benefits and have become instruments for increasing the awareness and understanding of health care issues, improving dialogue and communications, changing areawide benefits coverage and options available for local businesses, and changing the patterns of care delivered by providers. Although coalitions are often formulated with a great diversity in member background, the primary activities for most coalitions center on alternative delivery systems, benefits design, data analysis, health education, planning, legislative activities, and competitive promotion. Some, for instance, have actually sponsored the development of PPOs and HMOs, while others have supported existing HMOs outside the local area in an effort to have them set up businesses in the coalition's area.

Are the health coalitions on the right track? To answer this question the Health Insurance Association of America (HIAA) and A. Foster Higgins and Company, Inc. conducted a national survey of employers of all sizes. As of April 1989, their data suggest that health benefits costs continue to escalate, although per employee costs of providing benefits vary widely among employers. These differences can be attributed to the scope and level of benefits offered, the risk profile of the group enrolled, local prices for medical services, the level and effectiveness of employee participation in the managed care alternative, and the claims administration and plan management

---

[15] A. Foster Higgins and Company, Inc. "Foster Higgins Survey: Singing a Different Tune." *HMO Managers Letter*, 8(3):5, February 11, 1991.

[16] David F. McIntire. "Employers Ask for More from HMOs." *The Internist*, 26(9):12, October 1985.

arrangements.[17] The percentage increases also varied by managed care option, as shown in Table 7-1. Conventional insurance products increased by 11 percent between 1987 and 1988, while the increases for all HMO models were lower. Staff and group models had the lowest increase, 8 percent; and PPOs the highest, 17 percent. Using the conventional plans as a base, all HMO models had lower 1990 single-coverage premiums than the traditional indemnity/Blues plans; conventional plans cost $148, while IPA models at $125 cost the least, and group and staff model HMOs and PPOs cost $123 and $139, respectively. More important are the costs for family coverage, since most enrollees are included under this option: the premium for traditional plans was $319 in 1990; staff and group model HMOs had the lowest cost, $311 in 1990; PPOs had the highest cost, at $345; and IPAs were second highest at $316. Based on these data, employers, on average, should choose to offer staff or group model HMOs as their first choice, since they cost the least for both single and family coverage and have had the lowest premium increases. The least effective method of controlling costs appears to be the PPO arrangement, which had the highest rate of increase every year since 1987 and the highest family-coverage cost.

Most large businesses now offer managed care options to employees in an effort to reduce their costs; however, several other activities have assisted in controlling some of the employer health services costs.[18] These include:

1. *Precertification of nonemergency admissions.* Case management at the work site may be used, requiring employees to check with a medical services advisor before scheduling a hospitalization. The advisor determines the appropriateness of the admission and whether the procedure can be performed on an outpatient basis, whether charges for the hospital selected are competitive, and whether the estimated length of stay falls within the standard range for the diagnosis.

2. *Industrial health clinics.* Company-run medical clinics have been reinstituted to control the costs of primary care delivery and emergency care.

3. *Unbundle health services.* Delivery contracts for many services—radiology, laboratory, podiatry, vision care, catastrophic services such as cardiovascular and oncology care, and the like—may be negotiated separately to obtain the lowest cost arrangement.

4. *Ambulatory surgery.* Whenever possible, same day surgery may be provided for diagnoses that are included on a list of approved procedures.

---

[17] "DATA WATCH: Health Benefit Cost Increases." *Business and Health,* 7(4):14, April 1989.

[18] Klett. "Corporate America Opens the Door to Managed Care," pp. 54–60.

TABLE 7-1 Monthly Premiums and Annual Premium Increases in Four Health Plans—1987 to 1989

Type of Plan	1987–1988		1988–1989	
	Single	Family	Single	Family
Monthly Premium:				
Conventional	$ 98	$209	$148	$319
Staff/Group Model HMO	93	203	123	311
IPA HMO	88	226	125	316
PPO	103	232	139	345
Annual Premium Increase:	%		%	
Conventional	11		29.5	
Staff/Group Model HMO	8		24.1	
IPA HMO	10		20.8	
PPO	17		23.2	

SOURCES: Cynthia B. Sullivan and Thomas Rice, "The Health Insurance Picture in 1990," *Health Affairs, 10*(2):106, Summer 1991; Health Insurance Association of America, "HIAA Employer Survey, 1988; Health Benefit Cost Increases," *Business and Health, 7*(4):14, April 1989.

5. *Second opinions.* Employers may require a second opinion for all specialty procedures and nonemergency admissions, although some data suggest that this process is not effective in controlling costs, since most physicians providing a second opinion tend to agree with the original physician.

6. *Employee education.* Employees are required to learn how managed care systems operate and how to most effectively receive quality care at the lowest cost to themselves and their employer. This may be accomplished through on-the-job training sessions, the use of benefits manuals, advice on shopping around for providers, computer systems, and telephone hot lines for information about programs, services, costs, deductibles, and providers, as well as prevention-oriented educational programs that help employees make rational life-style choices (weight loss, exercise programs, smoking cessation, stress control, drug-free living, AIDS prevention, etc.).

7. *Employee responsibility.* Reinforcing the belief that the employee is responsible for the maintenance of his/her own good health. Employers may assist by providing a smoke-free workplace, wellness training programs, and fitness assessments, among other programs.

EMPLOYER ATTITUDES TOWARD HMOs

Several studies have revealed some significant issues regarding employer/HMO relationships. These findings suggest that most employers that offer HMOs to employees do so primarily because of their cost-effectiveness, although several of these studies have indicated that employers were split on whether HMOs were higher or lower in cost than other health plans.[19] For example, Louis Harris and Associates found that between their 1980 and 1984 surveys of employer attitudes, the number of employers stating that HMOs decrease the cost of employee health care rose from 13 percent to 30 percent, and 72 percent of the employers in 1984 felt that HMOs were better than the traditional system in controlling their employees' health care costs. In 1980, however, 51 percent of the respondents stated that HMOs had no effect on costs; by 1984, this percentage had increased to 63 percent, but almost one-fifth of the employers with relatively high HMO enrollments (20 percent or more of their employees) reported that their employee health care costs had increased rather than decreased. Hay Associates[20] found, in 1982, that when first offered to employees, the premiums for HMO plans were higher than their incumbent plans, but that after a few years the premiums for the non-HMO plans increased more rapidly than the HMO premiums, to the point where all health plan premiums were competitive.

Initially, employers are attracted to HMOs because of the possibility of reducing health benefits costs, but in many instances and for a variety of reasons, such reductions are not achieved. The intervening variables might involve the relative number of employees who opt for HMO coverage, the characteristics of those who choose the HMO versus other options, the strength and level of the competitors, the place in time—whether the HMO is a new offering or has been offered for several years along with other health plans— and, of course, the ability of the HMO to hold down costs by changing the behavior of its providers.

Several of the studies reported that some employers experienced adverse selection; that is, the healthier employees and their dependents joined the HMO to the disadvantage of the other health plans. Harris and Associates, for instance, found in their 1984 survey that 17 percent of the employers found some adverse selection; and 48 percent in an informal telephone survey by Hewitt Associates of 30 geographically dispersed large employers in 1986 said that their regular plan had experienced adverse selection due to HMO enrollment.[21] The issue of selection by enrollees has been and continues to be

---

[19] Tanniru R. Rao and Maryam Chin, "Employer Attitudes Toward Health Maintenance Organizations," *Health Care Management Review*, 7(1):59, Winter 1982; Hewitt Associates, *What Do Employers Think About HMOs?*, Lincolnshire, Ill., Hewitt Associates, Research Staff, January 1987, p. 5; and Louis Harris and Associates, Inc., *A Report Card on HMOs*, pp. 125 and 147.

[20] Mark Reisler. "Business in Richmond Attacks Health Care Costs." *Harvard Business Review*, 63(1):148, January/February 1985.

[21] Hewitt Associates, *What Do Employers Think About HMOs*, pp. 6–7; and Louis Harris and Associates, *A Report Card on HMOs*, p. 125.

a major concern for all insurers, employers, and the Federal Government. Blue Cross/Blue Shield executives have complained that HMOs regularly enroll the healthier people and leave those with substantial medical problems for BC/BS enrollment, which results in higher BC/BS premuims. Federal Government officials have expressed concern that CMPs and qualified HMOs under Medicare risk contracts market to and enroll only the "young" elderly, who exhibit less ill health. For the employer offering dual or multiple choice, the selection problem may force some health plans to dramatically increase their premiums; for employers who pay the total premium, such actions substantially increase their costs for health benefits.

The overall employer assessment of HMOs, however, has been positive. In 1982, Hay Associates[22] reported that 85 percent of their sample of 235 employers were either very satisfied or satisfied with HMO medical services and they strongly approved of the HMO's marketing, enrollment, and administrative procedures, while only 2 percent were dissatisfied with the general performance of HMOs. In the Rao and Chin[23] study of 172 employers in a Midwest metropolitan area, most participants agreed that the structure of an HMO offers its administrators and participating physicians adequate incentives to provide quality care. Approximately half of the employers in the Hewitt study[24] stated that their overall perception of HMOs was positive, 30 percent said their experiences were negative, and 20 percent were neutral. Approximately 80 percent of the executives in companies offering an HMO option rated their experience as positive, with one-fifth reporting it had been very positive, and 66 percent stating it had been somewhat positive; 9 percent found their experience with HMOs had been somewhat or very negative.[25]

Several of the studies reported that employers were concerned about the qualifications of the doctors and the overall quality of care in HMOs. Returning to the Harris study,[26] in 1980, 52 percent of the business executives surveyed perceived the quality of physicians in the traditional system better than, not equal to, those in HMOs; only 37 percent responded that the HMO was superior to the traditional system. By 1984, the traditional system was still considered better than the HMO system, but HMOs had made gains, with 48 percent of the executives perceiving HMOs providing better quality of care. These results are mirrored in the Rao and Chin study,[27] in which employers expressed

---

[22] Reisler. "Business in Richmond Attacks Health Care Costs," p. 148.

[23] Rao and Chin. "Employer Attitudes Toward Health Maintenance Organizations," p. 59.

[24] Reisler. "Business in Richmond Attacks Health Care Costs," p. 148.

[25] Louis Harris and Associates. *A Report Card on HMOs*, p. 133.

[26] Ibid., p. 147.

[27] Rao and Chin. "Employer Attitudes Toward Health Maintenance Organizations," p. 59.

concerns about the quality of physicians and the lack of personal commitment by physicians. The issue of physician competence also was addressed by Harris and Associates;[28] although confidence in HMO doctors by employers increased, many senior executives believed that the traditional system had superior doctors even though the researchers could find very few differences in board certification and experience among physicians in prepaid health plans and fee-for-service physicians. These data suggest that there continue to be negative perceptions about the level of HMO quality even though these plans have placed great emphasis on educating the consuming public through advertising and promotional activities.

This, however, is not the only problem HMOs face vis-à-vis employers; some still feel that HMOs violate the sacrosanct principle of free choice because their members are forced to use only HMO-participating physicians. As costs go up, however, employers are less concerned with this issue, especially if the HMOs provide assurances that they will choose only the best physicians as providers in the system. Other employers, especially in areas with few managed care options, still feel that HMOs are outside the mainstream of American medicine and arouse very little interest and enthusiasm among business leaders, their employees, and physicians. This myth is quickly being dispelled as more HMOs appear and as more Americans join these plans. Business coalitions have been one of the most valuable tools in introducing managed care in some communities and in helping explain how these systems operate. But, the most difficult problem faced by HMOs is convincing employers that they will receive any direct benefit from offering the HMO to their employees. As previously noted, it is sometimes difficult to show that the HMO will provide cost savings, since HMO premiums are, in many instances, higher initially than the traditional plans; one point that might be made is that HMO premiums do not increase as quickly as the traditional programs.

Offering the HMO option may mean that the employer will now offer two or more competing plans and will assume the extra burden of keeping track of enrollment and administering each system. The employer that provides multiple health plans also may encounter adverse selection in some plans and effectively increase the company's total health benefits costs by posing a threat to the costs of the experience-rated indemnity and Blues plans, even though the HMO premiums may not increase. Finally, except for curative medicine, employers may have some concern about the HMO's ability to maintain the health of their employees and dependents and to provide preventive medical care; it may be difficult for the HMO to convince employers that the plan will contribute to increased employee productivity and low absenteeism.

---

[28] Louis Harris and Associates. *A Report Card on HMOs*, pp. 147–148.

Consumer Satisfaction: The Member's Viewpoint[29]

Earlier in this chapter the issue of consumer satisfaction was introduced as part of the review of HMO members' characteristics. In addition to the Louis Harris and Associates study reviewed in that discussion, there have been numerous research efforts to determine consumer satisfaction with prepaid plans, usually in a comparison with the traditional fee-for-service health plans. In 1981, Harold Luft analyzed most of the major studies in his book *Health Maintenance Organizations: Dimensions of Performance.*[30] His general framework was to categorize satisfaction issues into the following eight areas: access, continuity of care, finances, humaneness, information transfer, quality and competence, overall satisfaction, and behavioral correlates such as enrollment and out-of-plan use. The discussion that follows builds on Luft's work by adding several studies of these areas beginning in 1978. Interestingly, the conclusions drawn by Luft from the studies he reviewed have changed little since his book was published.

Levels of consumer satisfaction provide useful information about the structure, process, and outcomes of care and allow health plan managers to evaluate various competitive aspects of the delivery system. Satisfaction is predictive of future consumer behavior; for example, there is a higher probability that consumers will disenroll or change plans when the level of dissatisfaction increases. Moreover, consumer satisfaction is a valid, although indirect, measure of the quality of care provided by a health plan. It is used by health plan managers in conjunction with measures of the technical quality of care that clinicians use for an overall assessment of the quality of care. Items that are usually considered include

- Patient-doctor and patient-staff interactions
- Access to and availability of care, including appointment and office waiting time, parking arrangements, and emergency care
- Costs of care
- Use of paraprofessionals as primary care and first contact care givers
- Staff courtesy

The results of selected studies since Luft's review reveal the following points.

---

[29] This section draws on Robert G. Shouldice and Norah Singpurwalla, "Consumer Satisfaction and Quality of Health Services," *Medical Group Management Journal, 35*(3):8–9, 11, May/June 1988, by permission of the Medical Group Management Association.

[30] Harold S. Luft. *Health Maintenance Organizations: Dimensions of Performance.* New York, John Wiley and Sons, 1981.

REGULAR PHYSICIAN RELATIONSHIP

Those studies that sought to determine the level of satisfaction in a particular HMO showed that consumer satisfaction was highest for those members who had a regular physician in the program.[31] They also indicated that members can be satisfied with one aspect of care and dissatisfied with others, such as access to care for routine but unexpected problems. One survey,[32] designed "to determine the extent to which HMO members perceive problems with access to care and to examine the relationship between perceived access problems and patient satisfaction," revealed that 17 percent of its members reported that they or their families had experienced problems in accessing care. Those experiencing such problems were less satisfied with the access aspect of the HMO program than with other aspects. Their dissatisfaction was evidenced by outside use of services and failure to see a doctor when the need to see one was perceived.

Another study[33] was conducted to determine whether providers' perceptions of consumer satisfaction were accurate when compared to what consumers reported. Encouragingly, the results showed that *providers were aware* of which aspects of the HMO the consumers were satisfied with and which ones provoked dissatisfaction. Aspects that most patients were satisfied with included costs, quality of care, and staff attitudes and behavior. A number of patients were dissatisfied with the "message center for contacting the doctor" and the "amount of time spent on the telephone with appointment or message center," but these patients represented a minority, 21 to 35 percent, respectively.

PHYSICIAN CONDUCT/HUMANENESS

Comparative studies of consumer satisfaction with alternative delivery systems versus fee-for-service systems yielded conflicting results. For example, in a setting that had both fee-for-service and prepaid patients with a single set of providers, overall satisfaction levels were not significantly different.[34] One

---

[31] Clyde R. Pope. "Consumer Satisfaction in a Health Maintenance Organization." *Journal of Health and Social Behavior, 19*(3):291–303, September 1978.

[32] Clyde R. Pope, Donald K. Freeborn, and Sylvia Marks. "Perceived Access to Care and Patient Satisfaction in a Prepaid Group Practice HMO." *Group Health Journal, 5*(2):22–27, Fall 1984.

[33] Donald K. Freeborn and Clyde D. Pope. "Client Satisfaction in a Health Maintenance Organization: Providers' Perceptions Compared to Clients' Reports." *Evaluation and the Health Professions, 4*(3):275–294, September 1981.

[34] James P. Murray. "A Comparison of Patient Satisfaction Among Prepaid and Fee-for-Service Patients." *Journal of Family Practice, 24*(2):203–207, February 1987.

particular aspect of satisfaction, however, "physician conduct/humaneness," revealed that the satisfaction level among prepaid patients was lower.

When matched patients in two different settings were compared, the results of a study by Sorenson and Wersinger[35] showed that although there was no difference in the overall satisfaction of patients in either setting, specific aspects of satisfaction revealed differences. For instance, significantly fewer HMO members reported having to wait too long to see their provider and having problems receiving emergency care. But significantly fewer HMO members also reported being satisfied with the medical care staff when asked "in your opinion, is your doctor and his/her staff interested in you as a person?"

AVAILABILITY AND ACCESSIBILITY

Rand Corporation researchers have used data gathered while conducting the famous Health Insurance Experiment (HIE) to compare levels of satisfaction with prepaid and fee-for-service medical care.[36] This study determined that the overall satisfaction level was the same for both the HMO and the fee-for-service system; but the people who were *assigned* to the HMO setting (as some were in the HIE) were less satisfied overall. With regard to consumer satisfaction with specific features of the program, those in the fee-for-service system scored their program higher in the areas of length of appointment waits (shorter); parking arrangements (better); availability of hospitals (better); and continuity of care (better). Prepaid consumers were more satisfied with the length of office waits and costs of care.

Caution should be exercised in generalizing the results of any of these studies because HMOs have different organizational arrangements. Also, consumer satisfaction levels may be tied to expectations that are too high for a particular system or for medical care. Or, it may be that dissatisfaction with a particular aspect of the program is temporary and is felt mostly by new members who are establishing new relationships and learning new procedures.

As noted previously, the nationwide survey by Hewitt Associates[37] on consumer satisfaction with alternative delivery systems reported generally that

---

[35] Andrew A. Sorenson and Richard P. Wersinger. "Aspects of Member Satisfaction Under Two Types of Health Delivery Systems: A Comparison of Prepaid Group Practice HMO Members and a Blue Cross/Blue Shield Matched Control Group." *Group Health Journal*, *1*(2):33–41, Summer 1980.

[36] Allyson Ross Davis, John E. Ware, Jr., Robert H. Brook, Jane R. Peterson, and Joseph P. Newhouse. "Consumer Acceptance of Prepaid and Fee-for-Service Medical Care: Results from a Randomized Controlled Trial." *Health Services Research*, *21*(3):429–452, August 1986.

[37] H. Taylor and M. Kagay. "The HMO Report Card: A Closer Look." *Health Affairs*, *5*(1):81–86, Spring 1986.

consumers were satisfied with their health care, plan coverage, and costs, and that most members intended to reenroll. In Wisconsin, 82 percent of the consumers enrolled in HMOs or PPOs said they were satisfied or very satisfied with their programs.[38] In Minnesota, the state health department reported that the number of written complaints against HMOs had increased in 1985, but the number was low—247 from 900,000 members in such plans. This information by itself, however, can be interpreted as meaning that there is a low level of dissatisfaction with HMOs.[39]

The rash of malpractice suits filed against HMO physicians and HMOs in the recent past may also be interpreted as a proxy indicator of enrollee dissatisfaction. It is expected that the number of lawsuits against HMOs will grow until court decisions establish basic principles of liability.[40]

The ultimate test of a system and satisfaction levels is the health plan's ability to maintain enrollment; low satisfaction will result in low enrollment or reenrollment and disenrollment. Satisfaction can be maintained and enhanced with good patient compliance with physician orders, good communication between physician and patient, and perceived continuity of care.[41]

Providers and administrators must be aware that an absence of complaints does not necessarily mean that there is no consumer dissatisfaction. Therefore, if HMOs and PPOs are to retain current members and attract new ones, it is imperative that consumer satisfaction be monitored. Both overall and individual attitudes and perceptions of satisfaction must be assessed. Standards should be established; measurements should then be made in the health center, both before and immediately after treatment, so that satisfaction can be compared with expectations. Tools to measure satisfaction should be created by the plan's management based on existing techniques or new, innovative approaches should be devised. For example, the patient-doctor interaction scale (PDIS) developed by Smith, Falvo, McKillip, and Pitz[42] that measures one attribute of satisfaction might be used. A format for satisfaction standards is provided in Table 7-2; several evaluation items are listed on the left. The health plan's administrative staff could then set goals, based on the

[38] K. R. Lamke. "Survey Finds Most Users Happy with HMOs, PPOs." *Milwaukee, Wisconsin Sentinal*, Sec. 1, p. 5, May 5, 1984.

[39] Walter Parker. "HMO Complaints Up, but Percentage Low." *St. Paul, Minnesota Evening Pioneer Press Dispatch*, C1, C3, January 10, 1986.

[40] "HMOs Are Objects of New Legal Theories." *HMO Managers Letter*, 5(3):4, February 8, 1988.

[41] J. K. Smith, D. Falvo, J. McKillip, and G. Pitz. "Measuring Patient Perceptions of the Patient-Doctor Interaction: Development of the PDIS." *Evaluation and the Health Professions*, 7(1):77–94, March 1984.

[42] Ibid.

TABLE 7-2 Sample Performance Standards Regarding Member Satisfaction

Items Evaluated	Sample Standard Percent of Sample "Satisfied"
1. *Access to care:*	
a. Emergency care (nonappointed) ....____ %	
b. Routine primary care (appointed) ....____	
c. Ability to receive specialty care ....____	
d. Hospitals used by health plan ....____	
e. Appointment waiting time ....____	
f. Office waiting time ....____	
g. Time spent on telephone with appointment or message center ....____	
h. Message center for contacting doctor ....____	
2. *Quality:*	
a. Technical knowledge, ability, and competence of doctors ....____	
b. Technical knowledge, ability, and competence of nurses/technicians ....____	
c. Staff spends enough time with patient ....____	
d. Staff thorough ....____	
3. *Information transfer:*	
a. Give enough information about medical problem ....____	
b. Give enough information about drugs prescribed ....____	
c. Give enough information about self-care at home ....____	
4. *Humaneness:*	
a. Doctors interested in patient ....____	
b. Nurses/technicians interested in patient ....____	
c. Nonclinical staff interested in patient ....____	
5. *Cost and Benefits:*	
a. Perceived value of services received to costs not paid by insurance ....____	
b. Level of benefits coverage provided ....____	
c. Level of copayments and deductibles ....____	

percentage of members sampled who responded that they were satisfied; a mean score or other method of numerically identifying an acceptable level of satisfaction would be inscribed opposite each evaluation item. A random sample of members would be questioned periodically. Responses could then be compared with the proposed standards and corrective actions taken where responses fell below expectations.

At this point in the discussion of consumer satisfaction, it may be useful to review Donabedian's[43] classic article regarding subscriber opinions. The

---

[43] Avedis Donabedian. "An Evaluation of Prepaid Group Practice." *Inquiry*, 6(3):7–8, September 1969.

studies that he reviewed offer a highly subjective, although informative, indication of subscriber viewpoints; they also support some general conclusions that are consistent with those drawn from the more recent articles previously described. The general impression is that a large majority of members are satisfied with whatever plan they belong to. Donabedian notes that there was general acceptance of three plans that differed significantly as to sponsorship and benefits. Although most members were satisfied, a small "hard core" of dissatisfied persons—approximately 10 percent of all members—had a negative view of almost all aspects of the plan to which they belonged, whether it was a prepaid group practice plan or another health insurance program.

The members who complained did so in almost all areas relating to care. They felt that the physicians were impersonal, that obtaining medical care was inconvenient, and that there was an atmosphere of a charity clinic and poverty medical care. Complaints concerned long waits and difficulty in obtaining home visits. Few complaints, however, concerned freedom of physician choice. Although more than 55 percent of the HMO complaints were related to certain "intrinsic" features of group practice, the remaining 45 percent were common to medical practice in general.[44]

It is important for the HMO manager to realize that a considerable portion of member complaints apply to medical care everywhere, although this should not be an excuse to avoid remedying most member complaints; to do otherwise would be harmful to a program that relies primarily on a word-of-mouth marketing strategy. Thus, it is imperative for HMOs to develop a mechanism for handling consumer complaints if they are to be competitive with the fee-for-service medical care system.

Another study reviewed by Donabedian reported that subscriber opinions were developed in part through their evaluation of medical care received, using two criteria: personal interest in the patient by the physician and technical competence. Members viewed prepaid group practice as promoting the technical quality of care but hampering the establishment of a satisfactory personal relationship with a physician. Members felt that quality was not measured by competent physicians but by the use of the technical, diagnostic, and consultative resources offered by the HMO. "Additionally, subscribers appreciate the absence of financial incentives. Labor Health Institute data indicate that subscribers tend to accept perceived limitations in care, so long as the quality of care is thought to be superior."[45] At the outset, there will always be some who will say they like the plan's quality of care, while, at the same time, will complain that they do not like the physician-patient relationship

---

[44] Ibid., p. 20.
[45] Ibid., p. 8.

or the perceived lack of personal attention. Some subscribers will bring into the plan a set of prejudices that precludes acceptance or approval of the plan.[46]

Several reasons have been suggested for this negative perception concerning the lack of personal interest and the system's unresponsiveness to subscribers' needs. Some felt that the doctors did not care about the patients because there were no financial, fee-for-service incentives for them to do so. Others stated that there appeared to be too many people—paraprofessionals, clerks, and others—between the patient and the physician. It may be that high medical staff turnover and the interchangeability of physicians make it difficult to establish deep physician-patient relationships.[47] Studies also show that only two-thirds of all HMO subscribers consider the HMO physician to be their family or regular physician.

Is consumer acceptance of, and satisfaction with, the HMO directly related to certain characteristics of the population served? Several studies have revealed that when given a choice among health insurance plans, subscriber selections were not strongly associated with demographic variables. Generally, preference for prepaid group practice was highest among persons between 30 and 60 years of age, with young children in the family, with generally better-than-average educations, and with average to moderately high income levels. Moreover, prepaid group practice plans won enthusiastic acceptance when continuity and quality of care were emphasized by the group, when obstacles between doctor and patient were removed, and when personal attention was given to the subscriber.

The attitudes of consumers are more than mirrors of accumulated experience; they are strong indicators of the plan's general acceptance and the degree to which it succeeds. "To some extent consumer acceptance of prepaid group practice plans is an expression of the absence of a prior patient-physician relationship or a breakdown of such relationships."[48]

Other Indicators of Member Satisfaction

Three rather subjective indicators are commonly used by HMO executives in evaluating the level of consumer acceptance and the extent to which HMOs meet the expectations of their subscribers. These include the frequency with which persons who are offered alternative choices (dual or multiple) select the HMO option, frequency with which plan members use services outside the

---

[46] Ibid.

[47] Ibid.

[48] Ibid., p. 10.

plan (leakages), and enrollee turnover (or disenrollment) rates. Although these indicators provide consumer opinion only, they do offer the HMO administrator some guidance on the need for changes in plan operation and for improving subscriber satisfaction with the plan. These indicators are described in the sections that follow.

DUAL CHOICE

HMO prototypes (the prepaid group practice plans on which the concepts of current HMOs are based) found that their initial marketing activities with employer groups and unions were enhanced by a dual-choice offering—two alternative health plans, allowing employees to choose the plan that was most suitable for them. Dual choice was the prepaid health plan's partial solution to the "free choice of physician" controversy.

Opponents of the HMO movement argue that, since the HMO represents a closed-panel practice of medicine, subscribers have little or no choice among physicians—that they receive care under the plan only through the physician panel, except in emergencies. This, it is contended, violates the right of free choice and impairs the patient's ability to obtain quality medical care. Thus, older HMOs have supported employers in their efforts to provide a dual choice in health plans—the HMO and another health insurance plan. The outcome has been that employees now can choose their health plan as well as their physicians.

But, for the HMO, multiple choice has had a negative impact. As the number of plans offered to employees increases, the likelihood that they will switch plans increases; this implies higher disenrollment and, thus, higher costs for all the health plans offered. From the employer's perspective, offering more than one health plan may mean increased administrative activities and higher premiums, since some adverse selection may occur. The lack-of-choice argument is less important today, however, because many fee-for-service subscribers have difficulty finding physicians who will accept them as new patients. Members of the HMO system not only are guaranteed a physician but are assisted in selecting one. The more important issue facing the industry may be the question of selection; will the self-selection process that is afforded employees in a dual- or multiple-choice situation create demographically unbalanced enrollment among the plans offered?

Employers, in most situations, are now offering multiple health plans; for instance, one or more Blue Cross/Blue Shield packages described as low versus high option, one or more indemnity insurance companies, one or more HMOs, and even a PPO arrangement. Initially, the HMO obtains permission from the employer (the health insurance policyholder of the subscribing group) to offer the HMO health plan in addition to the other health plans currently being offered. Employees are then given an opportunity to transfer to one of the several health plans—usually during an annual open enrollment period that lasts several weeks, at which time representatives of all the plans are available to assist employees in making their choice of plan.

When two competing health plans are *first* offered to a group, experience shows that enrollment is approximately equal in both plans. Over time, however, one of the programs usually achieves a substantially larger enrollment than the other. On the other hand, if dual/multiple choice is offered after one plan has been available for some time, the incumbent plan has a definite advantage. It may be several years before the HMO achieves parity in enrollment; then again, it may never reach the level of the incumbent plan's market share.[49]

Several studies concerning dual choice have been undertaken. One compared enrollment levels between Blue Cross and a Kaiser program; another described enrollment in Group Health Insurance (GHI) (Blue Cross/Blue Shield of New York City) and the Health Insurance Plan of Greater New York (HIP). Avedis Donabedian[50] reports that the results of both studies are similar; basically, people who choose HMOs do so because of the greater security these plans offer against the costs of illness. Those who select the alternative plan do so because it offers *greater physician choice.* The GHI/HIP study suggested that previous medical experience, in general, and prior relationships with a regular doctor, in particular, were important factors in the consumer's choice of plans; what friends and associates did or said also was an important factor influencing subscribers. Free choice, especially for physician care, was an important factor among the more educated and higher income families. A symbol of economic and social independence is the ability to afford free choice.

The Kaiser study showed that people joined the Kaiser program because of lower costs and better coverage. One might expect this in a dual-choice situation where the HMO program offers a wider range of benefits and greater economic security against additional charges. The HMO offering a dual-choice arrangement must take special care to plan for and manage potentially higher use situations, such as those that arise when enrolling large families whose health care needs may be greater; in those areas of the country that have greater medical care needs; and in those areas that have a higher percentage of young children.

There are several suggested reasons why employees do not select the HMO option. These include the limited geographical area in which a plan operates,

---

[49] Averam Yedida. "Dual Choice Programs." *American Journal of Public Health,* 49(11):1477, November 1959.

[50] Avedis Donabedian. *A Review of Some Experiences with Prepaid Group Practice.* Ann Arbor, Mich., School of Public Health, Bureau of Public Health Economics, University of Michigan, 1965, pp. 4–5, Research Series No. 12

lack of free choice of physicians and hospitals, philosophical opposition to HMOs as being components of a socialized medicine program, and potential gaps in coverage that are not found in the other available choices.[51] Because of the importance of using dual- and multiple-choice plan offerings to attract persons to the HMO, further discussion of dual choice as a marketing strategy is provided in Chapter 10.

Generally, choice of plans depends on the knowledge that a choice is available: knowledge of specific plan attributes; and the degree of importance of, or valuation placed on, each attribute to the subscriber's needs. This strongly suggests that evaluating the public health care needs and attitudes must be a major function of the HMO.

RISK VULNERABILITY HYPOTHESIS

Other data indicate that vulnerability to health and financial risks are basic factors affecting the awareness of a subscriber group to available alternatives when choosing between two or more health insurance plans. The hypothesis suggests that individuals who feel that they and their families are at high risk because of expected illness and financial losses due to large out-of-pocket costs prefer to join HMOs.[52] Rashid Bashshur and Charles Metzner state that persons in younger age groups, single persons, persons with no dependents, and those in lower income groups (measured by family income,

---

[51] Marie Henderson. "Federal Employees Health Benefits Program. II: Role of the Group Practice Prepayment Plans." *American Journal of Public Health, 56*(1):54–57, January 1966. See also Donald C. Riedel et al. *Federal Employees Health Benefits Program. Utilization Study.* Rockville, Md., Health Resources Administration, U.S. Department of Health, Education, and Welfare, 1975.

[52] The following sources offer discussions of this hypothesis: Rashid L. Bashshur and Charles A. Metzner, "Patterns of Social Differentiation Between Community Health Association and Blue Cross–Blue Shield," *Inquiry, 4*(2):23–44, 1967; _____, "Vulnerability of Risks and Awareness of Dual Choice of Health Insurance Plans," *Health Services Research, 5*(1):106–113, Spring 1970; A. Moustafa, Carl E. Hopkins, and Bonnie Klein, "Determinants of Choice and Change of Health Insurance Plans," *Medical Care, 9*(1):32–41, January–February 1971; Thomas W. Bice, "Risk Vulnerability and Enrollment in Prepaid Group Practice," *Medical Care, 13*(8):698–703, August 1975; Sylvester E. Berki et al., "Enrollment Choice in a Multi-HMO Setting: The Roles of Health Risk, Financial Vulnerability, and Access to Care," *Medical Care, 15*(2):95–114, February 1977; Richard Tessler and David Mechanic, "Factors Affecting the Choice Between Prepaid Group Practice and Alternative Insurance Programs," *Milbank Memorial Fund Quarterly/Health and Society, 53*(2):149–172, Spring 1975; A. C. Marcus, "Mode of Payment as a Predictor of Health Status, Use of Health Services and Preventive Health Behavior: A Report from the Los Angeles Health Survey," *Medical Care, 19*(10):995, October 1981; P. W. Eggers, "Risk Differential Between Medicare Beneficiaries Enrolled and Not Enrolled in an HMO," *Health Care Financing Review, 1*(3):91–99, Winter 1980; and Joan L. Buchanan and Shan Cretin, "Risk Selection of Families Electing HMO Membership," *Medical Care, 24*(1):39–51, January 1986.

home ownership, and neighborhood income levels) may be viewed as having less at stake economically, therefore, they feel less vulnerable to serious economic loss in meeting health needs. The opposite is true for older persons, those with higher incomes, those with dependents, and families with high economic needs and low income, who usually prefer prepaid health plans. Thus, these latter groups may be more aware of what the various health plans offer. If, however, the HMO is perceived to be a system that rations necessary health services, the risk vulnerability rationale may be diminished. Bashshur and Metzner[53] conclude that "it appears that persons with lower vulnerability or with decreased financial capacity to respond to felt vulnerability, and persons who are less involved in organizational activity, are those who are most likely to be unaware of alternatives available to them in such a situation of dual choice."

Other researchers, however, have reported mixed findings; for example, Luft[54] concluded that selection based on risk and utilization does occur, but that predicting the direction of the selection effect is difficult. He states that there are "three major determinants . . . : (1) the premium differential faced by the potential enrollee; (2) whether alternative plans require the enrollee to switch physicians or to obtain services in a different geographic setting; and (3) the type of options available." Most researchers agree that preexisting patient-physician relationships are most important—that individuals with strong relationships prefer to maintain them. If the HMO offers that opportunity, usually through an IPA arrangement, the patient will choose to join the plan, especially if it seems to be a better buy. Moreover, one must realize that as an HMO gains a following, patient-physician ties will be created as the healthy enrollees begin to use physician services, especially as they age. It is hypothesized that over the long term, the aging of HMO members will gradually create an increased use of services if all other conditions remain equal (out-of-pocket costs, premium differentials, and benefits).

LEAKAGES

Another indicator of consumer satisfaction is the extent to which HMO enrollees use services outside the plan in preference to similar services that are available within the HMO. The use of outside services may be related to prior physician-patient relationships, dissatisfaction with plan services, greater convenience,

---

[53] Bashshur and Metzner. "Vulnerability of Risks and Awareness of Dual Choice of Health Insurance Plans." See also Klaus Roghmann et al. "Who Chooses Prepaid Medical Care: Survey Results from Two Marketings of Three New Prepayment Plans." *Public Health Reports,* 90(6):516–527, November–December 1975.

[54] Luft. *Health Maintenance Organizations: Dimensions of Performance,* pp. 51–52.

and the type of health services desired, even though the use of outside services requires additional expenditures over the premiums paid to the HMO.

Leakages reduce the overall use of services per member, have an effect on the HMO's actuarial estimates, and thus directly affect premium levels. Some students of HMO management propose that sanctioning out-of-plan use (point-of-service options), or at least encouraging it, may help the plan remain financially competitive with other plans. In the short term, rates of ambulatory use will probably drop, but the plan may also experience a drop in members; losses in revenue through disenrollments will more than offset any savings due to leakages to outside providers.

MEMBER TURNOVER AND DISENROLLMENT RATES

Changes in health plan enrollment are of great interest to managers as an indicator of successful operation. Most enrollment efforts have concentrated on marketing issues and strategies and the HMO's plans to achieve its target levels. Less effort has been applied to understanding the effect of disenrollment and reenrollment on achieving desired total enrollment levels and projections. This is surprising when the detrimental effects of disenrollment are considered— the loss of premium income, the increased complexity in budgeting and planning for services, the increased cost of enrolling new members to offset disenrollees, and the general disruption of preferred long-term relationships between enrollees, the plan, and physicians.

Disenrollment is the number of members who enroll and subsequently disenroll within 12 months of enrollment. It consists of all disenrollments recorded within one year; deaths should not be included. Dividing the number of disenrollments by the number of total enrollments in a given 12-month period yields the disenrollment rate. It is also important to describe the type of disenrollment or resignation from the health plan—either voluntary or involuntary (sometimes referred to as mandatory disenrollment).

Voluntary disenrollment is a conscious, intentional, and deliberate decision by the member to leave the health plan. Studies of prepaid group practice plans identified dissatisfaction with plan attributes, inaccessibility of services, and certain sociodemographic characteristics of the plan's population as the most common reasons for voluntary resignations. Involuntary disenrollment, on the other hand, occurs when members change jobs or locations and are unable to transfer their health plan coverage, or when their current employer drops the HMO coverage. Involuntary resignations may also occur with Medicaid populations enrolled in HMOs—those who lose eligibility to participate in the Medicaid program, and those who are members of CMPs or risk-contracting HMOs that decide to terminate their HCFA contracts. Obviously, the HMO manager should be concerned with the reasons for both categories of disenrollment and should develop methods to address the problems.

A review of the literature regarding voluntary resignations identifies the following reasons for such action.[55]

1. Of greatest importance are economic factors, especially increases in the subscriber's portion of the premium that is not covered by the employer or union or increases in out-of-pocket costs. Disenrollments rise significantly with increases in relative premiums.

2. Competitive forces. As the number of plans increases, so does the likelihood that members will switch plans. Plans attempt to attract new members by offering new or combinations of features and by differentiating their plan from others, thus increasing enrollments/disenrollments.

3. Demographic characteristics, including age, sex, and marital status of enrollees. For instance, among the under age 65 population, one study reported higher voluntary disenrollments by nonwhites, single members, younger-than-average members, and individuals describing their occupation as "professional." It is hypothesized that many of these disenrollees are young, upwardly mobile, professional, single individuals who are changing jobs or moving to other locations. Other studies of non-Medicaid, commercial enrollees suggest that demographic characteristics play no part and are irrelevant in determining levels of disenrollment.

4. Several studies report that disenrollees are healthier than the average member and, therefore, are low users of plan services—an indicator of potential disenrollment. These members may have failed to create a traditional patient-physician relationship, therefore, service use within the plan was low, which contributes to overall general dissatisfaction with plan services and subsequent disenrollment. Some studies suggest that the HMO may experience adverse selection when healthier members disenroll. Conversely, other studies

---

[55] Stephen H. Long, Russell F. Settle, and Charles W. Wrightson, Jr., "Employee Premiums, Availability of Alternative Plans, and HMO Disenrollment," *Medical Care, 26*(10):927–938, October 1988; Charles W. Wrightson, James Genuardi, and Sharman Stephens, "Demographic and Utilization Characteristics of HMO Disenrollees," *GHAA Journal, 8*(1):23–42, Summer 1987; Anthony M. Tucker and Kathryn Langwell, "Disenrollment Patterns in Medicare HMOs: A Preliminary Analysis," *GHAA Journal, 9*(1):22–41, Fall 1988; Stuart B. Boxerman and Virginia D. Hennelly, "Determinants of Disenrollment Implications for HMO Managers," *Journal of Ambulatory Care Management, 6*(2):12–23, May 1983; William Gold, "Predicting HMO Disenrollment Behavior: Results of a Study of Demographic and Behavioral Characteristics of HMO Members," *Finance and Marketing in the Nation's Group Practice HMOs, Proceedings of the 31st Annual Group Health Institute, Washington, D.C., June 14–17, 1981*, Washington, D.C., Group Health Association of America, 1981, pp. 175–181.

have found no statistically significant connections between usage rates and disenrollment and no adverse selection as a result of disenrollments.

5. Dissatisfaction with plan attributes, including unusually long waits or delays in obtaining appointments, staffing patterns, hours of operation, the use of nonphysician providers, inability to obtain services because of facility location, and hours of operation.

6. The presence of multiple, alternative health insurance coverages available through working spouses provides a powerful disincentive to continue HMO coverage, especially if a family is unhappy or dissatisfied with the HMO's services.

7. Misunderstandings. In plans that enroll Medicare recipients, disenrollment usually occurs because of misunderstandings, especially that the enrollee would have to leave his/her current physician and switch to HMO physicians (the lock-in feature of HMOs). Disenrollees also do not like being treated by different doctors each time they visit the facility, which leads to the perception that the quality of their health care will be poor. Some Medicare enrollees leave the plan because their doctor has left. Unlike the under age 65 enrollees, Medicare disenrollees are high users of services; it is reasoned that high users have more contact with the HMO delivery system and thus quickly recognize areas with which they are dissatisfied—or they may resist case management pressures that limit their ability to self-refer to specialists.

Standards should be developed against which the plan can evaluate consumer attitudes. For example, Long, Settle, and Wrightson[56] provide a method for addressing the loss of enrollees due to the relative increase in HMO premiums, the most important reason for disenrollment of commercial enrollees. As part of their study methodology, they devised a method to measure changes in out-of-pocket monthly premiums for individual or family HMO coverage, relative to the change in premiums for other insurance options that were available. This relative price index could be calculated to determine the possible effect on disenrollment because of increases in premiums. The index is the difference between the change in the employee's contribution rate (i.e., the subscriber's portion of the premium for HMO coverage) and the change in the weighted average of the premiums for all other employer-sponsored health plans that are available to the employee. According to this study,[57] "the weights are defined to reflect the relative attractiveness of the alternative forms of coverage, that is, the weight for a specific alternative equals the number of fellow employees

---

[56] Long, Settle, and Wrightson. "Employee Premiums, Availability of Alternative Plans, and HMO Disenrollment," pp. 928–929.

[57] Ibid., p. 929.

subscribing to that alternative divided by the total number of fellow employees subscribing to [that plus all other] alternative forms of coverage. If the premium for a subscriber's own plan remains unchanged relative to the average premium for the alternatives, this variable equals zero; if a plan becomes more expensive relative to the alternatives, this variable takes on a positive value; and if a plan becomes relatively less expensive, this variable assumes a negative value."

Thus, plan managers would like to see an index with a negative, zero, or only slightly positive. As an example, the value of the index is created below for a hypothetical situation.

Given:
1. The employer provides three alternative health plans from which employees may choose; all plans provide exactly the same coverage/benefits package of services.
2. Of 200 employees, 60 choose plan X, 100 choose plan Y, and 40 choose plan Z, the HMO option.
3. Out-of-pocket contribution rates (monthly premiums paid by the employee) change by + $2.00 for plan X, − $1.00 for plan Y, and + $5.00 for the HMO plan Z.

Therefore:

4. The weights would equal 0.375 for plan X (60 divided by 160) and 0.625 for plan Y (100 divided by 160). Note that the number of individuals choosing a non-HMO plan is divided by the total choosing all non-HMO plans.
5. The change in the weighted average premiums for the alternative plans available to a subscriber of the HMO plan Z would equal $0.125 (or ($2.00 × 0.375) + (− $1.00 × 0.625)).
6. Thus, the index for the HMO plan Z would be $5.00 minus $0.125 or $4.875.

Comparing the index to an HMO-specific standard, the HMO manager could decide to modify plans for such a substantial, $5.00, out-of-pocket rate increase. For instance, the authors found in one HMO they studied that a $5.00 increase in an employee's monthly premium (relative to the average change in the employee's premium for all other available plans) led to a two-thirds increase in the HMO's disenrollment rate (or 69.7 subscribers per 1,000).[58] Disenrollment rates were lower for smaller monthly increases in relative premiums; for example a $1.00 per month increase resulted in 46.2 disenrollees per 1,000 when all other characteristics remained equal, or a rate of 4.62 percent. By defining an acceptable range of values for the index and monitoring the actual level of the index, the HMO manager should be able to make premium adjustment decisions vis-à-vis disenrollment more effectively.

---

[58] Ibid., p. 927.

Over the past 20 years, most HMOs must have had satisfied customers, because they had low turnover rates—from less than 1 percent to a high of 3 percent. The Kaiser programs have experienced current growth rates of up to 16 percent annually, with only a 2 percent disenrollment rate. Group Health Cooperative of Puget Sound has a disenrollment rate of less than 2 percent. Based on these data, HMO managers should continually monitor both enrollment and disenrollment rates to obtain broad estimates of consumer satisfaction with HMO programs. Levels of disenrollment below 3 percent can be considered acceptable. Higher levels suggest that the manager should evaluate programs and services to identify areas for improvement.

Special Consumer Groups

Throughout their history, HMOs have been concerned with the delivery of health services to special consumer groups—union or employer groups, groups of federal employees, Medicaid and Medicare recipients, underserved groups, or rural populations. P.L. 93-222 singled out several of these groups for special treatment, including medically underserved groups, rural groups, Native Americans, and domestic agricultural migratory and seasonal workers. In December 1973, the Secretary of Health, Education, and Welfare was authorized to reimburse qualifying HMOs for services rendered to Native Americans and migratory workers, as well as to set aside funds for and give preference to the development of HMOs in underserved and rural areas. In addition, as discussed in Chapter 5, several laws and their regulations addressed the provision of care to Medicare and Medicaid groups through HMOs. Because of the emphasis placed on these special groups, their attitudes and opinions and their special needs and desires must be considered. The following sections discuss two of these groups; two additional groups, Medicare and Medicaid recipients, are discussed in Chapter 5.

UNDERSERVED AREAS: THE RURAL POPULATION

The health care needs of people in rural areas are similar to those of people in urban areas. Their available health resources, however, are much more limited because of distance from, and lower per capita rates of, physicians. Limitations are most obvious in sparsely settled geographic areas and areas that are low in economic resources. While 90 percent of the nation's land continues to be inhabited by a little less than one-third of the nation's population, within this third are half of the nation's poor.

Poverty levels in rural areas can be better understood when one realizes that, among poor rural families, 70 percent exist on less than $5,000 per year.

Given the current planning constraints for HMO development, which set rural breakeven enrollment at a level of 20,000–30,000 subscribers and individual premiums at an average of $101.79 per month, it appears that HMOs are not the answer to the health problems of the rural poor. There are some examples of rural HMOs, however, that serve the nation's rural nonpoor—the Geisenger HMO of central Pennsylvania, Rural Health Associates of Maine, and the Northern Livingston Health Center in the Genessee Valley of New York, among others.

Many questions remain unanswered concerning an HMO's ability to develop and serve rural areas, and federal programs that aid in their establishment must deal with the following issues.

1. Developing and maintaining comprehensive service without sacrificing accessibility in terms of geographic access and family purchasing power and without denying rural consumers a realistic opportunity to share in decisions about matters that affect their health and their finances.

2. Establishing linkages between large and small centers to provide comprehensive services.

3. Maintaining a constant adequate flow of income from enrollees who get their income in lump sums once or twice a year rather than on a regular basis (weekly, biweekly, semimonthly, monthly, and so on); those who may be employed seasonally, sometimes with long periods of unemployment; those who may be affected by a general crop disaster in their area so that, although fully employed, they have little or no income in a given year; or those who may have subsistence-level incomes.

4. Maintaining an acceptable level of health services in rural areas with diminishing populations.

5. Overcomimg professional isolation and the poverty of social and cultural life in many rural areas to make them more attractive to professional health workers and their families.

6. Coping with development situations created by Medicare and Medicaid that make some of the present rural health care vendors unacceptable for participation under the program.

7. Developing more state Medicaid/HMO contractual relationships for rural populations.

8. Coping with the recurring threat of medical monopoly in rural areas.

9. Coping with high development and initial operating costs for HMOs serving rural areas that have great needs and that have been greatly underserved.

10. Developing total social programs for rural populations in addition to comprehensive HMO benefits packages, which singly will not bring community health to the area.

HMOs must be modified if they are to be effective in rural areas. During the planning stages, lower start-up enrollment and breakeven levels may be appropriate; initial enrollment levels in rural HMOs have been as low as 2,000–3,000 enrollees, and breakeven levels of operation may approach the 8,000–10,000 enrollment level rather than the urban 20,000–30,000 level. This suggests that the rural HMO must become even more efficient and cost-effective than its urban counterpart. Lower breakeven levels may require the following:

1. A less-comprehensive benefits package than that suggested by the HMO Act and its amendments, with a phase-in of additional benefits and point-of-service options as the plan increases its cash reserves.

2. Setting premiums at levels that will provide more funds for lower breakeven operation.

3. HMO catchment areas that will include larger geographic areas and, thus, longer travel distances and times for subscribers. HMOs may consider offering a transportation benefit, although, traditionally, rural families always have had to travel long distances for services.

4. Allowing HMO physicians to supplement either their own salaries or the plan's income by accepting fee-for-service patients. Tough management procedures would be necessary for control and for phasing out the fee-for-service practice as the capitated practice grows.

5. Planning by HMOs to include educational activities for major subscribers to explain the HMO concept and how to use the system, the efficacy of preventive health benefits, and why subscriber outlays for the HMOs will be larger than they were before joining the program.

6. Since the HMO would, in all probability, become the major health center for the region, the use of an existing hospital site would be most appropriate. This would require close coordination with the hospital and other local health providers.

7. The rural HMO must use all available federal and state support programs, including funds for categorical programs; funds created through negotiated contracts with Medicare and Medicaid agencies; funds for servicing federal employees, CHAMPUS recipients, migrant workers, and Native Americans; and contracts with the regional public health department to deliver both preventive and curative services. Although such funds are "soft money" that easily disappears, the federal and state programs could be used as an initial financial base, supplemented by subscribers who are not in funded projects. The goal of the rural HMO, however, should be to develop a mix of subscriber groups and fee-for-service activities rather than to depend on an enrollee population composed primarily of federal, state, and local government program recipients.

8. Management would have to use every available fiscal monitoring tech-

nique and stringent control procedures. Innovative fiscal programs are now available, such as those described in Chapter 11.

These eight points can be instrumental to the success of rural HMOs.

UNDERSERVED AREAS: THE URBAN POVERTY POPULATION

Are HMOs useful in providing services to poverty populations in major metropolitan areas? Before answering this question, several constraints placed on HMOs, concerning their participation with indigent populations, should be discussed. First, HMOs cannot be considered poor people's programs or poverty clinics; they must be able to maintain a mixture of subscriber groups and, indeed, a mix of indigent, commercial, and Medicare members to remain financially viable. The level of indigents usually accepted by an HMO should not exceed the level found in the general population. Second, poverty populations have a high need for health care, thus, are high users of health care facilities; they are considered high-risk groups, for which HMOs may not be willing to accept the financial risk. Finally, payments for services (benefits) may be limited, based on laws of and negotiations with state and federal assistance agencies.

The results of several Medicaid and Office of Economic Opportunity (OEO) programs indicate that if some restraint is used in the number of indigent persons enrolled in the HMO, there should be little or no added financial risk. Actuarial and underwriting activities certainly are an important aspect in the decision-making process concerning service to poverty populations, and somewhat greater resources must be made available for educational programs to teach this special group about the use of the system. The HMO should be able to deliver quality, comprehensive health services to indigent populations who are recipients of federal, state, and local government programs. No answer is currently available for providing services to those individuals who cannot pay premiums and for whom no government program has been established.

Consumer Participation Programs

Informed, knowledgeable, and active members can be a major asset for HMOs. They can help considerably in identifying problems and inadequacies in health programs and in ensuring that the solutions developed by the policymaking bodies are based on an awareness of consumer needs. In certain circumstances, members may help to determine overall policy and may participate in the strategic planning process. They most certainly are involved in opinion polls and patient satisfaction surveys. But members are involved less frequently in monitoring the delivery of health services and evaluating care from a clinical perspective in terms of accessibility, acceptability, comprehensiveness, and cost. Most importantly, consumers become spokespersons and salespersons for the HMO plan; they either encourage their friends to join the HMO or discourage them.

Consumer participation programs are developed around several basic elements:

1. A means of informing members about the HMO operation, programs, benefits and costs, choices, enrollment methods, complaint-handling procedures, and so on.

2. A program of member education and training that will lead to appropriate utilization of services and good health maintenance and prevention. Training sessions may be tailored to the orientation of enrollees who will participate on boards, consumer councils, or advisory committees.

3. A method of allowing members to augment their role as consumers in a free-market economy by participating in the decision-making process.

4. A mechanism for lodging and handling consumer complaints.

METHODS OF MEMBER PARTICIPATION

The first two of the aforementioned elements need little explanation. There are, however, several accepted methods for actual consumer participation and the handling of complaints. The consumer-model HMOs traditionally have been built on direct member involvement in the policy and decision-making processes through board of trustee representation. Although formal membership on a board does not ensure significant involvement, it does make the opportunity for participation explicitly clear and direct. HMOs like the Columbia Medical Plan, now a part of the Blue Cross-sponsored Free State HMO in Maryland, have established a consumer advisory council that provides input to the policymaking bodies of the plan. The advisory council has been successful in restructuring the benefits package as well as some operational aspects of the outpatient facility. Direct representation on internal management committees is another method of consumer participation. This form, used by Group Health Association of Washington, D.C., is one of the most effective ways for subscribers to share their insights with those who are directly responsible for the plan's day-to-day operation. It is also a valuable method for training and informing consumers and for providing immediate feedback to the subscriber group.

THE MEMBER COMPLAINT AND GRIEVANCE
RESOLUTION MECHANISM

Title XIII of the Public Health Service Act (P.L. 93-222, Section 130(c)7) requires that, to qualify as an HMO, a health plan must be organized to provide meaningful procedures for hearing and resolving grievances between the HMO and members of the participating organization. This and good management dictate that the development of a complaint mechanism is of great importance to the smooth operation of the health plan.

Studies of HMOs suggest four basic points for a responsive grievance system:

1. Providing information to members about the existence and procedures of the complaint mechanism

2. Identifying and broadly publicizing a primary entry point for complaints

3. Providing information to the complainant about each stage of referral undertaken by the complaint department and making available additional levels of referral and/or appeal

4. Establishing a standing grievance committee

There is critical need for mandatory arbitration regulations concerning all grievances in the health care industry, including a requirement for informal discussions, consultations, or conferences between the enrollee and the HMO within 30 days after the complaint is filed. If the problem is not resolved, mandatory hearings should be scheduled within 90 days after filing, so that grievances may be resolved before they become court cases.

Summary

HMO consumers are becoming more active in the development of health care policy and the evaluation of the health services product. This is the outcome not only of greater general consumer awareness but also (and more importantly) of the increasing number of individuals with health insurance, higher disposable incomes, higher living standards, and improved communications. Member participation is or will be felt in the areas of which health care product will be provided, the cost of care, method of financing, adequacy of manpower, quality of practice, organization of the delivery mechanism, policy formulations, and facility management.

A classic study conducted by Jerome L. Schwartz (see footnote 2) in six consumer cooperatives and six private physician health plans concluded that consumer participation changes with the age of the plan. An early tradition of cooperation can set the mode for participation; the size of the membership affects participation; and the influence of ordinary members is diminished when complex decisions are required to run large organizations. Moreover, Schwartz found that members who were active were usually from higher socioeconomic levels in the community.

Enrollment in HMOs by June 1990 exceeded 36 million people in some 614 health plans.[59] Membership growth rates dropped from an annual 15 to 20 percent to approximately 10 percent in 1988–1989. More than half (62 percent) of all HMO members are under age 40, 55 percent have household incomes exceeding $25,000, 63 percent are married, 66 percent are employed in organizations with 500 or fewer employees, and 52 percent do not have children under the age of 18. Over the last few years, the average age of HMO members has dropped. More white collar than blue collar workers enroll in HMOs.

The major purchasers of HMO products—businesses and unions—have been instrumental in helping HMOs develop, especially through their business or health coalitions. Employers are attempting to use managed care systems to help contain the 15 to 20 percent annual increases in health insurance premiums. Data for 1988 and 1989 suggest that HMOs had the lowest premium increases, while PPOs exhibited the highest increases. This suggests that HMOs are the best mechanism for employers in controlling increasing premium costs while PPOs are the least effective mechanism. PPOs, however, are growing more quickly than HMOs, possibly because of the health insurance industry's activities to expand more profitable lines of business.

Employers hold relatively positive attitudes regarding the HMOs they offer to employees; however, employers may face problems when sponsoring several health plans. It may be difficult to show any cost savings from offering the HMOs to employees, since HMO premiums may initially be higher than the traditional plans—but premiums may not increase as quickly for the HMOs. Offering the HMO option may mean that employers must track two or more health plans rather than just one, and the plans may face adverse selection, which could increase the employer's total health benefits costs. Finally, employers may not be convinced that the preventive benefits of the HMO will contribute to increased employee productivity or reduced absenteeism rates.

Four other indicators can be used in evaluating the level of consumer acceptance and the extent to which HMOs meet the expectation of subscribers—frequency of electing the HMO option under dual/multiple choice, subscriber opinion, frequency of use of outside services (leakages), and sub-

---

[59] Marion Merrell Dow, Inc. *Marion Merrell Dow Managed Care Digest, HMO Edition*. Kansas City, Mo., MMD, 1990, pp. 24–25.

scriber turnover or disenrollment rates. Generally, two competing health plans will achieve approximately equal enrollment during the first enrollment period, with one taking a definite lead over the other in the long run. People choose the HMO option because of greater security, lower costs, and better coverage, and the alternative plan because of greater physician choice. There is no appreciable adverse selection by enrollees in prepaid health plans, although non-HMO health plans are concerned that they are gradually enrolling more high-use members than their HMO counterparts. Choice of plans depends on the knowledge of availability of choice, the attributes and drawbacks of each plan, and the degree to which each attribute is of importance to the subscriber. Choice may also be influenced by the subscriber's perceived level of vulnerability to loss because of illness, but other factors—such as the premium level, a required switch of physicians, and the types of options available—may also have an effect on the potential subscriber's choice of health plans.

Overwhelmingly, members are satisfied with services provided by HMOs, with only some 6 to 8 percent expressing dissatisfaction; HMO members are more satisfied with the cost of the plan and the benefits and coverage than are members of traditional fee-for-service programs. Dissatisfaction with HMOs centers on the length of waiting times, the ability to see specialists, the level of physician conduct/humaneness exhibited by plan providers, difficulty in obtaining home visits, and problems common to medical practice in general. Prepaid group practice is perceived by patients as promoting the technical quality of care but hampering the establishment of a satisfactory personal relationship with the physicians. Use of outside services (i.e., leakages from the system) has been estimated at 15 to 37 percent of all services provided to plan subscribers. This outside use may be related to prior physician-patient relationships, dissatisfaction with plan services, greater convenience, and the type of health services desired—especially specialty care. Member opinions concerning the plan also are mirrored in its turnover rate. Levels of disenrollment below 3 percent are considered acceptable.

Service to underserved rural and urban poverty populations has presented special problems for HMOs. It is apparent that HMOs cannot be the single answer to the health problems of rural and urban poverty populations. HMOs were not developed to exclusively serve the needs of either the very poor or the very wealthy; they are more appropriately suited to provide health care to a cross-section of a community. With much care and planning, HMOs have successfully met the needs of these underserved groups together with other sectors of the community; however, there still is no solution to the problem of providing services to individuals unable to pay the premiums and for whom no governmental programs have been established.

HMO consumer participation programs are developed around four elements—a method of informing members of HMO procedures and policies, an education and training program, a method of participating in the decision-making process, and a consumer complaint system. Methods of participation include board of trustee representation, consumer advisory councils, and external management committees. Grievance resolution mechanisms are required by the HMO Act. Although various complaint mechanisms are used by HMOs, the use of a grievance committee and mandatory arbitration are limited to very few plans. Mandatory arbitration could be a method to settle grievance and malpractice problems before they become court cases.

References

Boxerman, Stuart B., and Virginia D. Hennelly. "Determinants of Disenrollment, Implications for HMO Managers." *Journal of Ambulatory Care Management, 6*(2): 12–23, May 1983.

Buchanan, Joan L., and Shan Cretin. "Risk Selection of Families Electing HMO Membership." *Medical Care, 24*(1):39–51, January 1986.

Davis, Allyson Ross; John E. Ware, Jr.; Robert H. Brook; Jane R. Peterson; and Joseph P. Newhouse. "Consumer Acceptance of Prepaid and Fee-for-Service Medical Care: Results from a Randomized Controlled Trial." *Health Services Research, 21*(3):429–452, August 1986.

Donabedian, Avedis. "An Evaluation of Prepaid Group Practice." *Inquiry, 6*(3):3–10, 20–25, September 1969.

Enthovan, Alain, and Richard Kronick. "A Consumer-choice Health Plan for the 1990's." *New England Journal of Medicine, 320*(2):94–101, June 12, 1989.

Gabel, Jon; Steven DiCarlo; Cynthia Sullivan; and Thomas Rice. "Employer-sponsored Health Insurance, 1989." *Health Affairs, 9*(3):161–175, Fall 1990.

Klegon, Douglas. "The Role of Consumer Attitudes and Preferences in the HMO Planning Process." *Journal of Health Care Marketing, 1*(3):20–31, Summer 1981.

Klett, Suzanne V. "Corporate America Opens the Door to Managed Care." *Medical World News, 27*(1):52–54, 59–63, 67–68, January 13, 1986.

Koba Associates, Inc. *HMO Consumer Complaint Mechanism.* Rockville, Md., Health Maintenance Organization Service, U.S. Department of Health, Education, and Welfare, 1974.

Long, Stephen H.; Russell F. Settle; and Charles W. Wrightson, Jr. "Employee Premiums, Availability of Alternative Plans, and HMO Disenrollment." *Medical Care, 26*(10):927–938, October 1988.

Louis Harris and Associates, Inc. *A Report Card on HMOs: 1980–1984.* Menlo Park, Calif., Henry J. Kaiser Family Foundation, 1984. Study No. 844003

Luft, Harold S. *Health Maintenance Organizations: Dimensions of Performance.* New York, John Wiley and Sons, 1981, Chapters 3, 11, and 12.

Pope, Clyde R. "Consumer Satisfaction in a Health Maintenance Organization." *Journal of Health and Social Behavior, 19*(3):291–303, September 1978.

Pope, Clyde R.; Donald K. Freeborn; and Sylvia Marks. "Perceived Access to Care and Patient Satisfaction in a Prepaid Group Practice HMO." *Group Health Journal,* 5(2):22–27, Fall 1984.

Rao, Tanniru R., and Maryam Chin. "Employer Attitides Toward Health Maintenance Organizations." *Health Care Management Review,* 7(1):57–66, Winter 1982.

Schwartz, Jerome L. *Medical Plans and Health Care.* Springfield, Ill., Charles C Thomas, Publisher, 1968, pp. 1–8, 44–64, 219–252.

Sorenson, Andrew A., and Richard P. Wersinger. "Factors Influencing Disenrollment from an HMO." *Medical Care, 19*(7):766–773, July 1981.

Sullivan, Cynthia B., and Thomas Rice. "The Health Insurance Picture in 1990." *Health Affairs, 10*(2):104–115, Summer 1991.

U.S. Department of Health, Education, and Welfare, Health Maintenance Organization Service, Office of Consumer Education and Information. "Development of a Consumer Program in Health Maintenance Organizations; A Position Paper." Rockville, Md., 1972. Mimeographed.

Wrightson, Charles W.; James Genuardi; and Sharman Stephens. "Demographic and Utilization Characteristics of HMO Disenrollees." *GHAA Journal, 8*(1):23–42, Summer 1987.

8

CONTROL, QUALITY AND UTILIZATION OF SERVICES, AND ACCOUNTABILITY

Historically, prepaid group practice plans and their successors—HMOs and CMPs—have been "number two" in their struggle to gain acceptance and recognition over the dominant fee-for-service health services delivery system. These alternative delivery systems and managed care organizations have been placed under a microscope and have become highly visible entities, with various external publics scrutinizing them to determine whether they measure up to the traditional system.[1] Delivery and financing performance standards are being applied to MCOs with greater frequency to determine whether the MCOs measure up to their reputations of being better managers of input resources and of generating higher quality outputs. As a result, managed care administrators have been forced to monitor the allocation and utilization of resources, the quality of services provided, and the outcomes of their systems so as to control their organizations and to survive in this ever competitive and regulated environment.

This chapter addresses control issues, with special emphasis on the external environment and the regulators, qualification processes and accreditation, and state regulatory activities. An HMO control model is described, as well as the use of a management information system (MIS), the setting of standards, and the process of evaluation. Finally, utilization review, quality assurance, and risk management as part of the control process are examined.

---

[1] Some of these analyses include Avedis Donabedian, *A Review of Some Experiences with Prepaid Group Practice,* Ann Arbor, Mich., School of Public Health, Bureau of Public Health Economics, University of Michigan, 1965, pp. 1–74, Research Series No. 12; National Academy of Sciences, Institute of Medicine, *Health Maintenance Organizations: Toward a Fair Market Test,* Washington, D.C., NAS, May 1974, IM Publ. No. 74-03; and Harold S. Luft, *Health Maintenance Organizations: Dimensions of Performance,* New York, John Wiley and Sons, 1981.

The Need for Control

Control is a management function that is common to all organizations; it denotes the activities of monitoring and evaluating the use of resources, the process of converting resources into medical services, and the analyses of the HMO results achieved, especially health maintenance. As described by the classical management theorists, the application of control processes is one of the major functions of successful managers; control is required if the organization is to operate efficiently and effectively, allowing the appropriate use of staff and other resources and facilitating the achievement of organizational goals and objectives. For managed care, the major objective is to achieve a financing/delivery system that provides cost-effective health services to an enrolled population. Measures of success in meeting this objective include an analysis of (1) the cost of service delivery versus the premiums collected, (2) the levels of consumer satisfaction and enrollment in the program, (3) the quality of care, as defined by the process of delivery, and the clinical outcome, and (4) the disability, morbidity, and mortality of the enrolled population. Good managers, therefore, will initiate and implement an ongoing, internal control process for measuring program outputs to ensure that they are consistent with desired objectives.

Control is vital in all managed care organizations because of the external pressures placed on them through federal and state regulatory activities, especially the HMO qualification and the CMP certification processes. Both the qualification and certification processes apply federal standards to the operation of the health services organization to determine its level of functioning, especially its ability to control the quality of services and its financial stability. For HMOs and CMPs, these processes place substantial external pressure on the health plan to ensure that it is not only operating in conformance with federal standards but also that it is monitoring and controlling plan operations to maintain future compliance with the standards.

In like fashion, most states have either passed special HMO-enabling legislation or placed HMOs and PPOs under the purview of the insurance commissioner, using existing state insurance laws. Such laws and regulations force managers to control their operations and maintain compliance with state-mandated standards. Some HMOs elect to complete the process for accreditation of their programs. Managers of these HMOs recognize the value of evaluating and appraising their operations through generally accepted standards created by the accrediting body—a process of voluntarily controlling the HMO with the hope of improving its ability to achieve health plan objectives.

HMO members, as part of the HMO family, often are the most important players in pressing the organization to control its operations. This occurs as potential members choose whether or not to enroll in the health plan, or when those enrolled for a period ultimately choose to disenroll—the free market in a competitive environment in operation. Membership, being the engine that drives the HMO, is a gauge of the manager's success in controlling plan activities. The mechanical problems that can occur with this engine are expressed not only as loss of membership, but also as complaints, grievances, or, most seriously, lawsuits brought against health plan physicians and the HMO itself. Thus, like all other health services organizations, prepaid health plans also must be concerned with the potential threat of malpractice issues; risk management for the HMO implies not only the control and management of insurance risks, but also the possibility that professionals in the plan will commit a professional, clinical act that will place the health plan at high risk of a lawsuit. The application of quality assurance and utilization review procedures to internal standards and standard operating procedures is one method of controlling the level of risk.

One final introductory word concerns *control* as applied to managed care organizations. All effective control systems are open-loop systems, that is, managers and other personnel in the health plan take corrective action when the results of operations are different than those expected. In addition, the system is information-based, in that data are collected on the input of resources, the process of converting inputs into health services, and the output/outcome from the health plan. With such information or feedback, managers can compare results to expected inputs, processes, and outputs and initiate appropriate action, if necessary. The model, therefore, follows the design provided in Figure 8-1. Control of inputs implies that during the strategic planning and budgetary processes, the manager has created standards concerning resources. These then become the baseline against which available resources are compared. For example, Figure 8-1 identifies levels of professional and paraprofessional staffing, inpatient and outpatient facilities, supplies, and capital as measurements of resource consumption in HMOs. Because controlling the quality of care depends largely on the quality of the providers, another useful input measure is an initial assessment of the provider's licensure and an ongoing assessment of his/her maintenance of proficiency and capabilities through annual credentialing activities. One further input assessment might be a review of the accreditation, state licensure, and federal Medicare certification of hospitals used by the health plan.

In controlling operations, the conversion process is perhaps the most difficult to handle, since this activity is somewhat less measurable and sometimes less tangible. Generally, expectations about the operation—sequencing of tasks, flow of work, timely decision making, clear communications—form the basis for analysis. Documents that describe appropriate operations include job descriptions and specifications, strategic and short-range plans, budgets, standard operating procedures, organizational charts, and statements of the

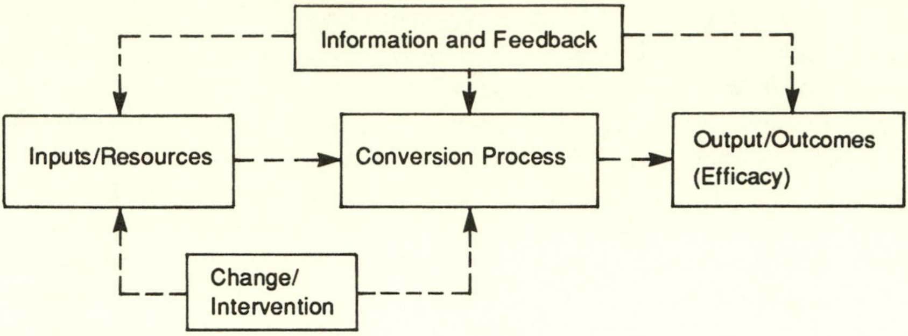

Areas where indicators/standards might be developed.

Inputs/Resources:
1. Physicians per 1,000 members
2. Paraprofessionals/physicians
3. Beds per 1,000 members
4. Office space (square feet) per physician
5. Supplies consumed
6. Capital consumed
7. Credentialing and licensure

Conversion Process:
1. Adherence to standard operating procedures and clinical protocols
2. Work systems for functions of the health plan, such as claims processing; management of inpatient utilization; electronic data processing; and budgeting and accounting, including financial record keeping, strategic planning, marketing and enrollment activities, account maintenance, and administrative and medical decision making
3. Specific job design and job specifications
4. Integration of work effort and communication channels, usually included in job descriptions and graphically exhibited on organizational charts
5. Decision making and delegation to subordinates, and methods of accountability
6. Suitability and timing of tests, treatment, and follow-up

Output/Outcomes:
1. Inpatient rates per 1,000 members per year
2. Ambulatory services per 1,000 members per year
3. Prescriptions per member per year
4. Average length of stay
5. Enrollment, reenrollment, and market share
6. Profitability and/or surplus from operations
7. Performance of stock companies
8. Medical records reviewed
9. Morbidity of members
10. Loss ratio by plan overall and by special member groups
11. Clinical outcomes of inpatient and outpatient services
12. Physician productivity (visits per time period)
13. Member satisfaction studies
14. Severity of illness
15. Paid hours per patient visit

FIGURE 8-1 HMO control system—measurements and interventions.

goals and objectives of the firm and the individual work units. Subjective measurements of managerial methods, practices, styles, and communication should be included in controlling the conversion process.

Finally, output and outcome measures can focus attention on both the quality and quantity of the work completed, services provided, and satisfaction with the health plan. The measurements that are most familiar include inpatient rates per 1,000 members, encounter rates by members, market share, numbers of enrollees, and so on. Significant measures of outcome and quality of services may also be used; these include comparing the actuarial estimates of rates of disease with actual rates of disease, comparing loss ratios of premiums collected to costs of services provided, and reviewing medical records of clinical outcomes for both inpatient and outpatient services provided to members. The ultimate measures of the MCO's success should include analyses of the financial success of the plan, its ability to provide quality services and maintain membership, and its maintenance of members' health, measured by both medical outcomes and patient satisfaction. Successful operation also requires control of the health plan's functions (insurance, financial, marketing, enrollment, etc.) and the medical services delivery functions; control of both functions is critical.

External Control: Accreditation

HMOs with a serious commitment to improving and controlling the quality of services may utilize the services of an extramural body that can objectively evaluate the performance of the HMO against standards applied to similar organizations. The ultimate goal of such activities is to improve performance through peer reviews that have as their basic feature the education and self-study of one's organization. Such reviews in managed care have been accomplished by one of three accrediting bodies: the Joint Commission on Accreditation of Healthcare Organizations (JCAHO), the Accreditation Association for Ambulatory Health Care (AAAHC), and the National Committee for Quality Assurance (NCQA). Each of these accrediting bodies uses similar survey standards and survey procedures, and each has a policy of limiting public disclosure of survey results.

JOINT COMMISSION ON ACCREDITATION OF HEALTHCARE ORGANIZATIONS

As the dominant accrediting institution in the health services industry, the Joint Commission on Accreditation of Healthcare Organizations was originally organized in 1913 by the American College of Surgeons; in the late 1940s, it merged with the American College of Physicians, the American Hospital Association, the American Medical Association, and the Canadian Medical Association. This merger was incorporated in 1951 as the Joint Commission on Accreditation of Hospitals (JCAH), with the hospital accreditation program starting in June 1952.[2]

In 1975, the American Group Practice Association (AGPA) and JCAH, along with the Group Health Association of America (GHAA) and the Medical Group Management Association (MGMA), formed the Accreditation Council for Ambulatory Health Care (AC/AHC). AC/AHC created an accreditation manual and a series of quality assurance educational conferences that were offered to freestanding ambulatory care organizations. But, by 1979, JCAH decided to dissolve the AC/AHC and its other councils to streamline and increase consistency among its accreditation efforts. Because of a loss of autonomy, AGPA, GHAA, and MGMA then severed their relationship with JCAH, and, along with the American College Health Association and the Free Standing Ambulatory Surgical Association, created the Accreditation Association for Ambulatory Health Care, Inc. (AAAHC).[3] In 1987, JCAH changed its name to JCAHO. JCAHO continues to offer accreditation to freestanding and hospital-sponsored ambulatory care centers, including ambulatory care clinics and surgery centers, emergency care centers, group practices, and primary care and urgent care centers. JCAHO accredited health maintenance organizations until mid-1989, when this program was terminated.

In the 1988 edition of the Joint Commission's *Accreditation Manual for Hospitals (AMH)*, the commission provides seven standards that are used to survey hospital-sponsored ambulatory care services. In addition, the commission has approved standards that are described in the *Ambulatory Health Care Standards Manual, 1988*, which have been used for accreditation purposes since January 1988. These standards address 16 areas that have an impact on the quality of services delivered. Finally, JCAHO has further identified five areas where HMOs are specifically examined. The seven standards in the *AMH* require that:

1. Ambulatory care services are provided safely, effectively, and in a manner designed to assure the quality of care.
2. Personnel are prepared for their responsibilities in the provision of ambulatory care through appropriate education and training.

---

[2] Arthur G. Isack. "Accreditation Council for Ambulatory Health Care." *Journal of Ambulatory Care Management, 1*(4):31–45, November 1978.

[3] Heather R. Palmer, *Ambulatory Health Care Evaluation—Principles and Practices,* Chicago, Ill., American Hospital Association, 1983, pp. 7 and 49; and Isack, "Accreditation Council for Ambulatory Health Care," pp. 33 and 50.

3. There are written policies and procedures that guide the provision of care.

4. The facilities used in the provision of care are designed and equipped to assure safe and effective care.

5. A medical record is maintained for every patient who receives ambulatory care.

6. Quality control mechanisms are established.

7. The quality and appropriateness of care are monitored and evaluated and identified problems are resolved.[4]

The *Ambulatory Health Care Standards Manual* applies to almost all ambulatory settings, including HMOs. It is designed to allow the user to perform a self-evaluation of services offered. As such, it is an effective management tool in determining the level of functioning and the quality of services that are being provided by the organization. JCAHO is quick to point out that self-evaluations should be conducted on a routine basis to continually assess areas needing improvement. In addition to evaluating HMOs, JCAHO suggests that five additional areas be examined: access to care, management structure, continuity of care, technical quality of care, and member satisfaction.[5]

Access to care is the patient's ability to make appointments with providers, including referral physicians, within a reasonable period of time and to be seen at all hours of the day, including emergency visits. *Management structure* suggests that the HMO has an effective quality assurance (QA) program, appropriately credentials its providers, ensures that its members are educated about the system, and provides a safe environment for the patient. *Continuity of care* is the HMO's process of maximizing the coordination of all care by ensuring that effective linkages exist between providers and that there are appropriate discharge planning procedures for patients who have been hospitalized. *Technical quality of care* addresses the actual technical or clinical competence of providers who deliver appropriate care according to professional standards. Further, the HMO must provide effective health education and preventive measures. Finally, *member satisfaction*, including both individual members and employers, and disenrollment analyses are also used to judge the quality of care.

JCAHO was relatively active in HMO accreditation between 1987 and 1989. During 1987, it contracted with the Prudential Insurance Company and Travelers Health Network of South Carolina to review the performance of their HMOs; standards were applied to determine appropriate structure and administrative and clinical processes. This project involved surveying up to 26 of the Prudential HMOs nationwide, as well as training 12 Prudential senior-level

---

[4] Joint Commission on Accreditation of Healthcare Organizations. *Accreditation Manual for Hospitals, 1988.* Chicago, Ill., JCAHO, 1988, pp. 67–73.

[5] Elizabeth Flanagan. "Five Standards for Evaluating HMO Quality." *Hospitals, 61*(3):88, February 5, 1987.

employees (vice presidents and medical directors) to help their HMOs maintain compliance with the standards. In April 1988, PruCare of Orlando, Florida, a 30,000-member group practice model HMO, became the first HMO to be accredited by JCAHO's new managed care standards; it received a three-year accreditation. In May 1988, the Blue Cross Association reached an agreement with JCAHO to review the quality of care in its 96 affiliated Blue Cross HMOs, covering 4.5 million members, over a three-year period. Keystone Health Plan West, Inc., Blue Cross of Western Pennsylvania's 48,000-member HMO, became the first HMO in Pennsylvania to receive a full three-year accreditation by JCAHO. Keystone is one of the 41 HMO-USA members that, as of July 1989, received JCAHO accreditation; HMO-USA is the national network of BC/BS HMOs located in some 200 cities across the country. In addition to these organizations, JCAHO has reviewed, but not accredited, HMOs for a few other clients, including the 11 Medicaid-contracting HMOs in Ohio and the Florida Health Care Plan, Inc., which is a 20,000-member staff model HMO in Daytona Beach, Florida.

The process of accreditation is similar in all accrediting organizations. Initially, each HMO voluntarily decides whether to attempt the process that ends with accreditation of its programs and facilities. Contact with the accrediting body provides an indication of suitability for accreditation. The accrediting organization makes available standards and a self-assessment manual to assist the organization in determining its readiness for a site visit. After submitting the self-study material to the accrediting organization, a determination is made to provide on-site reviews by volunteer reviewers. Depending on the accrediting organization, the team members may include physicians, registered nurses, administrators, lawyers, and the like. Site visits take two to three days, and the review may encompass all aspects of the HMO's operation. The visit may be concluded with a final (exit) meeting, with the reviewers providing some feedback to the health plan. Usually, the findings of the reviewers are provided to the accrediting body's accreditation committee, which then determines whether to accredit and the length of the accreditation. Written notification is then provided to the health plan. Most accreditation processes provide for an appeal if the accreditation decision is unfavorable.

ACCREDITATION ASSOCIATION FOR AMBULATORY HEALTH CARE, INC.

As previously noted, when JCAH dissolved its Accreditation Council on Ambulatory Health Care in 1979, the Accreditation Association for Ambulatory Care was created by the former AC/AHC members—the Group Health Association of America, Medical Group Management Association, and American Group Practice Association—and the American College Health Association and the Free Standing Ambulatory Surgical Association. Since AAAHC's founding, GHAA withdrew its membership to pursue evaluations of the quality of qualified HMOs but remains fully supportive of AAAHC's other efforts. The board of the association has been subsequently increased to include the American Academy of Facial Plastic and Reconstructive Surgery, the National Association for Ambulatory Care, and the American Society of Outpatient Surgeons.

Since 1979, AAAHC has accredited more than 100 HMOs and 300 ambulatory care centers, representing 2 million enrollees with 6,000 physicians.[6] AAAHC begins by examining the HMO's application before surveying to ensure that standards can be applied. Basically, the organization must be a formally organized and legally constituted entity that has been providing ambulatory health care services for at least six months, it must comply with applicable state and federal laws and regulations, and it must be under the direction of a physician or group of physicians who accept responsibility for services rendered. Standards cover 18 areas that are similar to those used by the Joint Commission, although they are written in general terms to allow an organization to meet the intent of the standards conducive with its particular situation. Usually, site surveys are conducted by three-member teams composed of two physicians and an administrator selected from a pool of 200 volunteers nationwide. If successful, the organization receives a one- to three-year accreditation, similar to that of JCAHO.

AAAHC has accredited CIGNA HealthPlan, Inc.'s staff, network, and group model HMOs, and has begun to accredit CIGNA's 19 IPA model HMOs; these IPA health plans cover approximately 1.2 million enrollees. CIGNA was the first multistate HMO to seek accreditation from AAAHC, with HMOs in Arizona, California, Florida, and Texas the first to be surveyed.[7]

THE NATIONAL COMMITTEE FOR QUALITY ASSURANCE (NCQA)

NCQA was incorporated in 1979 with the objective of developing standards specifically for HMOs. Original support was from the Medical Directors Division of GHAA and the American Medical Care and Review Association (AMCRA). Initial impetus came from a perceived need to evaluate the quality of care provided by federally qualified HMOs and partly because of an expressed need by the HMO industry for an HMO-specific quality assurance review methodology. NCQA attempts to satisfy HMO providers, through the accredita-

---

[6] Julie Johnsson. "HMOs Seek AAAHC Accreditation to Bolster Marketing, Recruiting." *Contract HealthCare*, p. 29, May 1988.

[7] Ibid.

tion process, that their delivery system is operating with an effective quality assurance program. It also attempts to provide federal and state governments, employers, and other purchasers with information about the level of quality services that are provided by the HMO.[8] As one might expect, the emphasis of NCQA is on the clinical aspects of service delivery, with physician members of the GHAA Medical Directors Division or physicians from IPAs or other managed care plans acting as reviewers. The reviewers try to determine whether there is an actual change in the HMO's delivery of care rather than just the existence of a QA structure. Additionally, they examine the number and work load of primary and specialty care physicians to determine the availability of care, ancillary support services, and hospitals that contract with the HMO. Some attempt is made to review convenience (for example, appointment availability and specialist referrals), credentialing procedures, and standards for obtaining continuing medical education. Additionally, enrollee acceptability of services is gauged by examining the grievance procedures and patient satisfaction survey results.[9]

Since 1980, NCQA has designed, developed, and applied an HMO-specific methodology for the examination of quality assurance programs. It has selected and trained 82 physicians who are HMO clinicians, and has conducted 60 assessments of HMOs. Many of these reviews were financed by the Office of Prepaid Health Care, Health Care Financing Administration, DHHS through three separate contracts; many occurred in the state of Pennsylvania. NCQA has been approved by the states of Pennsylvania and Kansas to review all HMOs that are licensed in those states. While these two states already have laws mandating external reviews, many other states either have or are expected to have similar laws; obviously, NCQA would like to be approved to conduct these reviews. Some reservations have been expressed, however, concerning the autonony and independence of NCQA as a fair and impartial reviewer, since by the composition of its support organizations, GHAA and AMCRA, it appears to represent the wishes and opinions of the HMO industry. Thus, NCQA has taken great precautions to ensure that its reviews are as objective and credible as possible. It has been actively seeking input from employers to determine their concerns regarding these reviews. Employers, it appears, feel that NCQA should generally not be concerned with governance and organizational structure but should instead address the entire process of identifying QA problems in HMOs and act as a clearinghouse of HMO quality, documented by an annual review process. Employers would like to see the results of surveys made public,

---

[8] National Committee for Quality Assurance. *Organizational Manuscript*. Washington, D.C., NCQA, Revised February 1986, pp. 1–2.

[9] Ibid., p. 12.

although accrediting organizations have always held that the results of surveys should only be provided to the surveyed organization. In 1989, nine Michigan HMOs joined an alliance of automakers and autoworkers to develop HMO quality guidelines. NCQA directed the project, using the guidelines that were developed to evaluate the performance of participating HMOs.[10]

QUALIFICATION AND CERTIFICATION

Although federal HMO qualification and CMP certification were discussed in Chapters 2 and 5, respectively, the process is reviewed here to create a perspective. As a review and accreditation process, qualification and its look-alike CMP certification activity follow procedures defined by the Health Care Financing Administration's Office of Prepaid Health Care (OPHC), which is responsible for administering them. There is a four-step application process that takes 100 to 120 days to complete once OPHC receives the completed application. After the HMO or CMP completes the 40-page application, OPHC performs a desk review in the areas of finance, marketing, law, health services, and management. Analysts then prepare a written report of their findings, highlighting issues and questions that can be discussed during a site visit. A team of up to six technical specialists in these areas spends two full days interviewing staff at the HMO and reviewing on-site documentation to verify information in the application. Although the team usually is composed of OPHC personnel, occasionally experts from the HMO field are asked to participate in the on-site reviews. Each reviewer prepares a final report that is submitted to the qualifications officer, who then prepares a comprehensive report and recommendation for the senior staff of OPHC. The director of OPHC's Office of Qualification can make three decisions—to "qualify" the HMO, provide a "60-day notice of intent to deny qualification," or decide on "denial of an application for qualification or eligibility." In the second situation, OPHC is implying that there are some barriers to qualification, but these problems usually can be resolved within a two-month period. In the last situation, the director informs the HMO of the deficiencies found and schedules a meeting to clarify the issues of concern and to determine what can be done to receive qualification. The HMO must then wait four months before reapplying.

Early qualification applications were free to the HMO, but because the federal program's qualification work load has increased and funds have become more limited, a fee for qualification is now required (like other accreditation programs). Additionally, as debate about the continuing need for the HMO Act increases, Congress may choose to terminate and dismantle,

---

[10] Howard Larkin. "Currents." *Hospitals,* *63*(11):54, June 5, 1989.

or sunset, the act as the current HMO amendments expire. If and when this occurs, some arrangements will have to be made to either continue the federal qualification process or to move to voluntary accreditation, such as the programs described above. The latter concept is gaining acceptance in the field.

OTHER REVIEW OPTIONS

In addition to the option of using one of the accreditation organizations and/or applying for federal qualification or certification, HMOs may have other options available to them. In some states, the licensing requirement includes quality review processes; Maryland, for instance, requires an active QA review process *initially* and *annually* for all HMOs in the state. The results of such state reviews are open to the public, unlike the more confidential processes of the accrediting bodies and federal agencies. Open disclosure allows the public to be aware of the HMOs that offer high-quality care, and it may allow HMOs to make comparisons of quality with other HMOs, adding to the intense competition among managed care organizations.

Another review option occurred when Congress granted sweeping powers to peer review organizations (PROs) to assess the quality of care rendered to HMO members; therefore, PROs may provide HMOs with quality review assistance. PRO review of HMOs was originally mandated by Congress in 1985 but was amended in the 1986 Omnibus Reconciliation Act to allow HMO-sponsored organizations to review HMOs. A second amendment required HCFA to allow such organizations, called quality review organizations (QRO), to bid for contracts to review HMOs in at least half of the states in the nation. The first round of bidding produced only one experienced bidder, Quality Quest, a peer review organization designed to review Medicare HMOs and CMPs, cofounded by the Foundation for Health Care Evaluation (a Minnesota PRO) and InterStudy (the HMO research group). Quality Quest has activities in Illinois, Missouri, and Kansas, while the Foundation for Health Care Evaluation provides Medicare HMO and CMP reviews in Minnesota, with assistance provided by InterStudy.[11] Another PRO, the Keystone Peer Review Organization in Pennsylvania, began its two-year cycle on January 1, 1987, with a second cycle beginning January 1, 1990.

Review by the PROs includes services rendered on or after April 1, 1987. Initially, PROs had to contend with a backlog of reviews, which may have added to their start-up difficulties, and HMOs had some problems in retrieving their

---

[11] Stephen H. Siegel, Phyllis M. Albritton, and Michael C. Thornhill, "PRO Review: Strategies for HMOs," *Group Health Association Journal,* 9(1):14–16, Fall 1988; and M. R. Traska, "Quality Quest Gears Up for HMO/CMP Review," *Hospitals, 61*(22):60, November 20, 1987.

older medical records. Not all HMOs, however, are included in PRO reviews; only HMOs and CMPs with risk contracts must submit to these reviews as a condition of such contracts. Those that do qualify find the review onerous; inpatient, outpatient, and other services provided by the health plan are reviewed for quality, completeness, timeliness, and appropriateness of care provided—including the appropriate level of care. Three levels of reviews have been created: limited, basic, and intensified. If the evaluation by the PRO finds that the HMO or CMP has an acceptable internal quality assurance program (based on the 1985 Quality Assurance Guidelines), its review may be at the limited or basic level. Intensified reviews are implemented only as a remedial measure, but they are an administrative nightmare for the health plan because of the data required by the PRO. If the PRO identifies a deficiency, the HMO/CMP is notified and given 30 days to comment. If the HMO/CMP does not respond or if the response is deemed unsatisfactory, the PRO may request a corrective action plan, due within 10 to 30 working days of the request, based on the complexity of the deficiency. If the health plan fails to develop or implement a corrective plan, the PRO may recommend sanctions to the Secretary of Health and Human Services that a civil monetary penalty be imposed on the HMO/CMP, or that official notice be published of the HMO's/CMP's substandard health care services. The PRO may also recommend to HCFA that it terminate or not renew the HMO's/CMP's Medicare contract. Sanctions and penalties on the health plan are severe and escalate quickly, unlike those that are imposed on other Medicare providers, especially hospitals. The HMO/CMP field has voiced reservations about the form and process of review procedures and the increased costs of such reviews. Consequently, these costs, along with limited capitation payments under the TEFRA program, have been the major reason for HMOs/CMPs to terminate or not renew their at-risk contracts with HCFA.

WHICH APPROACH: ACCREDITATION, QUALIFICATION, CERTIFICATION, OR PRO?

Many HMOs are motivated to be accreditated or reviewed by a federal agency or other outside agency for a number of reasons: as a marketing tool with employers and federal agencies such as Medicare, to enhance recruitment of physicians, to attract enrollees, to provide assurances that the HMO is well managed, and to obtain a Medicare at-risk contract, among others. Employers, enrollees, and governmental agencies, as the ultimate users of the information that might be obtained from accreditation or other reviews, need assurances that the review process is unbiased, timely, fair, and veracious. Even the prestigious JCAHO has been accused of apparent cursory reviews and delayed responses in its accreditation activities of hospitals. A *Wall Street Journal* article suggested that JCAHO may have allowed hospitals with significant violations to remain accredited and allowed others to remain accredited for various periods before being notified of review results, despite state inspections that revealed problems that caused subsequent state action to close these facilities.[12] During the interim, patients were placed in potential peril because of deficiencies that were not made public by the commission.

Although some employers rely on federal qualification as a means of determining which HMOs offer high-quality care, most feel accreditation fails to provide them with the information they are seeking about the quality of services and financial stability of the health plans. Many employers feel that accreditation should be only one of several factors, along with enrollee satisfaction and adequate grievance procedures, for them to consider when deciding whether to offer employees a new health plan. And many HMO managers hold the opinion that the quality assurance guidelines used by PROs for reviews are too onerous and the sanctions too harsh. While, on the one hand, the accreditation and qualification processes may not provide the depth of analysis and timeliness needed to assure ongoing high-level operations (and quality of services), on the other hand, the PRO reviews may be too rigorously applied, the process may be too difficult to carry out, and the cost to the health plan may be too high. Employers and other purchasers need to see evidence of outcomes rather than merely an accreditation certification. An appropriate quality/accreditation review process should be one that can be consistently applied across all HMOs and universally used to compare one HMO with others.

Since JCAHO decided to terminate its HMO accreditation activities in mid-1989, the other accreditation bodies have escalated their activities to assume the accreditation and qualification process of HMOs once the HMO Act sunsets. Whether the field will see a dominant accrediting organization emerge is still questionable.

Utilization

Control processes require that data regarding the operation of the health plan be collected through a management information system (MIS), which data can be used by the management team to steer the health plan to success. Although MIS requirements will be discussed later in this chapter, data regarding operating HMOs are provided in this section to describe the performance of an MIS in financing and delivery.

Data on utilization of physician and hospital services and pharmaceuticals can be obtained from several sources, including studies performed by the

---

[12] Walt Bogdanich. "Small Comfort—Prized by Hospitals, Accreditation Hides Perils Patients Face." *Wall Street Journal,* October 12, 1988, Section A, p. 1.

Group Health Association of America, InterStudy, the Office of Prepaid Health Care (Health Care Financing Administration, DHHS), and Marion Laboratories.[13] Each has developed its own methodology for collecting data. Because there are substantial definitional problems in the managed care field, for the purposes of this text the following definitions are used.

1. AMBULATORY TERMS:

   a. *Physician Visit:* A face-to-face contact between an HMO member and a physician who exercises independent judgment in the care and provision of health services.

   b. *Nonphysician Visit:* A face-to-face contact between an HMO member and a nonphysician provider who exercises independent judgment in the care and provision of health services.

   c. *Ambulatory Visit (Encounter):* A face-to-face contact between an HMO member and any provider (physician or nonphysician) who exercises independent judgment in the care and provision of health services.

2. HOSPITAL TERMS:

   a. *Hospital Days per 1,000 Members or People:* Rate of use of hospital services, obtained by dividing the total days of care provided during a year by the total population under consideration, and then multiplied by 1,000.

   b. *Hospital Days per 1,000 Cumulative Member Months:* A more precise measurement of hospital-day use, this rate is obtained by dividing the total days of hospital care provided during a year by the cumulative total of member months during that period, and then multiplied by 1,000. The cumulative member months (CMM) for 50,000 members continuously enrolled for 12 months would be 50,000 times 12, or 600,000 CMM.

   c. *Average Length of Stay (ALOS):* The average stay of inpatients during a specific period is derived by dividing the number of

---

[13] Greater reliance can be placed on the Marion data because these data are collected from all HMOs in the United States and compared against data reported to state insurance commissioners, while both InterStudy and GHAA's data are from plans that elect to participate; for example, only 33 percent of all HMOs in operation as of December 31, 1986, representing 58 percent of the nation's HMO enrollment, responded to the GHAA survey. Likewise, InterStudy's data are from 239 of 608 plans (39 percent of all HMOs) in 1987. It would appear, therefore, that the Marion data are the most reliable in representing all HMOs in the United States. Additionally, the strict reporting requirements for qualified HMOs add validity to the Office of Prepaid Health Care's data.

inpatient days by the number of admissions during the period, usually a year.

d. *Admissions per 1,000 Members or People:* The number of patients, excluding newborns, accepted for inpatient services during a year, divided by the total population under consideration and then multiplied by 1,000.

e. *Discharges per 1,000 Members or People:* Although the number of admissions to hospitals may differ slightly from those that are discharged, it will be assumed here that admissions and discharges are the same.

3. POPULATIONS:

a. *Members:* Anyone enrolled in an HMO and entitled to receive benefits; members may also be called enrollees.

b. *Commercial Members:* HMO members under age 65 are usually enrolled by virtue of employment (commerce).

c. *Medicare:* Individuals who are Medicare recipients and are enrolled in an HMO, usually through risk or cost contracts with the Health Care Financing Administration. For the purposes of this section, it will also be assumed that Medicare and "over age 65" are the same, unless otherwise noted.

d. *Medicaid:* Individuals who are Medicaid recipients and are enrolled in an HMO.

UTILIZATION OF PHYSICIAN SERVICES

Data on the use of physician services by HMO members for 1986 through 1989 are provided in Tables 8-1, 8-2, and 8-3. The conclusion that might be drawn is that members of HMOs use approximately 3.4 to 4.0 physician visits per member per year (PMPY), and that members of qualified HMOs use somewhat more physician visits than all HMOs—approximately 3.8 to 4.7 visits PMPY.

UTILIZATION OF NONPHYSICIAN SERVICES

The *Marion Managed Care Digest* provides information about nonphysician visits—services provided by nursing personnel, technicians, physician extenders, and so on. In Table 8-2, Marion reports that nonphysician visits averaged 3.7 PMPY for both 1986 and 1987, but increased to 3.8 visits in 1988, with a low of 2.1 in 1989.

Researchers for the *Marion Managed Care Digest* caution that there may have been some confusion regarding the definitions of *physician visits* and

TABLE 8-1   Utilization of Physician Services by HMO Model, 1986, 1987, 1988, and 1989: Under and Over Age 65

	1986 Marion			InterStudy		
HMO Model	<65	>65	All	<65	>65	All
Staff	—	—	3.7	3.7	6.7	3.9
Group	—	—	3.8	3.3	6.4	4.0
IPA	—	—	3.6	3.8	7.4	3.9
Network	—	—	3.9	4.1	8.7	4.1
U.S. Total	—	—	3.7	3.7	7.2	4.0

	1987 Marion			InterStudy		
HMO Model	<65	>65	All	<65	>65	All
Staff	—	—	4.0	3.2	7.4	3.7
Group	—	—	3.5	3.6	6.6	3.9
IPA	—	—	3.6	3.9	7.4	4.1
Network	—	—	4.0	3.9	7.4	3.9
U.S. Total	—	—	3.7	3.8	7.2	4.0

	1988 Marion			GHAA		
HMO Model	<65	>65	All* (Est.)	<65	>65	All* (Est.)
Staff	3.4	5.1	3.5	3.4	7.1	3.6
Group	3.6	4.8	3.7	3.4	5.9	3.8
IPA	3.7	4.8	3.8	4.0	7.4	4.1
Network	4.1	7.3	4.3	3.9	6.4	3.9
U.S. Total	3.7	5.0	3.8	3.7	6.9	4.0

	1989 Marion		
HMO Model	<65	>65	(Est.) All*
Staff	3.3	6.8	3.4
Group	3.3	6.4	3.4
IPA	3.4	6.4	3.5
Network	3.2	4.9	3.3
U.S. Total	3.3	6.2	3.4

*All physician visits in 1988 and 1989 were computed by applying the ratio of over age 65 to under age 65 enrollees in the survey. For 1988, of the total 33,715,500 enrollees, 1,661,547, or approximately 5 percent, were over age 65. For 1989, the ratio of total enrollees (35,031,160) to under age 65 members (1,515,745) shows that approximately 4.3 percent were over age 65.

SOURCE: Marion Merrell Dow, Inc., *Marion Managed Care Digest. HMO Edition*, Kansas City, Mo., MMD, 1987, pp. 32–33, 1988, pp. 24–25, 1989, pp. 24–25, 1990, pp. 24–25; Group Health Association of America, *HMO Industry Profile, Vol. 2, Utilization Patterns*, Washington, D.C., GHAA, 1988, pp. 23 and 29, 1990, p. 41; and InterStudy, *Trends in HMO Hospital and Ambulatory Utilization, 1981–1987* Excelsior, Minn., InterStudy, 1989, pp. 25–26.

TABLE 8-2   Utilization of Nonphysician Services and All Ambulatory Visits by HMO Model, 1986, 1987, 1988, and 1989: Under and Over Age 65

	Total Ambulatory Visits Per Member								
	Marion Managed Care Digest		InterStudy			GHAA			
HMO Model	Nonphysician Visits	All*	<65	>65	All*	<65	>65	All	
1986									
Staff	4.4	8.1	6.3	9.9	5.9	4.2	8.2	5.0	
Group	4.7	8.5	4.9	9.7	6.4	4.2	8.8	4.5	
IPA	3.2	6.8	4.6	8.5	4.8	4.2	8.1	4.6	
Network	3.7	7.6	4.5	8.7	4.8	4.6	8.2	4.9	
U.S. Total	3.7	7.4	4.9	9.1	5.2	4.3	8.3	4.7	
1987									
Staff	4.9	8.9	5.9	9.9	5.7	4.8	8.5	4.9	
Group	4.2	7.7	5.5	9.7	6.0	4.7	8.7	4.3	
IPA	3.4	7.0	4.9	8.5	5.1	4.8	10.0	5.3	
Network	3.5	7.5	4.5	8.7	4.6	4.5	6.6	4.5	
U.S. Total	3.7	7.4	4.5	9.1	5.1	4.7	9.0	4.9	

	Marion Managed Care Digest								
	Nonphysician Visits			Total Visits					
	<65	>65	All*	<65	>65	All*	<65	>65	All
1988									
Staff	3.7	3.8	3.7	7.1	8.5	7.2	5.1	9.9	5.3
Group	3.8	3.5	3.8	7.4	8.3	7.5	4.7	8.3	4.7
IPA	3.6	10.2	3.9	7.3	15.0	7.7	4.9	7.7	5.1
Network	5.8	7.1	5.9	9.9	14.4	10.2	4.8	8.9	5.0
U.S. Total	3.8	5.7	3.8	7.4	10.7	7.6	4.9	8.9	5.0
1989									
Staff	2.6	2.9	2.6	5.9	9.7	6.0			
Group	1.9	1.6	1.9	5.2	8.0	5.3			
IPA	3.6	10.2	3.9	7.3	15.0	7.7			
Network	2.5	4.3	2.6	5.7	9.2	5.8			
U.S. Total	2.1	3.0	2.1	5.4	9.2	5.5			

*Estimated.

NOTES: 1988 and 1989 data for InterStudy and 1989 data for GHAA were not available. See Table 8-1 for data on utilization of physician services.

SOURCE: Marion Merrell Dow, Inc., *Marion Managed Care Digest. HMO Edition*, Kansas City, Mo., MMD, 1987, pp. 32–33, 1988, pp. 24–25, 1989, pp. 24–25, 1990, pp. 24–25; Group Health Association of America, *HMO Industry Profile, Vol. 2, Utilization Patterns*, Washington, D.C., GHAA, 1988, pp. 23 and 29, 1990, pp. 12 and 40; and InterStudy, *Trends in HMO Hospital and Ambulatory Utilization, 1981–1987*, Excelsior, Minn., 1989, pp. 25–26.

TABLE 8-3 Annualized Incurred Physician and Total Visits per Member for Type A* and Type B* Federally Qualified HMOs

A. Physician Visits—Office of Health Maintenance Organizations:

	Commercial Members		Medicare Members		Medicaid Members		Total Members	
	A	B	A	B	A	B	A	B
1985	3.8	3.3	10.2	8.1	3.6	3.5	—	4.6
1st Q. 1986	3.9	2.3	8.8	7.7	4.1	3.6	—	4.7
2nd Q. 1986	4.1	—	11.1	—	4.1	—	—	—
3rd Q. 1986	4.0	—	9.7	—	5.6	—	—	—
Average 1986	4.0		9.9		4.6			

B. Physician Visits—InterStudy and GHAA

	Commercial Members	Medicare Members	Medicaid Members	Total Members
1986 InterStudy	3.7	7.2	—	3.8
1987 InterStudy	3.7	7.3	—	3.9
1988 GHAA	3.7	7.1	3.7	4.0
1989 GHAA				

C. Total Ambulatory Visits—Office of Health Maintenance Organizations:

	Commercial Members		Medicare Members		Medicaid Members		Total Members	
	A	B	A	B	A	B	A	B
1985	4.4	4.5	12.3	10.1	4.6	5.6	—	4.6
1st Q. 1986	4.7	4.6	10.8	9.3	4.7	5.5	—	4.7
2nd Q. 1986	4.9	—	14.1	—	4.8	—	—	—
3rd Q. 1986	4.6	—	11.5	—	4.7	—	—	—
Average 1986	4.7		12.1		4.7			

D.1. Total Ambulatory Visits—InterStudy and GHAA

	Commercial Members		Medicare Members		Medicaid Members		Total Members	
	Inter-Study	GHAA	Inter-Study	GHAA	Inter-Study	GHAA	Inter-Study	GHAA
1986	4.4	4.3	9.2	7.3	—	5.1	4.6	4.7
1987	4.6	4.3	10.1	7.3	—	4.1	4.8	4.7
1988	—	4.9	—	9.0	—	5.2	—	5.0

D.2. Total Ambulatory Visits—Marion Managed Care Digest

	Commercial	Medicare	Total (Est).
1988	7.4	10.7	7.6
1989	5.4	9.2	5.6

*Type A plans are federally qualified HMOs that have not achieved a net operating profit for three consecutive quarters plus a positive net worth, while Type B plans have achieved financial stability by meeting these criteria. As of April 1987, there were 281 Type A and 184 Type B plans, for a total of 465 federally qualified HMOs.

SOURCE: U.S. Department of Health and Human Services, Office of Health Maintenance Organizations, *Statistical Data for Type A and B Federally Qualified HMO Populations of the United States of America*, Washington, D.C., DHHS/OHMO, Loan Branch, Division of Compliance, 1985 and 1986; InterStudy, *Trends in HMO Hospital and Ambulatory Utilization, 1981–1987*, Excelsior, Minn., 1989, pp. 25–26; Marion Merrell Dow, Inc., *Marion Managed Care Digest. HMO Edition*, Kansas City, Mo., MMD, 1989, pp. 24–25, 1990, pp. 24–25; Group Health Association of America, *HMO Industry Profile, Vol. 2, Utilization Patterns*, Washington, D.C., GHAA , 1988, pp. 29 and 31; 1990, pp. 40 and 49.

ambulatory encounters in their questionnaire, which may have resulted in some double counting of the total visits provided in Table 8-2. Results of this double counting are shown in the Total Visits column. These figures are not comparable to those provided by GHAA and InterStudy and are discussed later in this section. But for the present, the conclusion is that *nonphysician visits* by HMO members will continue to be provided at a rate of 3.0 to 5.7 visits PMPY—a rate comparable to the use of physician visits by HMO members.

UTILIZATION OF PHYSICIAN SERVICES BY ELDERLY MEMBERS

These same sources and tables provide information on physician visits by HMO members under and over age 65. It might be concluded from the information shown that the overall use of physician services by over age 65 HMO members was from 5.0 to 6.2 physician visits PMPY (Table 8-1), although mature, federally qualified plans probably experienced a somewhat higher use rate by elderly members—7.1 to 11.1 (Table 8-3) physician visits PMPY.

UTILIZATION OF NONPHYSICIAN SERVICES BY THE ELDERLY

Medicare members' use of nonphysician services, as reported by Marion, showed approximately 5.7 nonphysician visits PMPY in 1988 and 3.0 in 1989 (Table 8-2).

ALL AMBULATORY UTILIZATION

If the Marion data for all ambulatory visits are not considered (because of the possible problem with double counting described previously), use by HMO members was approximately 4.7 to 5.2 ambulatory visits of all types PMPY (Tables 8-2 and 8-3). If only over age 65 members are considered, the data from GHAA , InterStudy, and Marion suggest that these members used from 8.3 to 10.7 ambulatory visits PMPY. The conclusion that might be drawn is that total ambulatory visits by all HMO subscribers should be around 5 visits PMPY; by over age 65/Medicare members, 9 visits PMPY; and by Medicaid members, about the same rate as total members—5 visits PMPY.

HOSPITAL UTILIZATION

Three measures of hospital use are provided in Tables 8-4 and 8-5, although the most important measurement is hospital days per 1,000 members or 1,000 cumulative member months. Hospital days per 1,000 members according to the

TABLE 8-4 Average Hospital Days per 1,000 Members by HMO Model, 1986, 1987, 1988, and 1989: Under and Over Age 65

HMO Model	Marion			1986 GHAA			InterStudy*		
	<65	>65	All	<65	>65	All	<65	>65	All
Staff			379.6	330	1,728	428	369	1,785	428
Group			382.5	345	1,714	452	328	1,630	441
IPA			402.0	394	1,703	417	397	1,962	469
Network			363.8	400	1,706	434	441	1,949	451
U.S. Total			388.3	375	1,710	440	394	1,855	455

HMO Model	Marion			1987 GHAA			Interstudy*		
	<65	>65	All	<65	>65	All	<65	>65	All
Staff			370.4	325	1,767	442	363	1,895	443
Group			368.6	319	1,735	404	354	1,708	474
IPA			381.7	379	1,667	429	389	2,007	440
Network			372.0	345	1,315	382	420	2,085	460
U.S. Total			377.2	356	1,641	417	388	1,945	449

HMO Model	1988 Marion			1989 Marion		
	<65	>65	All	<65	>65	All
Staff	380.3	1,753.6	—	362.3	1,704.1	—
Group	353.7	1,655.0	—	344.5	1,704.1	—
IPA	364.2	2,091.7	—	387.0	2,197.9	—
Network	361.0	1,486.3	—	348.1	1,884.6	—
U.S.Total	364.0	1,946.0	—	372.8	1,924.4	—

*CMM or cumulative member months.

SOURCE: Marion Merrell Dow, Inc., *Marion Managed Care Digest. HMO Edition*, Kansas City, Mo., MMD, 1987, pp. 32–33, 1988, pp. 24–25, 1989, pp. 24–25, 1990, pp. 24–25; Group Health Association of America, *HMO Industry Profile, Vol. 2, Utilization Patterns*, Washington, D.C., GHAA, 1988, pp. 25, 29, and 31; and InterStudy, *Trends in HMO Hospital and Ambulatory Utilization, 1981–1987* Excelsior, Minn., InterStudy, 1989, p. 8.

three sources provided in Table 8-4 range from a low of 377.2 days per 1,000 in 1987 to a high of 455 per 1,000 in 1986 (for all classes of HMO members). From Table 8-5, it appears that HMOs provide approximately 400 days per 1,000 of all members.

All sources listed in Table 8-5 consistently report that commercial, or under age 65 members, use less than 400 days per 1,000 members—ranging from a low of 356 to a high of 394. Over age 65 or Medicare members use substantially more hospital services; all sources report that this group uses 1,641 to 1,945 days per 1,000 members. Note that Medicare members, compared to all other

TABLE 8-5   Average Length of Hospital Stays (ALOS), Average Inpatient Days per 1,000 Members (or per Cumulative Member Months), and Discharges per 1,000 Members: All and Federally Qualified HMOs

ALOS in All HMOs— 1986, 1987, and 1988

	Total			Medicare			Medicaid		
Source	*1986*	*1987*	*1988*	*1986*	*1987*	*1988*	*1986*	*1987*	*1988*
GHAA	4.8	4.7	4.8	6.9	7.0	7.0	4.4	4.1	4.2
InterStudy	4.8	4.8	–	7.2	7.3	–	–	–	
U.S. Population: Government (All short-stay hospitals)	6.3	6.3	6.7	8.5	8.6	8.0	–	–	
U.S. Population: AHA (Community hospitals)	7.1	7.2	7.2	–	–	–	–	–	

ALOS in Federally Qualified HMOS—1985 and 1986

	Commercial		Medicare		Medicaid		Total	
Type	*A*	*B*	*A*	*B*	*A*	*B*	*A*	*B*
1985	4.4	–	7.1	9.5	3.6	7.8	4.5	–
1st Q. 1986	4.3	–	7.6	10.4	3.5	6.8	–	–
2nd Q. 1986	4.2	–	6.9	–	4.2	–	–	–
3rd Q. 1986	4.1	–	7.2	–	4.7	–	–	–
Average '86	4.2	–	7.2	10.4	4.1	6.8	–	–

Average Hospital Days per 1,000 in HMOS—1986, 1987, 1988, and 1989

	Total				Medicare			
Source	*1986*	*1987*	*1988*	*1989*	*1986*	*1987*	*1988*	*1989*
GHAA	440	417	438	–	1,710	1,641	1,932	–
InterStudy	445	449	–	–	1,855	1,945	–	–
Marion	388.3	377.2	–	–	–	–	1,946	1,925
U.S Population (All short-stay hospitals)	833.1	808.7	622.7	–	3,121	3,030	2,970	–

	Medicaid				Commercial			
Source	*1986*	*1987*	*1988*	*1989*	*1986*	*1987*	*1988*	*1989*
GHAA	482	483	529	–	375	356	358	–
InterStudy	–	–	–	–	394	388	–	–
Marion	–	–	–	–	–	–	364	372.8
U.S Population (All short-stay hospitals)	–	–	–	–	–	–	519	–

TABLE 8-5 *Continued*

Annualized Incurred Hospital Days per 1,000 in Federally Qualified HMOs—1985 and 1986

	Commercial		Medicare		Medicaid		Total	
Type	A	B	A	B	A	B	A	B
1985	349	322	1,935	1,832	352	475	–	410.6
1st Q. 1986	360	310	1,962	1,730	302	477	–	403.8
2nd Q. 1986	360	–	1,903	–	350	–	–	–
3rd Q. 1986	368	–	1,921	–	407	–	–	–
Average 1986	363	310	1,929	1,730	353	477	–	403.8

Discharges per 1,000—1986, 1987, 1988, and 1989

	Total				Medicare			
Source	1986	1987	1988	1989	1986	1987	1988	1989
GHAA	92	90	92	–	265	271	269	
U.S. Population	132.8	127.9	93.4	–	367.3	350.5	334.1	–

	Medicaid				Commercial			
Source	1986	1987	1988	1989	1986	1987	1988	1989
GHAA	118.6	122.6	128.9	–	85	82	82	–
U.S. Population	–	–	–	–	–	–	95.6	–

SOURCE: American Hospital Association, *Hospital Statistics,* Chicago, Ill., AHA, 1988, p. xxvi; _____, *Hospital Statistics,* Chicago, Ill., AHA, 1989, p. xxiv; U.S. Department of Health and Human Services, National Center for Health Statistics, *Health United States 1988,* Hyattsville, Md., DHHS/NCHS, 1989, p. 112; _____, *Health United States 1989,* Hyattsville, Md., DHHS/NCHS, 1990, p. 183; Marion Merrell Dow, Inc., *Marion Managed Care Digest. HMO Edition,* Kansas City, Mo., 1989, p. 24, 1990, pp. 24–25; U.S. Department of Health and Human Services, Office of Health Maintenance Organizations, Loan Branch, Division of Compliance, *Statistical Data for Type A and B Federally Qualified HMO Populations of the United States of America,* Washington, D.C., DHHS/OHMO, 1985 and 1986; Group Health Association of America, *HMO Industry Profile,* Washington, D.C., GHAA, 1988, pp. 5–9, 11, 15, 25, and 31; and _____, *HMO Industry Profile,* 1990 ed., Washington, D.C., GHAA, 1990, pp. 8, 10, 12 and 46.

HMO members, use *four to five times* the number of hospital days per 1,000 members. Data regarding Medicaid members' hospital use are limited.

Another indicator of inpatient use in Table 8-5 is the average length of stay (ALOS). Commercial members show a shorter length of stay, around 4.2 days, while Medicare members show a longer than average stay, 6.9 to 10.4 days. Data regarding Medicaid members are too variable to arrive at even a general conclusion regarding ALOS. Discharges or admissions per 1,000 population also are reported in Table 8-5. For HMOs, GHAA data suggest that all members have a rate of approximately 90 discharges from hospitals per 1,000 members, with

TABLE 8-6   Average Pharmaceutical Services Used by HMO Members and the Average Cost per Prescription Filled by HMOs: 1988

Model type	Number of plans	Prescriptions filled per member per year	Number of plans	Average ingredient cost/prescription
Staff	9	4.86	8	$ 9.50
Group	12	5.54	9	11.10
IPA	55	4.74	46	11.70
Network	14	4.94	14	12.20
U.S.Total	90	4.89	77	11.50

SOURCE: Marion Merrell Dow, Inc. *Marion Managed Care Digest. HMO Pharmacy Edition.* Kansas City, Mo., MMD, 1989, p. 12.

commercial members somewhat lower at 82 discharges per 1,000 members and Medicare members substantially higher at 265 to 271 discharges per 1,000 members.

PHARMACEUTICAL UTILIZATION

The *Marion Managed Care Digest* provides data regarding drug use in a sample of HMOs by model. In Table 8-6, the data suggest that, on average, HMO members use approximately five prescriptions per member per year at an average 1988 cost (of ingredients) of $11.50.

COMPARISON OF UTILIZATION IN HMO AND FEE-FOR-SERVICE (FFS) SETTINGS

Hospital services account for approximately one half of all health expenditures in the United States; therefore, a reduction in hospital services would offer the greatest potential for cost savings in health spending. HMOs and other managed care organizations have attempted to maximize savings by reducing overall hospital utilization.

Generally, HMO members use considerably less services than the U.S. population as a whole. HMOs have lower physician-to-population and hospital bed-to-population ratios than the general population in the United States. HMOs tend to staff their health centers in the range of 1 physician to 1,000–1,100 members (see Table 6-5, Chapter 6). Conversely, in the United States generally, the range of physicians to population averages 1 physician to 420 people. Given the financial incentives to provide additional services and the abundance of physicians in FFS, significant pressure is created for the delivery of more health services—some of which may be unnecessary. Similar relationships occur in the availability of hospital resources; for example, although the ratio of beds to population in the United States is 5.8 per 1,000, HMOs planning for hospital services or that own and/or operate hospitals use a ratio of 1.5 to 2.0 beds per 1,000 enrollees. Some researchers suggest that cost savings in HMOs are due in part to the more limited availability of providers in those settings as compared to FFS—a reverse of Roemer's Law;[14] Roemer suggests that if hospital beds are available, they will be filled. As a reverse of this law, the HMO clearly needs and plans for fewer beds than FFS and, consequently, uses fewer hospital days per 1,000 population than do FFS systems. Whether the lower use of hospital days can be attributed to the availability of fewer beds, a change in physician admitting behavior, unique characteristics of HMO members, or all three factors, HMOs appear to be achieving their objectives of equal or better quality care than the FFS system, using fewer resources. Some experts suggest that HMOs achieve these results (that is, shorter average length of stay in hospitals, fewer inpatient days, and fewer of their members admitted to hospitals than the U.S. population as a whole) by choosing other alternatives to inpatient care, by admitting only critically ill members, by enrolling lower risk people who will need less hospital care, and by more effective management techniques, including preadmission authorization. Whatever the reasons, HMOs use fewer hospital resources than the traditional FFS system without compromising the quality of services and medical attention to members who need care.

Other writers suggest that HMOs substitute outpatient services for hospital services. If, indeed, this does occur, one would expect that the use of physician services in HMO settings would be higher than that experienced in the U.S. population as a whole; however, all HMO members averaged approximately 3.8 to 4.0 physician visits per member per year while the general population averaged 4.7 physician visits per person per year in 1987.[15] Similarly, physician visits by HMO members over age 65 ranged from 5.0 to 7.2 visits per member

---

[14] Milton I. Roemer. "Bed Supply and Hospital Utilization: A National Experiment." *Hospitals*, 35(22):36–42, November 1961.

[15] Data reported from the National Health Interview Survey (U.S. Department of Health and Human Services, National Center for Health Statistics, *Health United States, 1988*, Hyattsville, Md., DHHS/NCHS, 1989, p. 106) for physician contacts was adjusted to remove telephone contacts. Physician contacts in 1987 were reported to be 5.4 per person; telephone physician contacts were 0.7 per person, with the remaining 4.7 visits comparable to those physician services provided by HMOs. It is interesting to note that some experts compare physician use by HMO members to the U.S. population physician services, based on the results of the National Ambulatory Medical Care Survey (National Center for Health Statistics, Hyattsville, Md., U.S. Department of Health and Human Services, Public Health Service, 1986). In this survey, for 1985, U.S. citizens generally used approximately 2.7 visits to physicians, but *only* in the physicians' offices and not including emergency rooms, hospital outpatient departments, at home, and so on. They then fallaciously conclude that HMO members use more physician services than do people in the United States generally.

per year, while the National Center for Health Statistics reported that people over age 65 in the general population used 7.8 visits per person per year in 1987.[16] The rate of use of physician services by all HMO members and the under age 65 population in HMOs was less than the U.S. population as a whole—from one visit annually for all members to almost three visits annually for the over age 65 members. It might be stated that the rate of physician services for all HMO members is generally similar to that found in the U.S. population as a whole; however, over age 65 HMO members appear to use substantially fewer physician services than the general U.S. population. These lower HMO member use rates may be explained by changes in physician practice patterns, educational efforts to change patient behavior in the system, incentives for both physicians and members to be wise users of health services, membership selection through selective marketing techniques, and the like.

The result, however, is substantial reductions in health plan costs for HMOs. The magnitude of these savings can be seen in the following example. Assuming that the HMO saves approximately half the hospital days over the traditional FFS system and that the all-inclusive cost of a hospital day is $800, at 400 days per 1,000 members, the HMO achieves a $320,000 savings yearly for 1,000 members. If plan members use one physician visit less than FFS individuals, and each visit is $30, then the HMO saves $30,000 for these physician services. Total yearly savings per 1,000 HMO members for hospital and physician services only would be $350,000. For 50,000 members the HMO would experience a $17.5 million savings annually over traditional FFS systems. Obviously, the HMO will have other costs that may reduce these savings, but it is realistic to assume that HMOs do provide the potential for cost-effective delivery of services with reasonable quality assurances. A more detailed discussion of studies concerning utilization in HMOs and the economic consequences of such use of services is provided in Chapter 11.

Evaluation: MIS, Standards, and Rules-of-Thumb[17]

Because managed care systems, especially HMOs, are sensitive to even the smallest change in the use of benefits and services, HMO managers have a special need to understand, evaluate, and control HMO operations. Systems for data collection and the development of standards of operation based on rules-of-thumb about general HMO operations provide assistance in these control

---

[16] Ibid.

[17] This section is adapted from "Controlling HMO Operation" by Robert G. Shouldice, *Medical Group Management,* *34*(4):8–12, July/August 1987.

TABLE 8-7 Sample HMO Operating Standards

Factor	Range or Value	Reference Chapter
Utilization		
1. Physician Visits PMPY	a. All Members: 3.8 to 4.0	8
	b. Commercial: 3.7	8
	c. Federally Qualified, All: 4.6	8
	d. Over Age 65: 5.0 to 7.2	8
	e. Medicare: 7.2	8
	f. Medicaid: 3.6 to 4.6	8
2. Nonphysician Visits PMPY	a. All Members: 3.8	8
	b. Commercial: 3.7	8
	c. Over Age 65: 5.7	8
3. All Ambulatory Visits PMPY	a. All members: 5.0	8
	b. Commercial: 4.3 to 4.6	8
	c. Federally Qualified, All: 4.7	8
	d. Over Age 65: 9.0	8
	e. Medicare: 9.5	8
	f. Medicaid: 5.0	8
4. Hospital Days/1,000 Members	a. All members: 400	8
	b. Commercial: 356 to 394	8
	c. Federally Qualified, All: 400	8
	d. Over Age 65: 1,750 to 2,000	8
	e. Medicare: 1,750 to 2,000	8
	f. Medicaid: 475	8
5. Average Length of Stay (days)	a. All Members: 4.8	8
	b. Commercial: 4.5	8
	c. Medicare: 7.2 to 10.4	8
6. Discharges/1,000 Members	a. All Members: 90	8
	b. Commercial: 83	8
	c. Medicare: 265 to 270	8
	d. Medicaid: 120	8
7. Prescriptions Filled PMPY	All Members: 4.89	8
Financial		
8. Average Ingredient Cost/Rx	All members: $11.50	8
9. Distribution of Expenses	a. Physicians: 35% to 45%	11
	b. Hospital: 25% to 35%	11
	c. Administation: 12% to 15%	11
	d. Other: 10% to 15%	11
10. Reserves	0 to 25% of premiums	11
11. Actual Income PMPM	$68 (1986 Federally Qualified HMOs)	11
12. Actual Expenses PMPM	$71 (1986 Federally Qualified HMOs)	11

TABLE 8-7   *(Continued)*

Factor	Range or Value	Reference Chapter
13. Premium Income as a Percentage of Total Income	80% to 90%	11
14. Actual Total Income as a Percentage of Actual Total Expenses	At least 100%	11
15. Health Care Expense Ratio: Health Care Expense/Total Health Care Revenue	80% to 90%	11
16. Net Worth: Net Worth Plus Subordinated Liabilities, Minus Intangible Assets	Positive	11
17. Operating Margin: (Premium-Benefits)/Premiums	11.8%	11
18. Return on Sales: After-Tax Net Income/Premium Revenues	2.1%	11
19. Return on Equity: After-Tax Net Income/(Reserves/Equity)	29.5%	11
20. Return on Total Assets: After-Tax Net Income/Total Assets	7.6%	11
21. Average Collection Period (in days): Accounts Receivable/Average Daily Sales or Premiums/365	17.9 days	11
22. Current Ratio (times): Current Assets/Current Liabilities	1.0 to 1.5	11
23. Debt/Equity Ratio (times): Total Debt/(Reserves/Equity)	2.9	11
24. Debt Service Coverage (times): (After-Tax Net Income plus Interest Expense plus Depreciation)/Debt Service Requirement	3.0	11
25. Profit Margin: Net Income/Total Revenue	Positive	11
26. Incurred but not Reported Expenses	50% of outstanding claims collected at end of second month following services, 85% collected after the third month, and 98% collected after the fifth month	11
27. Cash Management	Cash and liquid assets available equal to two months operating expenses	11
Staffing and Personnel Performance		
28. Average Weekly Workload and Amount of Time Spent with Patients	HMO physicians, on average, work 48.9 hours per week, provide 44.3 patient care hours per week, provide 103 office visits per week, and provide 24.9 hospital visits per week	6

TABLE 8-7 *(Continued)*

Factor	Range or Value	Reference Chapter
29. Physician to Member Ratio	1:1,000 to 1:1,100	6 and 8
30. Family Practice to Member Ratio	1:2,500	6
31. Nonphysician FTE Staff per MD	5 to 5.3	6
32. Business, Clerical, and Administrative FTE Personnel per Physician	1.35	6
32. FTE Paramedical Personnel (Excluding Radiology and Laboratory) per Physician	3.5	6
33. Ratio of Full-time Employees to Members	1 Employee to 2,097 members	6
34. Ratio of Business and Finance Personnel to Members	2.75 employees, plus 1 employee for every 3,125 new members	6
35. Ratio of Data Processing Staff to Members	2 employees, plus 1 employee for every 10,000 new members up to 50,000 members	6
37. Paid Hours per Patient Visit		11
Facilities, Supplies, and Equipment		
38. Hospital Beds per 1,000 Members	1.5 to 2.0	8
Insurance and Actuarial/Underwriting		
39. Claims to Loss Ratio (Claims/Loss)	<85%	11
40. Annual Premium Increases	<or = 8%	7
41. Average Monthly Single Member's Premium	$90–$95 (1988)	7
42. Average Monthly Family Premium	$203–$225 (1988)	7
Marketing		
43. Consumer Satisfaction with Services	>90%	7
44. Dissatisfaction with Waiting Time	<30%	7
45. Employers Stating that HMO Decreased Their Employee Health Care Costs	>30%	7
46. Employers Stating that HMO Created Adverse Selection for Their Regular Health Plans Offered	<20%	7
47. Employers Satisfied with HMO's Medical Services	>85%	7
48. Percent of All Medical Services Used Out-of-Plan	<15%	7
49. Percent of Members Using at Least One Visit Out-of-Plan	<20%	7
50. Annual Disenrollment Rate	<3%	7

activities. Data collected over the last decade have become the basis of several rules-of-thumb that managers can use to gauge their operations in comparison to other HMOs in the managed care field. They are the very basis of all budgeting activities and many actuarial analyses. These values may also be helpful during the strategic planning and development phases of HMO activity, while setting assumptions, and during the negotiation of HMO capitation rates with providers. Based on the data provided earlier in this chapter and in other sections of this text, standards for evaluating HMO performance may be developed. The items in Table 8-7 provide a starting point for developing individualized HMO operating standards; they should be used by managers only as guides. The reference chapter is provided to help direct the reader to a more complete discussion of the factor.

In the section that follows, a method for assessment using operating standards is described.

ASSESSMENT, EVALUATION, AND MANAGEMENT INFORMATION SYSTEM (MIS)

As part of the control process, managers periodically assess the operations of the health plan's activities. Assessment is an ongoing process that provides an opportunity to question whether the organization is meeting expected objectives and whether corrective actions need to be taken. As shown in Figure 8-1, the assessment component of the control process includes several steps. Initially, management will develop goals and objectives for the health plan. These will be implemented through the identification of standards and indicators of performance that help describe appropriate and acceptable levels of performance; in Figure 8-2, this is described as expected performance. In effect, these levels are identified during the planning process for inputs, the conversion process, and outputs. Note that sample indicators are provided earlier in this chapter, in Figure 8-1.

As health plan activities commence and services are provided, performance data and the results of operation are collected via a management information system. These data are compared against the expected standards initially set during the planning stage. Evaluations and appraisals then occur; management questions whether the results and levels of performance meet the expectations and organizational standards. In some situations, expectations will be met and even exceeded; in those cases, the standard may appear to be set at appropriate levels and management may want to set higher performance standards to provide a modest incentive for staff to continue improving performance. Where operations fall short of expectations, management will want to ascertain the cause and take corrective action.

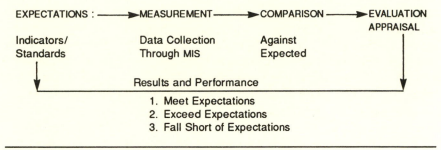

FIGURE 8-2   The assessment component of control.

An effective evaluation component of a control system must be supported by a management information system that allows for efficient and timely data acquisition and analyses. A management information system is a network of communication channels that acquires, retrieves, processes, and redistributes data that are used to manage and in support of evaluation and decision-making processes.[18] It is used to accumulate data to meet the internal and external needs of the organization. This is accomplished by processing data generated by the subsystems within the health plan and center. These include the financial management system, medical records system, membership and enrollment records, patient information system, and so on. It may be a fully computerized processing activity or computer-assisted manual system. But most importantly, it must be built around the needs of managers to manage and control operations. Specifically, it must meet two distinct requirements.[19]

1. Provide an integrated data base for the collection of all patient treatment information and member-related data that are needed to provide and monitor patient services. These data should include:

    a. Quality assurance
    b. Facility and staff planning
    c. Relationships with providers and institutions
    d. Patient and physician education
    e. Member and employer group relations
    f. Member group premium negotiations

---

[18] Patricia A. Neal. *Management Information Systems for the Fee-for-Service/Prepaid Medical Group.* Denver, Colo., Center for Research in Ambulatory Health Care Administration, 1983, p. 12.

[19] Ibid., pp. 13 and 14.

2. Provide reporting that meets distinct management needs in the following areas:

    a. Management of each functional area
    b. Financial management and planning
    c. Management reporting to meet outside reporting requirements
    d. Marketing intelligence and analyses

Although there are many MIS vendors in the managed care field, and many more "home grown" systems, most management information systems are based on several subsystems. A useful MIS will allow each of these subsystems to operate independently, but will also provide interface among the subsystems.[20] These include a:

1. HMO membership system
2. Claims processing and reporting system
3. Patient accounts receivable system
4. Utilization reporting system
5. Financial information system
6. An integrated patient information system
7. (Clinical) quality assurance system
8. Patient satisfaction system

With this lineup of subsystems, one might wonder if the results are worth the cost involved in their operation. Managers should determine the cost-benefit of the MIS by considering the businesses carried on by the HMO, the functions managed, the various processing alternatives available, and their costs. Obviously, the HMO will need accurate and timely data if it is to survive; therefore, a minimum set of data elements will need to be collected and analyzed, on which action will be taken. If the health plan is to perform a credible quality assurance program, data elements associated with its operation must be included in the MIS. Like all other plan activities, however, management must determine the minimum and optimum MIS activity that will provide for successful operations.

Quality of Care

Although the primary concern of medical care personnel has always been the delivery of quality medical care, several related forces have pushed the quality

---

[20] Ibid., p. 31.

issue higher on their lists of priorities. The first is the growing number of malpractice suits. In particular, the Darling and Brune cases clearly established the necessity for providing the highest level of care for all patients, at all times, and ensuring that this high level of care be one of excellence, not merely one of local practice.[21]

The second force is the demand for high standards of care by enrollees and the major buyers of HMO products. HMO members, their employers, the Federal Government and third party fiscal intermediaries, and affiliated insurance companies will more frequently use the measurement of quality, not just price, as a major criterion for purchasing HMO health coverage. More importantly, consumers can, by dropping out of a plan, register their dissatisfaction with the care rendered or, through formal review procedures and malpractice actions, become involved in evaluating the levels of care provided by a plan. Philosophically, the HMO and other managed care programs are continually faced with the conflict between controlling utilization and the probability that such control compromises the quality of care.

A third force is public concern about quality in the health care industry, where reductions in revenues may squeeze quality—especially in HMOs, where one of the corporate objectives is controlling costs while maintaining competitive premiums. If we are to see increases in quality over existing levels, HMOs will need to increase revenues while holding the line on costs, even though the field is experiencing inflationary forces. It is natural, then, that a discussion of quality be included in a chapter concerning control of HMO activities.[22]

Major criticisms about the quality of care provided by HMOs have concerned health plan proponents. These arguments suggest that HMOs use poorly trained doctors who join an HMO because it offers a safe, comfortable place to make a living; that HMOs provide less than adequate amounts of care because of capitation payments that reverse the physician's traditional fee-for-service incentive; that HMOs use mostly moonlighting residents or foreign-trained

---

[21] *Darling v. Charleston Community Hospital*, 33 Ill. 2d 326, 211 N.E. 2d 253, 1965; and *Brune v. Belinkoff*, 354 Mass. 102, N.E. 2d 793, 1968.

[22] This discussion provides only a brief review of the conceptual framework that has evolved in the quality assessment and assurance area. For an excellent review of quality-of-care issues, see Mary Helen Shortridge, "Quality of Medical Care in an Outpatient Setting," *Medical Care, XII*(4):283–300, April 1974; Avedis Donabedian, *A Guide to Medical Care Administration, Vol. 2—Medical Care Appraisal—Quality and Utilization*, New York, American Public Health Association, 1969; _____, *Explorations in Quality Assessment and Monitoring, Vol. I—The Definition of Quality and Approaches to Its Assessment*, Ann Arbor, Mich., Health Administration Press, 1980; _____, *Explorations in Quality Assessment and Monitoring, Vol. II—The Criteria and Standards of Quality*, Ann Arbor, Mich., Health Administration Press, 1982; _____, *The Methods and Findings of Quality Assessment and Monitoring, An Illustrated Analysis*, Ann Arbor, Mich., Health Administration Press, 1985.

physicians to provide care; that HMOs place blocks between the patient and the physician by using deductions, copayments, and the like, and by subjecting members to long waits to obtain appointments once in reception rooms; that HMOs drop the really tough cases as soon as they become expensive, or prohibit high-risk people from joining the plan; and that HMOs provide adequate general care but send members with major illnesses to outside-the-plan specialists.

Some of the answers to these criticisms can be found in the literature; other arguments may be valid but the evidence of their proof is weak or not available. Indeed, most early studies of HMOs "which measured quality in terms of the structure, process, and outcome of care, provided a generally consistent picture. In terms of the structural measures of quality—the facilities, services, staffs, and monitoring systems—HMOs often appeared to be superior to fee-for-service practices. This advantage was largely because they were organized settings and were relatively new. Thus, HMOs often had built-in review systems (especially in individual practice associations) and prepaid group practices shared medical records. The newness of many HMOs meant they were more likely to have younger and more highly trained physicians than the community average."[23]

DEFINITION AND MEASUREMENT OF QUALITY

It might be stated that, if an organization, whether it is a capitated health plan or some other service-oriented plan, consistently provides a product or service that is perceived by the purchaser as being of low quality for high cost, it will lose customers (e.g., members) to the point where the product must be improved or the organization will fail. For some HMOs, this point has become fatally clear; others have become very conscious of their product's quality. But what is quality? Avedis Donabedian, who has written the seminal works on quality, suggests that to answer this question, one must first identify what it is that the HSO wants to accomplish—its objectives of health care and, more importantly, what *should* be achieved. He feels that quality of care is therefore defined as "that which has the greatest likelihood of achieving an organization's objective of care with the most efficient use of resources."[24] As discussed in Chapter 7, one of the most important objectives of an HMO

---

[23] Harold S. Luft. "HMOs and the Quality of Care." *Inquiry,* 25(1):147, Spring 1988. It is of interest, however, to note that Luft feels that the generally favorable findings for HMO quality may have changed. He states on page 148 of his article that "the conventional wisdom now is that HMOs are able to provide comprehensive coverage at lower total cost while maintaining adequate quality of care." The rationale for such a statement is not convincing, however.

[24] Avedis Donabedian. "The Quality of Care in a Health Maintenance Organization: A Personal View." *Inquiry,* 20(3):218, Fall 1983.

is member or purchaser satisfaction and the caring component; Donabedian concurs that client satisfaction is one of the first objectives of care. He indicates that although an HMO will usually consider as its objectives the promotion, safeguarding, and restoration of health, it is difficult to precisely define "health." Thus, as an objective of care, one must look at client satisfaction and understand that clients are influenced by the stability and nature of their interpersonal relationships with their health care practitioners, the service setting of the organization, the ease of access to care when care is determined as being needed, and the empathy of physicians. Although health and quality are difficult to define, a member will be primarily satisfied with the organization's attempt to promote and restore health if perceptions of these characteristics are favorable.

Donabedian supports his consumer satisfaction hypotheses regarding measurements of quality of care by referring to the classic work by Friedson. In his studies of prepaid group practice, Friedson found that enrollees understood the distinction between technical quality and personal concern by the health professional, and that both are considered equally important with regard to their perception of quality care.[25] Donabedian asserts that technical expertise obviously is important, but if there seems to be a lack of personal interest or concern, patients question the doctor's resolve in using his/her expertise on their behalf. Conversely, patients do not believe that care is of high quality if the technical expertise is not acceptable, even if the health practitioner is seemingly concerned about the patient. The second objective, then, which is as important as members' satisfaction, is that of technical quality and the clinical competence of practitioners. Technical quality has, historically, been defined by the public health outcome measures of the incidence and prevalence of disease, morbidity, mortality, and disability. In fact, the actuarial studies that underlie HMO premiums are substantially based on these data, drawn from rate tables—descriptions of the rates of disease by classes of people. These efficacy or "outcome" measures provide only a limited view of the health of populations; as shown in Figure 8-1 earlier in this chapter, there are other outcome or output measures that increase our ability to describe the success of the HSO in achieving its clinical and managerial objectives. Additional measures of clinical and technical competence can be identified when assessing inputs and the process of converting those inputs into health services. Again, several such input and conversion process factors are provided in Figure 8-1. Input measures include physician-to-population ratios, physician office space per practitioner, and credentialing of providers. Process measures involve an analysis of the use of resources by providers

---

[25] Ibid., p. 219.

and include such indices as adherence to standard operating procedures and clinical protocols or algorithms, job design, and the managerial and operational functions of planning, decision making, communications, and the like. For clinical evaluations, medical records are the primary source documents for data. Usually, a group of physicians will periodically review records chosen for review because of potentially unacceptable or red-flag events known as "sentinels" or sentinel events. This approach assumes that physician reviewers are using implicit criteria, or explicit criteria recorded in written protocols. In either event, the assumption is that providers have consensus criteria that describe good or high-quality medical practice. Such criteria should help to maximize successful outcomes and health plan objectives, with the most efficient use of resources, as Donabedian maintains.

CLINICAL AND PRODUCTION EFFICIENCY AND APPROPRIATENESS

As can be observed from the list of input and process measures provided in Figure 8-1, some are clinical while others are organizational or production in nature, involving the entire system of delivery. Indeed, Donabedian suggests that attaining objectives (e.g., providing high-quality care) requires efficiency in both the clinical and production functions of the HMO. "Clinical *efficiency* pertains to the manner in which a practitioner manages the clinical problems of each patient."[26] This concept goes directly to the heart of a managed care system—the development of a case management plan or strategy of care for each patient under the practitioner's control. It involves the careful selection of resources and the sequencing of those elements to create for the patient a unique strategy that is also clinically most efficient and the one that represents the highest quality. A correlate may be *appropriateness,* where a particular diagnostic and therapeutic course of treatment is only appropriate given the circumstances of the patient under care.

"Production efficiency pertains to the way in which an organization as a whole produces the goods and services out of which the practitioners construct the strategies of care that they implement, in collaboration, of course, with their co-workers and patients."[27] While clinical efficiency is under the control of the practitioners, production efficiency is directed and controlled by the HMO's managers, although it is affected by the practice patterns of the physicians and requires their cooperation. Measurements of production efficiency should include an analysis of the effectivness of standard procedures, integration

---

[26] Ibid., p. 220.

[27] Ibid., p. 221.

of work efforts, effectiveness of communications, ability to make appropriate decisions, and the like.

METHODS OF QUALITY ASSESSMENT

Given an understanding of the definition, role, and dimensions of quality assessment, what methods can be used by MCOs to create an effective and efficient quality assessment program? Table 8-8 provides some answers to this question. Note from the previous discussion that three primary areas have been identified for quality assessment—technical or clinical competence; the general system of clinical and production efficiency and management; and consumer preference and satisfaction. Some examples of methods that fall under each of these areas are provided.

Technical and Clinical Competence: First, time-proven, predominately inpatient techniques might be used, including implicit and explicit reviews, with medical records for review identified through the use of sentinels and/or tracer conditions.[28]

Implicit reviews are carried out by physicians and other experts who intuitively can recognize good care vis-à-vis input, process, and outcome analyses. Usually, this process is performed by a group whose collective judgment is better than that of the individual; it is somewhat informal, without the use of written criteria or standards, although case selection may follow sophisticated identification techniques.

Explicit reviews apply specific criteria to the medical record or observe the actual delivery of care. Professionals write standards and clinical algorithms that then can be used by the paraprofessional staff to evaluate care. This provides for clear, precise analyses, but it also may oversimplify or even allow for irrelevant review. Explicit reviews are performed by PROs, although the criteria may be applied by professionals rather than by nonmedical staff— peers who may use intuition and implicit processes at the same time.

The use of *sentinels* is a method of identifying or "flagging" medical records or patients for review. As noted previously, reviewers using this technique identify a class of unacceptable events or outcomes. Using both implicit and explicit processes, the reviewers then perform detailed investigations of the cases. In some instances, these reviews will entail a search for exceptional levels of morbidity or mortality by disease category, or statistical outliers (especially financial outliers identified through the DRG payment mechanism) in rates of utilization and requests for payment for services. These

---

[28] Donald M. Berwick and Marian Gilbert Knapp. "Theory and Practice for Measuring Health Care Quality." *Health Care Financing Review, Annual Supplement,* December 1987, p. 50.

TABLE 8-8   Quality Assessment Methods for MCOs

A. *Technical or Clinical Competence Reviews*
   1. Implicit methods
   2. Explicit methods
   3. Sentinel events

B. *General Systems (Clinical and Production Efficiency)*
   1. Accreditation process
   2. Federal HMO qualification and CMP eligibility activities
   3. Systems analyses
   4. Management audits
   5. Relation, decision, and activity analyses

C. *Consumer Preference and Satisfaction Reviews*
   1. Health center visit—exit interview
   2. Mailed opinion questionnaire
   3. Observations using rating forms

sentinel events lead the reviewer to areas where further study is needed. But, the sentinel events may themselves become indicators of quality when the professionals identify them as outcomes that should be avoided. Some examples of sentinels are the measurements and indicators shown in Table 8-9. Another method of chart identification involves the use of tracer conditions such as hypertension or diabetes. These symptoms are commonly occurring elements of many diseases or conditions. By tracing their occurrence through the delivery of services, reviewers determine whether adequate care was provided.

General Systems Reviews: Most managers realize that quality assessment is multidimensional in nature. In addition to the traditional methods described above, the role of reviews and quality control at all stages of service delivery must be recognized. It is important not only to evaluate the outcome of the system, but also to design the delivery activities for reinforcing quality at each step in providing services. Each individual involved in the process must be responsible for maintaining a high level of quality at that particular step in providing care. Recognition by employees and medical staff of this "quality responsibility" develops as a part of the organization's *culture*—the "way we do things around here." Culture develops at the top of the organization, through example, commitment, and mandate of the top executives. These managers provide assistance to employees and staff to continually improve quality, and together with other members of the organization, establish clear goals regarding quality that are then embraced by all employees. Finally, managers need to recognize and understand the relationships between input, process, and outcomes. These relationships define the multidimensional nature of quality

TABLE 8-9 Examples of Indicators of Potential Quality Problems*

A. HEALTH CENTER/AMBULATORY SERVICES :

1. *Technical/Clinical Indicators:*
   a. Deaths in centers; Ideal is 0.
   b. Follow up of abnormal Pap Smears; Ideal is 100%.
   c. Medication dispensing errors; Ideal is 0.
   d. Remake of glasses; Ideal is 0.
   e. Patients with verified hypertension who receive physician assessment and follow-up; Ideal is 100%.
   f. Patients with abnormal laboratory test results contacted and appropriate follow-up; Ideal is 100%.
   g. Tuberculin testing performed on new pulmonary patients; Ideal is 100%.
   h. Pediatric patients (age 15–24 months) who have been screened for anemia and have had a tine test; Ideal is 100%.
   i. Psychiatry patients on lithium have lithium blood levels drawn at least every three months; Ideal is 100%.
   j. Unplanned direct admissions to the hospital from the health center; Ideal is 0.

2. *Member Satisfaction Indicators:*
   a. Routine physician-appointment availability; Ideal is appointment available within one week of inquiry.
   b. Members who refused treatment or left before being seen; Ideal is 0.
   c. Waiting time in the examination room; ideal is 10 minutes.
   d. Amount of time on telephone hold; ideal is 30 seconds.

3. *System and Management Indicators:*
   a. Informed consent forms correctly completed; Ideal is 100%.
   b. Injury to patients during treatment; Ideal is 0.
   c. Patients who commit or attempt to commit suicide; Ideal is 0.
   d. Patients who arrive after office hours who had a scheduled appointment earlier that day; Ideal is 0.
   e. Patients who have missed appointments or are lost to follow-up. Ideal is 0.
   f. Frequency with which the medical record accompanies the patient. Ideal is 100%.
   g. Length of time the medical records are out of the records room. Ideal is 3 to 4 days.

B. HOSPITAL INPATIENT SERVICES

1. *Technical/Clinical Indicators:*
   a. Premature deliveries (earlier than 37 weeks). Ideal is 0.
   b. Unscheduled return to the operating room. Ideal is 0.
   c. Cesarean sections performed. Ideal is not more than 20% of births delivered by Cesarean section.

2. *System and Management Indicators:*
   a. The number of missing and/or incomplete charts. Ideal is 0.
   b. Timely discharge planning. Ideal is 100%.
   c. Precertification and approval of planned admissions. Ideal is 100%.
   d. Application of length of stay standard to all admissions. Ideal is 100%.

*Adapted from Elizabeth Flanagan, "Indicators of Quality in Ambulatory Care," *Quality Review Bulletin*, *11*(4):130–137, April 1985; Eileen M. Oswald and Inge K. Winer, "A Simple Approach to Quality Assurance in a Complex Ambulatory Care Setting," *Quality Review Bulletin*, *13*(2):56–60, February 1987; Julie Johnsson, "Mid-sized HMO Tracks Quality Without Spending a Fortune," *Contract Healthcare*, June 1988, pp. 30–32; and Julie Micheletti, Thomas J. Shlala, and Ann T. Freedman, "Restructuring Quality Assurance Programs in HMOs and Other Competitive Medical Programs," *Quality Review Bulletin*, *14*(3):80–85, March 1988.

assessment and help to maintain high levels of quality through analyses of system delivery. These relationships, themselves, may even become proxy indicators of the quality of care.

The health plan manager may also use one or more other general system review activities, including HMO accreditation or the CMP eligibility process. But more importantly, analyses of the general systems and delivery components of the health plan are vital to understanding organizational deficiencies. Peter Drucker, a prolific writer on management, suggests that managers use relationship, decision, and activity analyses to help pinpoint problems and arrive at solutions. By observing relationships among employees, by understanding by whom and how decisions are made in the organization, and by charting the activities or tasks that are completed by employees, the manager is better able to ensure that quality is maintained and enhanced. At a minimum, managers should facilitate the development of standard procedures that define the way activities will be carried out. These standard operating procedures (SOPs) will become the standards by which the organization's activities can be measured. SOPs assist in ensuring effective communications, integrating work effort, and facilitating decision making.

Consumer Preference and Satisfaction: The quality assessment methods that have been reviewed so far include technical and systems analyses. A third area where quality assessments are performed is identified in Table 8-8— consumer preference and satisfaction. As discussed in Chapter 7 and earlier in this chapter, member satisfaction is as important as the other technical components of quality assessment. Several methods of data collection are used, the most important of which is questionnaires that elicit data regarding the patient's assessment of outcome, ambiance, interpersonal relationships, staff morale, humaneness of providers, and the like. These data may be elicited immediately after delivery of ambulatory services through an exit interview, mailed questionnaires after other services are provided (such as an inpatient stay), or observations made by staff members of such issues as attractiveness of facilities, number of patients waiting to see providers, noise levels, ability to protect the patients's privacy, use of waiting time for patient education, and parking availability at different hours of operation.

The assessment process should be effective and efficient and should provide measurements of quality without the need for excessive use of manpower or sophisticated data tracking systems. The management information system needed to assemble data may be as simple as a complete and comprehensive medical record and the periodic use of member questionnaires. As health plans grow in enrollment and delivery sites, however, data systems increase in complexity and cost. IPA model HMOs, for example, create the most complex situation for quality assurance activities because of the many ambulatory delivery sites involved. But, initially, MCO managers should attempt to develop quality assurance programs that use indicators of potential quality problems and require limited data and inexpensive management information systems. These quality assessment and assurance systems tend to use standards, indicators, monitors, sentinels, and the like, to effectively and efficiently monitor the quality of activities. Table 8-9 provides some indicators that can be used in an efficient quality assessment program.

The health plan first decides which indicators to use and then assigns an ideal level of operation. A data collection system is put into operation to assist in measuring activities against these indicators. Corrective actions may include changing goals and objectives, changing SOP and indicator values, or correcting deficient activities of employees and the medical staff. Note that the emphasis of the sample indicators in the table is placed on ambulatory health delivery; this is not to indicate the relative importance of either delivery site. Rather, hospitals have a long record of applying QA/UR activities to managed care and traditional patients, while ambulatory sites have little experience in applying quality assurance techniques to their operations. The ambulatory indicators in Table 8-9 are intended to show that an efficient QA system can be developed for health center operations.

Experiences of Group Model HMOs with Quality of Care

Donabedian suggests that the quality of medical care in a prepaid group practice plan, for example, a group model HMO, can be evaluated by using several dimensions, including the effective use of medical care services by the enrollee, the types and kinds of physicians and hospitals used by the health plan, the physicians' performance, and the effects of the services on the health of the subscribers—or outcome measurements, as described in the preceding section.

The question of whether prepaid group practice enrollees use medical care services more effectively is answered by a review of several studies. Donabedian concludes from two studies that relatively few (15–30 percent) of the subscribers to prepaid group practice feel that being a member of such a plan has affected their use of medical care services. In addition, Donabedian states that "the available evidence indicates that prepaid group practice enjoys no superiority in the establishment of a perceived relationship between patient and physicians."[29] Long-term patient-physician relationships are considered to enhance the quality of health care. Another measurement of quality, according to Donabedian, may be the use of preventive services. In his studies, there was little evidence to show that the use of preventive services was higher by prepaid group practice subscribers. There is some suggestion, however, that members in prepaid plans were more likely to delay less in seeking medical care when ill (i.e., less than one day after illness began). In addition, there is substantial evidence that prepaid group practice plans reduce the disparity between high and low socioeconomic groups in the use of health care services.[30] Delays in seeking medical care and disparity between high and low socioeconmic groups are evidence of a poorly functioning health delivery system, resulting in the lack of appropriate care.

The second dimension of quality reviewed by Donabedian was the type and kind of physicians and hospitals that are used by prepaid group practice plans. Qualified physicians and accredited hospitals may be considered proxy indicators of the level of health care quality. The studies reviewed by Donabedian suggest that the specialty care that was used by prepaid group practice subscribers was provided by qualified specialists (diplomate or equivalent). But prior to 1970, prepaid group practice physicians were least likely to use accredited hospitals. Reasons given were that prepaid physicians had difficulty obtaining privileges in accredited hospitals or that there were few accredited hospitals in the regions where the study plans were operating. Since the passage of Title XIII of the Social Security Act and the rapid expansion of HMOs, most, if not all, now use accredited hospitals for inpatient care.

Another proxy method for identifying quality, according to Donabedian, is to review how physicians actually manage cases. He states that evidence shows that prepaid group practice appears to exert some control in reducing unjustified surgery and, to that extent, contributes to the quality of care. ". . . the manner in which a group is organized, staffed, and equipped appears to be fairly closely related to the quality of physician performance as judged by a review of case records supplemented by interviews with the managing

---

[29] Avedis Donabedian. "An Evaluation of Prepaid Group Practice." *Inquiry, 6*(3):21, September 1969.

[30] L. S. Rosenfeld, Avedis Donabedian, and J. Katz, "Unmet Needs for Medical Care," *New England Journal of Medicine, 258*:369–376, February 20, 1958; Theodore J. Colombo, Ernest W. Saward, and Merwyn R. Greenlick, "Group Practice Plans in Governmental Medical Care Programs. IV, *American Journal of Public Health, 59*(4):641–650, April 1969; and Clifton R. Gaus, Norman A. Fuller, and Carol Bohannon, "HMO Evaluation: Utilization Before and After Enrollment," Paper Presented at the Annual Meeting of the American Public Health Association, Atlantic City, N.J., November 15, 1972, pp. 6–11.

physicians."[31] Thus, a review of practice patterns by the medical group may be important.

The last dimension of quality described by Donabedian is measurement of the health and well-being of the subscribers. Results of studies concerning morbidity and mortality of the general population are inconclusive. Donabedian noted, however, that in two studies comparing the population of the Health Insurance Plan (HIP) of Greater New York with the population of New York City and an Old Age Assistance (OAA) recipient group, prematurity and prenatal mortality rates were significantly lower in HIP, and the mortality for OAA recipients also was lower for those patients in the HIP programs than for the New York City population. Further data that have been systematically studied regarding matched groups of HMO and non-HMO populations are provided later in this chapter. The favorable showing of prepaid group practice plans may not represent what occurs in most prepaid group practice populations, but data suggest far-ranging health policy implications if these results are validated by future studies. Indeed, several experts suggest that the reasons for better outcomes from prepaid group practice plans may be the result of using medical group practices rather than the prepaid component of the system. Thus, the medical care industry may achieve valuable results through the greater use of medical groups along with traditional fee-for-service.

Although an analysis of HMOs by these four dimensions shows a somewhat positive performance for prepaid group practice plans in comparison to other forms of health insurance and delivery, much more research and study are necessary to accurately determine both the positive and negative quality issues in prepayment practices. Positive forces include the use of unit medical records for members throughout their association with the prepaid plan, allowing for continuity of medical care. Unit medical records also provide a mechanism to facilitate peer review—each new physician the patient sees is provided with the record of all preceding physician services rendered. As an informal peer review mechanism, this process tends to provide both a retrospective and prospective check on HMO physician services. It should be supplemented by the development of regular, continuous monitoring of care that includes the formulation of standards and formalized case reviews by a quality assurance committee of the medical staff. The use of a managing primary-care practitioner—the assignment of an enrollee to a physician who will "watch over" all care provided to the patient—is a well-used and appropriate quality control mechanism in prepaid group practice. The concept of the managing physician is akin to the family doctor concept, which was lost to increased specialization by physicians in the United States. This concept is now

---

[31] Donabedian. "An Evaluation of Prepaid Group Practice," p. 23.

recognized as the first level in a good personal health care system. In addition to controlling medical delivery, the HMO system also may provide greater control and coordination of the physical health care resources made available to the physician. More appropriate use of available buildings, equipment, supplies, and even ancillary personnel may make the physician's services a better "product." It is well understood that the coordination effort of the HMO makes the availability of an HMO service an advantage of the system and that subscribers have fewer and shorter delays for services when ill or injured. The HMO physician's control of services has reduced to some extent the inappropriate and unjustified use of surgery or other health care services. Finally, control of physician appointments by the group practice favorably affects the quality of care.[32]

Alternatively, there are several forces that may lower the quality of HMO care. Herbert Klarman suggests that "Ancillary services may be wasted if ordered by the physician without discrimination. Excessive referrals may lead to a wholesale evasion of responsibility for the care of the patient. . . Finally, the peer review that actually takes place in the group setting may be overrated."[33] By the use of capitation payments, HMOs change physician incentives from providing more services to controlling or reducing unjustified services. Unfortunately, in its cost-controlling efforts, an HMO, especially an investor-owned HMO, may inadvertently achieve this goal by inappropriately reducing the amount of quality services provided, although evidence does not support this potential capitation effect.

Other quality control devices that may be considered by the group model HMO manager include some of the following.

1. *Physician Group Contract:* In developing capitation levels between the HMO and the physician group practice, the first step should be to determine appropriate utilization levels of service to be provided. Described as a range, the appropriate utilization of services can be converted to dollars of services. For example, physician group X, associated with the Healthville HMO, determines that an appropriate utilization rate for appendectomy surgery is from

---

[32] As noted above, several researchers and authors have suggested that many of these advantages (control of utilization of services, accessibility of care, equality, satisfaction, and so on) are not the result of a capitation payment alone but that organized multispecialty group practice arrangements with mostly salaried physicians may be a more significant variable. See, Clifton R. Gaus, Barbara S. Cooper, and Constance G. Hirschman, "Contrasts in HMO and Fee-for-Service Performance," *Social Security Bulletin, 39*(5):3–14, May 1976; and Luft, "HMOs and the Quality of Care."

[33] Herbert E. Klarman. "Economic Research in Group Medicine." In: *New Horizons in Health Care; Proceedings of the First International Congress on Group Medicine, Winnipeg, April 26–30, 1970.* Winnipeg, Can., the Congress Secretariat, 1970.

4.2 to 6.8 per 1,000 members. Group X will be providing services to 1,000 members, and the average cost for physician services for an appendectomy in its geographic area is $300. Thus, the range of physician cost to be built into the capitation rate for this service would be from $12,600 to $20,000 per year. Inappropriate levels of care could then be described as levels above or below this range.

Renegotiation of the physician group contract would take into consideration such matters as the group's ability to work within the appropriate range established, the record of consumer grievances, ombudsman reports, peer evaluations, evaluation of interviews with physicians managing the group practice, local professional standards review organization analyses, and staff admitting privileges at local hospitals. Establishing standards of care and acceptable utilization levels similar to the aforementioned example is very important for those health care delivery programs that are reviewed by local professional standards review organizations. To cope with this kind of review, many providers have developed treatment protocols or patient-treatment algorithms. The protocols provide a description of the treatment program for all of the specific services provided by the health plan. Each treatment program describes the utilization rate and length of hospital stay, if indicated, and then a description of the step-by-step treatment of the condition. Added to this information is the level of consumption (i.e., the average range of utilization for each service by the HMO's service area population) and an average cost. With this information, capitation rates can be developed quickly.

2. *Formal Peer Review:* The HMO's contract with the physician group should define the physician's responsibility for monitoring quality, especially for the establishment of quality standards. Naturally, the unit medical record serves as the written evidence. Observations of how medicine is actually practiced should become a part of the formal peer review process. Advanced quality assurance systems using such programs as those previously described should be used. These systems will be built around formal peer review, medical record review, and observation analysis.

3. *Health Ombudsman:* An individual may be appointed to answer or find answers to specific member complaints, to follow through on complaints, to monitor spot checks, and to be generally available to help consumers find their way through the HMO. To be effective, the ombudsman should report to the HMO board through the executive director.

4. *Grievance Procedure:* The complaint-review mechanism is discussed in detail earlier in this chapter.

5. *Reinsurance:* Congress recognized the need to protect newly developing HMOs from financial disaster caused by large and unusual expenses or losses created by accepting unmanageable risks. All HMOs now use a reinsurance

mechanism to avoid the unanticipated consequences of providing less or lower quality care to protect their reserves. On the other hand, passing the complete risk for providing health care to an outside insurer could be an indication of the HMO's inability to provide adequate service. Older HMOs, with relatively large reserves, have found that the use of reinsurance is not only unnecessary, because of their ability to cover losses from accumulated reserves, but that it can be more costly than self-insuring, because of large reinsurance premium payments to outside insurers.

Quality Performance of All HMO Models

A review of current evidence regarding the experience of HMOs in maintaining quality in their organizations is appropriate. In 1980, Cunningham and Williamson[34] reviewed more than 90 articles covering many of the studies performed through that date; some of their findings are:

- A 1955–1957 study of obstetric care by the Health Insurance Plan (HIP) of Greater New York showed that premature births were significantly lower for health plan patients than for patients of private physicians. Another HIP study compared elderly public assistance patients enrolled in HIP to those receiving medical care from other sources; the mortality rate for HIP enrollees was 14 percent lower than for non-HIP patients.

- A survey in Alameda County, California found that women enrolled in the Kaiser Health Plan received more Pap tests than women covered by other types of insurance.

- A study conducted in the Los Angeles, California city schools showed that parents belonging to HMOs took their children in for preventive medical care more often than those who were covered by fee-for-service plans. This was especially true for lower income parents.

- The University of Michigan conducted a study in Hawaii comparing HMOs with other providers. Higher quality of care was noted in prepaid plans; the HMOs proved to be more efficient in directing patients to appropriate specialists. Hospitalization rates were lower without sacrificing quality. HMO pediatricians received higher scores than fee-for-service pediatricians for histories, physical exams, laboratory testing, and completeness of immunizations. Overall physician performance was rated slightly higher for prepaid plans than for the others.

---

[34] Francis C. Cunningham and John W. Williamson. "How Does the Quality of Care in HMOs Compare to that in Other Settings?" *Group Health Journal*, *1*(1):4–13, Winter 1980.

- A Johns Hopkins study in Baltimore, Maryland showed that low-income children who were members of the East Baltimore Medical Plan received more preventive care, such as vaccinations and physicial exams, than children receiving health care elsewhere. Although it was found that children belonging to the HMO received more care overall than those who were not HMO members, no significant differences were found among adults.

- The Seattle (Washington) Prepaid Health Project compared the quality of care for urinary tract infections provided by Group Health Cooperative of Puget Sound (an HMO) and a Blue Shield plan. The study used a physician performance index to rate the quality of care. GHC's score for laboratory testing was double that of independent practitioners. There was greater use of urinalysis and urine cultures in the HMO, and the HMO recorded more extensive histories and provided more complete physical examinations. The therapeutic index was higher for the HMO.

Since 1980, several comparative studies have been completed with results similar to the pre-1980 studies—suggesting that HMOs generally have equal or better technical or clinical quality than the traditional system of delivery. Several of these studies are reviewed below.

- In 1981, Frechette and Russo[35] published the results of a study conducted by the Massachusettes Department of Public Health comparing the quality of maternity care for members of the Harvard Community Health Plan, a Boston-based HMO, and private fee-for-service practices. All deliveries took place at the Boston Hospital for Women Division of the Brigham and Women's Hospital. Over a nine-month period, 5,003 consecutive deliveries were reviewed. Of these deliveries, 12.8 percent, or 640, were HMO patients and 62.6 percent, or 3,134, were private patients; the remaining 24.6 percent received prenatal care in clinics and were not included in the final analyses. The findings suggest that the overall outcomes of care of both the HMO and FFS patients were similar. The percentages of occurrence of stillbirths, neonatal deaths, one minute Apgar scores less than 6, low birth weights, and short gestations were comparable in both groups. Although outcomes of care in both populations did not vary, there were differences in the process of

---

[35] Alfred L. Frechette and Pearl K. Russo. "A Comparison of the Quality of Maternity Care Between a Health Maintenance Organization and Fee-for-Service Practices. *New England Journal of Medicine, 313*(11):784–787, March 26, 1981.

care; the rate of cesarean sections was 3 percent lower in HMO patients, which may suggest that some unnecessary surgery for FFS patients had been performed. Also, the length of stay (LOS) of the 623 HMO patients averaged 0.4 days less than the LOS of the fee-for-service patients, resulting in an overall reduction of 249 patient days during the period of the study.

- Francis et al.[36] reported in May 1984 on comparisons of HMO and fee-for-service patients with colorectal cancer. HMO patients received a greater amount of care from the first contact through diagnosis than fee-for-service patients, including more physician visits and more endoscopies. The interval between diagnosis and surgery, however, was shorter for the fee-for-service patients. Access to care, rates of surgery, chemotherapy and radiation, and lengths of hospital stay showed no significant differences between the two groups, and there was no difference in general health at 3 and 12 months after surgery. Survival rates were similar for both groups.

- Wright, Gardin, and Wright[37] studied (in 1984) the care provided to two groups of patients at the same hospital by the same obstetricians—some covered by an HMO and others insured in the fee-for-service system. The results suggested that HMO patients visited their physicians less often than fee-for-service patients, and lengths of hospital stays were shorter for HMO patients; however, based on outcome measures, there were no significant differences between the two groups.

- A study reported by Ware et al.[38] in 1986 provided a comparison of health outcomes at an HMO with that of FFS patients. Conducted in the Seattle, Washington metropolitan area, the study included 1,673 individuals, ages 14 to 61, who were randomly assigned to Group Health Cooperative of Puget Sound or a fee-for-service insurance plan. The participants were provided with free care for three to five years. Initial health assessments were used at the beginning and throughout the study. "For non-poor individuals assigned to the HMO who were

---

[36] Anita M. Francis et al. "Care of Patients with Colorectal Cancer—A Comparison of Health Maintenance Organization and Fee-for-Service Patients." *Medical Care, 22*(5):418–425, May 1984.

[37] Charles H. Wright, Hershell Gardin, and Carla L. Wright. "Obstetric Care in a Health Maintenance Organization and a Private Fee-for-Service Practice: A Comparative Analysis." *American Journal of Obstetrics and Gynecology, 149*(8):848–856, August 15, 1984.

[38] John E. Ware, Jr., et al. "Comparison of Health Outcomes at a Health Maintenance Organization with Those of Fee-for-Service Care." *Lancet, 1*(8488):1017 and 1021, May 3, 1986.

initially in good health there were no adverse effects. Health outcomes in the two systems of care differed for high- and low-income individuals who began the experiment with health problems. For the high-income initially sick group, the HMO produced significant improvements in cholesterol levels and in general health ratings by comparison with FFS care. The low-income initially sick group assigned to the HMO reported significantly more bed-days per year due to poor health and more serious symptoms than those assigned free FFS care, and a greater risk of dying by comparison with pay FFS plans." The authors concluded that even though there were striking reductions in the medical costs at GHC, they observed increases only in bed days and serious symptoms, and these differences were confined to the low-income, initially sick group. Thus, for the economically advantaged, there are two good reasons for joining an HMO—substantial cost savings and gains in health status. Low-income groups in the study, however, appeared worse off at GHC. The authors suggest that HMOs might be predisposed to underserve, and poor people may be less likely to overcome this obstacle. Since the HMO places greater reliance on the patient for follow-up and compliance with medical regimens, poor people may be less likely to assume this responsibility.

- Yelin, Shearn, and Epstein[39] compared the health care use and outcomes of a group of patients with rheumatoid arthritis receiving care in a group model HMO and fee-for-service settings. In 1982, one half of all 114 board eligible or certified rheumatologists in northern California were randomly sampled. Participating physicians provided the names of all patients with rheumatoid arthritis presenting during a one-month period; 812 of these patients were interviewed. Then, in 1984, 745 were again interviewed; 569 received care in FFS settings and 176 in a prepaid group practice. In both 1982 and 1984, the researchers found that both groups of patients received similar amounts of care. Both FFS and prepaid patients achieved similar outcomes, as measured by symptoms of illness, functional status, and work disability. The researchers found that FFS patients reported poorer overall health status. It was concluded after two years of follow-up study that patients in prepaid group practice received similar medical care inputs and achieved outcomes at least as good as those in FFS.

---

[39] Edward H. Yelin, Martin A. Shearn, and Wallace V. Epstein. "Health Outcomes for a Chronic Disease in Prepaid Group Practice and Fee-for-Service Settings." *Medical Care, 24*(3):236, March 1986.

- Siu, Lebowitz, Brook, Goldman, Lurie, and Newhouse[40] (in 1988) conducted a randomized trial where families were assigned to either the Group Health Cooperative of Puget Sound or to fee-for-service care (this study was part of the Rand Health Insurance Experiment). The researchers attempted to determine whether HMOs selectively avoid discretionary hospitalizations by enrolling healthier populations. The medical records of 122 fee-for-service enrollees and 122 HMO enrollees were reviewed by researchers who were blinded to the system. The results showed that the rate of discretionary surgery was lower in the HMO, while the rate of nondiscretionary surgery was equivalent in the two systems. Rates of both discretionary and nondiscretionary medical admissions were lower for the HMO. The researchers found no observable adverse effects on health from lower rates of nondiscretionary hospitalization, either because the net effect on health was small or because the HMO substituted appropriate ambulatory services. Finally, they concluded that HMO reductions in hospitalization rates did not occur "across the board"; discretionary surgery was selectively avoided.

- In 1988, McCusker, Stoddard, and Sorenson[41] studied the ability of HMOs to contain health plan costs by controlling and reducing hospital services for their terminally ill patients; since terminal illness is very costly due to high hospitalization costs, it was hypothesized that total HMO costs could be reduced by limiting hospital care to these patients. The researchers examined hospital utilization and costs in a matched-pair comparison of HMO members and nonmembers under age 65 in Monroe County, New York who died of cancer between 1976 and 1982. They found that the HMO used somewhat fewer hospital days and had lower hospital costs than non-HMO members, but the differences were not statistically significant. Interestingly, they also found greater variance in the costs of care for nonmembers than for HMO members. The researchers concluded that they found no cost-saving effects for HMOs in terminal cancer care in this matched-study design.

Harold Luft,[42] a strong critic of HMO operations, stated that HMOs generally

---

[40] Albert L. Siu, Arleen Lebowitz, Robert H. Brook, Nancy S. Goldman, Nicole Lurie, and Joseph P. Newhouse. "Use of the Hospital in a Randomized Trial of Prepaid Care." *Journal of the American Medical Association, 259*(9):1343, March 4, 1988.

[41] Jane McCusker, Anne M. Stoddard, and Andrew A. Sorenson. "Do HMOs Reduce Hospitalization of Terminal Cancer Patients?" *Inquiry, 25*(2):263–270, Summer 1988.

[42] Harold S. Luft, "Assessing the Evidence on HMO Performance," *Milbank Memorial Fund Quarterly, Health and Society, 58*(4):501–521, 1980; and _____ . "How Do Health Maintenance Organizations Achieve Their Savings?" *New England Journal of Medicine, 298*(22):1336–1342, June 15, 1978.

have equal or better resources than fee-for-service organizations, sometimes have a greater number of better trained physicians, and are more likely to use accredited hospitals. In a 1978 paper, he questioned the ability of HMOs to achieve cost savings while maintaining quality, although he later concluded that there is no evidence that HMOs are sacrificing quality for cost containment.

These conclusions are certainly supported by the studies described above, and the same conclusion was drawn by another prolific writer, David Mechanic. In a 1985 article regarding cost containment and quality of care, Mechanic[43] reviewed several recent studies, some of which showed significant differences in utilization of services (i.e., lower hospital days, etc.) between HMOs and the traditional system because of limits on access to facilities and providers; he concluded that "there is little overall evidence. . . that these variations in [use and] access of outpatient care have the significant impacts on health that some believe them to have."

Summary

HMOs and other managed care organizations require strong control processes to ensure the maintenance of high-quality services and to live up to their reputations as better managers of medical resources. Control for HMOs, like other organizations, denotes monitoring the use of resources, conversion of these resources into medical services, and evaluation of the results achieved. It is an essential management function not only because of the internal need for cost control and high performance and quality, but also because of the external pressures created by federal and state regulatory activities to perform effectively. In addition, HMO members play an important role in pressuring the organization to control operations, especially when they choose to enroll or disenroll because of dissatisfaction. Intense dissatisfaction may be exhibited by threats of malpractice or grievances against the health plan and its providers.

Like other organizations, control models used by HMOs are information-based. Data are collected on actions of the health plan staff, including input of resources, the process of converting inputs into health services, and the output or efficacy of the system. Early during the strategic planning and budgeting process, standards and indicators of success are designed and created. These then are used to measure HMO operations.

The HMO manager may obtain some assistance in evaluating and controlling operations from independent organizations such as accrediting bodies and

---

[43] David Mechanic. "Cost Containment and the Quality of Medical Care: Rationing Strategies in an Era of Constrained Resources." *Milbank Memorial Fund Quarterly/Health and Society,* 63(3):453–475, Summer 1985.

through the qualification process. Several accrediting institutions are available, including the Joint Commission of Health Care Organizations, the Accreditation Association for Ambulatory Health Care, Inc., and the National Committee for Quality Assurance. Each applies standards of operation, delivery, and management that have a direct impact on the quality of services. In addition, HMOs can seek federal qualification, while CMPs must be certified prior to negotiating a Medicare risk contract with HCFA. Both qualification and certification follow HCFA-defined procedures that evaluate the organization's ability to manage its activities, deliver high-quality services, market effectively, operate within the legal and regulatory environment established by Congress and HCFA, and be financially stable. These evaluations are provided to health plans that request such activities, but all HMOs may be required to participate in state licensure and quality assurance review processes, which may be required initially and annually thereafter.

In 1988, Congress mandated that professional review organizations (PROs) assess the quality of care rendered to HMO members. Limited to those HMOs and CMPs with Medicare risk contracts, the review includes inpatient, physician, and others services provided by the plan for quality, completeness, timeliness, and appropriateness of care. Health plans that show problems with their internal quality assurance program are required to undergo intensified reviews. If deficiencies are not corrected in a timely fashion, the PRO may recommend to the Secretary of Health and Human Services that the health plan's contract with HCFA be terminated. Obviously, the field has voiced strong reservations regarding the review process and the levels of review; some feel that the administrative and financial burden will force many plans to abandon their risk contracts when they come up for renewal.

The ambulatory field generally, and the HMO industry specifically, have experienced problems with utilization definitions. To assist in standardizing terminology, the term *physician visit* is defined as a face-to-face contact between a physician and an HMO member and does not include nonphysician providers. *Nonphysician visit* refers to care by providers in the health center other than physicians. *Ambulatory visit* is defined as a combination of physician and nonphysician visits.

The use of physician visits by an HMO member, as reported by several sources, ranged from 3.4 to 4.0 on average for years 1986 through 1988. Federally qualified HMOs report that on average, members used 4.6 visits PMPY. Nonphysician visits added another 2.1 to 3.8 visits PMPY to the total ambulatory services that HMO members used per year. In comparison to the rates of ambulatory use by the general U.S. population, HMO members consistently used fewer services—from one visit less annually for "all" members to almost three visits annually for those over age 65. The results were similar for inpatient services; HMO members in all age groups had a shorter length of hospital stay (HMO ALOS was 4.8 versus the U.S. population of 7.2 days in 1987), and used fewer inpatient days per 1,000 enrollees (under age 65 members used approximately 400 days per 1,000 members while the U.S. population used approximately double that figure). The over age 65 HMO members used some 1,950 hospital days per 1,000 versus 3,030 days per 1,000 population for the U.S. population. Likewise, HMOs admitted fewer of their members to hospitals than generally experienced in the United States. These differences were explained by several hypotheses. Some experts suggest that HMOs limit availability and access to physicians and hospital beds. Others suggest that HMO physicians choose alternative treatment modalities than those in fee-for-service, that they admit only the critically ill to hospitals, and use better and more effective case management techniques. Critics of HMOs suggest that they selectively market and enroll populations with lower risks for service. HMO managers feel that they are more effective in managing the total system of delivery and provision of care. They also cite their educational efforts to change physician and patient behavior in the system and the incentives for both physicians and members to be wise users of health services.

Whatever the reasons for these results, HMO managers have a critical need to understand, evaluate, and control operations. In this process, the development of standards becomes one of the first steps in the monitoring and control activity. Data from operating health plans may provide the basis for standards, although care must be used when a particular HMO measures its activities against standards created industrywide. Some of these standards include the distribution of expenses, the actual income and expenses per member month, premium income as a percentage of total income, the plan's net worth, its operating margin, return on equity, average collection period, debt service coverage, profit margin, incurred but not reported expenses, annualized incurred patient days, average length of hospital stay, physician visits per member, and the like. All standards used relate to input, conversion process, or outcome from service delivery. The assessment process using these standards requires the collection of performance data via a management information system. Such a system must provide a data base for collecting all patient treatment information and member-related data that are used to monitor patient services; it must further provide for reporting that meets management needs in the managerial functional areas, in finance and planning, for outside organizations such as lending institutions and the Federal Government, and marketing intelligence and analyses.

HMOs have been criticized about the level of quality of health care services. Most research concerning HMO care shows a favorable quality profile; this is logical, since health plans, whether prepaid or fee-for-service, would cease to exist if care was perceived by patients to be consistently poor. There are sufficient data to draw conclusions about two aspects of quality in HMOs—

consumer satisfaction and technical or clinical quality of care. As discussed in Chapter 7, 92 to 94 percent of HMO members are satisfied with services provided by the health plan, especially with the cost of the plan and the benefits and coverages. Dissatisfaction usually is expressed with the length of waits, ability to see specialists, level of physician humaneness, and difficulty in obtaining home visits. With regard to clinical aspects, nearly all studies show that HMOs generally have equal or better technical or clinical quality than the traditional fee-for-service system of care. Forces that may positively affect the quality of care provided by an HMO include the use of a unit medical record, formal and informal peer review, use of the case-managing primary care physician, control and coordination of health care resources and more appropriate use of these services, and control by the medical group or physician panel of the appointment of new physicians to its group or panel. The major force that may negatively affect HMO quality may be the capitation incentive system, although the use of treatment protocols or algorithms to determine appropriate practice patterns and use levels may offset any negative aspects of capitated medicine. Quality control devices available to the HMO manager should be used and should include a strong HMO physician group contract; formal peer review, including a formal quality assurance and utilization review process; a health ombudsman; grievance procedures; use of reinsurance; accreditation of the health plan and its administrators; and the use of consumer evaluations of the program.

Quality assessment methods that are available include implicit reviews carried out by physicians, who intuitively recognize good or bad care and are operating as a group with collective judgment. Explicit reviews can also be used, where professionals create specific criteria that are systematically applied to medical record reviews or to actual observations of care being given. In addition, sentinel events flag activities, and tracer conditions identify charts that may then be scrutinized by implicit and explicit reviews. Such events might include exceptional levels of mortality or morbidity, statistical outliers in rates of payments and services, unexpected clinical outcomes, and the like. The assessment process should be effective yet efficient and require a data base collected through a management information system.

References

Accreditation Association for Ambulatory Health Care, Inc. *1987-88 Handbook*. Skokie, Ill., AAAHC, 1987.

Berwick, Donald M., and Marian Gilbert Knapp. "Theory and Practice for Measuring Health Care Quality." *Health Care Financing Review, Annual Supplement*, December 1987, pp. 49–55.

Caper, Philip. "Defining Quality in Medical Care." *Health Affairs,* 7(1):49–61, Spring 1988.

Card, William F., and R. Lehmann. "An Overview of the Methodology Used by the Joint Commission to Evaluate Medicare-Certified HMOs." *Quality Review Bulletin,* 13(12):415–417, December 1987.

Cunningham, Francis C., and John W. Williamson. "How Does the Quality of Care in HMOs Compare to that in Other Settings?" *Group Health Journal,* 1(1):4–25, Winter 1980.

Donabedian, Avedis. "The Quality of Care in a Health Maintenance Organization: A Personal View." *Inquiry,* 20(3):218–222, Fall 1983.

Gonnella, Joseph S., and Daniel Z. Louis. "Evaluation of Ambulatory Care." *Journal of Ambulatory Care Management,* 11(3):68–83, August 1988.

Group Health Association of America. *HMO Industry Profile. Vol. 2. Utilization Patterns.* Washington, D.C., GHAA, 1988.

InterStudy. *Trends in HMO Hospital and Ambulatory Utilization, 1981–1987.* Excelsior, Minn., InterStudy, March 1989.

Luft, Harold S. "HMOs and the Quality of Care." *Inquiry,* 25(1):147–156, Spring 1988.

Marion Merrell Dow, Inc. *Marion Managed Care Digest. HMO Edition.* Kansas City, Mo., MMD, 1987, 1988, 1989, and 1990.

McIntyre, David J., and Ronald S. Moen. "The Accreditation Question—A Call for Accountability." *Medical Group Management,* 34(5):21–24, September/October 1987.

Mechanic, David. "Cost Containment and the Quality of Medical Care: Rationing Strategies in an Era of Constrained Resources." *Milbank Memorial Fund Quarterly/ Health and Society,* 63(3):453–475, Summer 1985.

Neal, Patricia A. *Management Information Systems for the Fee-for-Service/Prepaid Medical Group.* Denver, Colo., Center for Research in Ambulatory Health Care Administration, 1983.

Rakick, Jonathan; Beaufort B. Longest; and Kurt Darr. *Managing Health Services Organizations.* Philadelphia, Pa., W. B. Saunders Co., 1985, pp. 298–333.

Siegel, Stephen H.; Phyllis M. Albritton; and Michael C. Thornhill. "PRO Review: Strategies for HMOs." *Group Health Association Journal,* 9(1):14–21, Fall 1988.

U.S. Department of Health and Human Services, Health Care Financing Administration, Office of Prepaid Health Care. "Quality Assurance Guidelines for Health Maintenance Organizations and Competitive Medical Plans." Rockville, Md., DHHS/HCFA/OPHC, July 25, 1986.

9

DEVELOPMENT AND EXPANSION ACTIVITIES

This chapter suggests a framework for bringing together the major components of the managed care organization (MCO) during its initial and expansionary stages. Several dimensions of the planning and development process are presented, various critical areas are discussed, and the many steps and problem areas faced by most developing or expanding MCOs are identified. Because much of the development activity in the managed care area today concerns expansion of services, service areas, and facilities, the issues of expansion and facility development are also discussed. Specific opportunities regarding joint ventures and other linkages among managed care and traditional organizations and their attending problems, including antitrust issues, are addressed.

Phases in Planning and Development: The Federal Model

The "Rules and Regulations" issued in 1977 by the Department of Health, Education, and Welfare to implement Title XIII of the Public Health Service Act—the Health Maintenance Organization Act—delineated the rules by which HMOs received federal funding and became federally qualified. These rules provided for the funding of HMOs through four phases of development—feasibility, planning, initial development, and initial operation. Although these phases are somewhat artificial divisions of the development process, it is useful to discuss them because they provide a framework for the planning and development processes and because of published development manuals that follow these phases.

FEASIBILITY PHASE

Managed care organizations begin as an idea, a concept, or an attitude of someone in the community that perhaps a new method of providing health care may be better and more useful than the present system or may be the most logical way to finance and deliver medical services. The feasibility phase in development or expansion initiates the somewhat expensive and complex process of establishing a new or expanded health delivery structure using existing components—providers, hospitals, pharmacies, and long-term-care facilities. Initial effort is directed toward the completion of a "feasibility study"—a rational method of providing the planner with information for making a "go" or "no go" decision. The study involves an examination of the critical issues that will determine the probable success or failure of the proposed HMO/PPO or expansion, and it should provide, ultimately, an analysis of the degree of risk (in monetary terms) that the project must face.

The feasibility study should assess the present and projected health needs of the community, the existing and projected resources in relation to such needs, and the interest in, or receptivity of the consumers, payers, and providers to an MCO. Although it is not anticipated that at this stage the study will be exhaustive, the thoroughness with which the study is conducted should have a direct impact on the potential success of the MCO. The feasibility study provides the structure and foundation on which each succeeding stage can be built, the basis on which feasible program goals and objectives can be set, and the basis on which plans and programs may be determined and funded. It also identifies the target population that may be served, the kind of services to offer, and the potential for competing in the existing market and for achieving the desired enrollment. A completed feasibility study should provide a firm and well-justified answer to the question of whether the proposed health plan and/or expansion of the existing program will be successful.

Initially, the planner will need funds to hire staff, to complete applications for financial assistance from lending organizations, and to assemble a planning team. The identification of initial funds and organization of the development team are the first stages in the feasibility study, as outlined in Figure 9-1. The team will, in all likelihood, be composed of the MCO advocate and others who have realized the need for such an organization. For expansion of the service area or new programs, the team will usually consist of the current administrative group. If possible, this team should be composed of individuals with skills that will be valuable during the feasibility phase—a doctor, a registered nurse, a health services administrator, a health planner, a service plan or indemnity insurance company executive, a banker and financier, and so on. The first task facing this team will be to outline the MCO's mission and objectives, its reasons for being, or, in the case of an expansion, the goals to

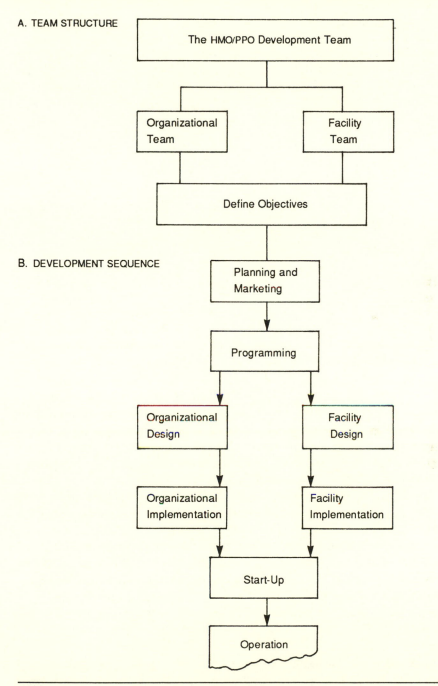

FIGURE 9-1 The HMO/PPO development process.

be attained by moving into new areas or programs. These objectives generally will cover the personal convenience of the providers and consumers, the needs of payers, especially businesses and government, the economies that may be realized in the MCO, the professional development of the health care staff, and the introduction of specific medical services to a particular community; statements regarding the use of fee-for-service and capitation arrangements in physician compensation mechanisms also should be included.

Answers to the following questions should enter into the development of objectives:

1. Which organizational model has been selected? Why was it chosen?

2. What is the degree of commitment of the local providers of care? Have any contributed time, money, or both to the project?

3. What is the level of the planner's knowledge of the HMO concept? What are the planner's skills concerning the management of developmental activities and operations?

4. Are there sufficient sources of information on which to base developmental decisions?

In addition, if expansion of the service area or program is a part of the feasibility analysis, the following questions would also apply:

5. Which organizational model will be used for the new area or program, since mixed-model health plans seem to provide the flexibility needed to compete in today's market? Are there potential problems using a mixed-model approach?

6. Can expansion be accomplished through purchase, acquisition, or venture activities with another organization?

7. Does the ultimate survival of the existing programs depend on service area or program expansion, or are there other methods available to assure the continuing success of the programs?

8. Does the current administrative structure contain the expertise needed to adequately manage a much larger organization? Will divisions or substructures be needed; will decentralization of certain administrative activities be necessary to maintain efficiency and economies in the health plans activities?

9. What methods can be used to assure coordination and integration of all the health plan programs and components, including the new ventures?

By now, the reader has probably recognized that planning and developing a new MCO, or expanding an existing one, is more than just the step-by-step process outlined in Figure 9-1. All of the activities shown must be completely

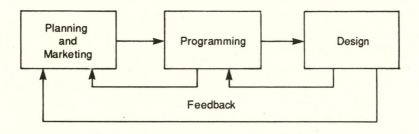

FIGURE 9-2 Feedback and interrelationships in the MCO development process.

carried out; but will they always occur in the order shown? No; most likely the MCO will have preexisting constraints placed on its developmental activities—a group practice may be converting to capitation, state laws and regulations may limit expansionary desires, existing HMOs and PPOs may create unreasonable competition in certain areas of the market, or the developer may own or have available existing facilities to house a health plan. These preexisting conditions should create the backdrop against which the planning activities take place; they should be considered along with all other data to help define goals and objectives and to redefine the mission if unsurmountable problems are encountered. Development consists of a circular set of activities; it is an iterative process in which all of the activities must be completed—some concurrently, but always with feedback and always with a review of current activities. For example, once data show that certain objectives cannot be carried forward, the planning team must modify these objectives to have a better fit with the circumstances in the marketplace. Figure 9-2 indicates that there are three major activities in the development process, each of which may be carried out concurrently, but each having an effect on the others.

For the MCO developer with an existing facility or facilities, planning, programming, and program design will be directly affected by the size, location, and layout of those facilities. The planning and development steps, beginning with team development through implementation and start-up, will be completed and evaluated against the facility constraints. A similar situation exists when an operating HMO decides to expand into PPO-like products; the current capitated physician group, for example, may need to be evaluated to determine whether it would be possible to accommodate discounted fee-for-service arrangements.

Because of the importance placed on the feasibility stage, the HMO planner may wish to follow the *Guide to Development of Health Maintenance Organizations* prepared for the Department of Health and Human Services by Birch and Davis Associates.[1] Although it was published in March of 1982, the *Guide* is still the most useful document that describes the step-by-step process of completing managed care feasibility and planning studies. It is based on the requirements of the federal HMO office, and describes the completion of five study issues—development of organizational arrangements and management, legal feasibility, market feasibility, health services delivery feasibility, and financial feasibility. The issues included in each phase are identified in Table 9-1, and each issue covers an area of risk that requires the planner's evaluation and decision. A "no go" decision in any one of these areas should be interpreted as a major impediment to successful development and operation. If a satisfactory solution cannot be devised, the planner should consider terminating the plans for a new HMO or for expansion. Normally, contingency arrangements can be made so that a satisfactory "go" decision will be possible.

One additional critical area of development noted in market analysis but not specifically identified by the *Guide to Development of Health Maintenance Organizations* is so obvious that it may be overlooked by the planner—evaluation of the health care needs and demand in the community. Experience has shown that, where there is a substantial unmet need or a lack of a formalized system of health care delivery and availability of acceptable health insurance products, there is a high probability that the HMO's development or expansion will be successful. Another of the study tasks requires that the planner show evidence of unmet need and demand in the service area; there must be a demonstrated lack of adequate primary care. This insufficiency can be measured by four criteria, the first being the primary consideration.

1. *Lack of health care services:* Requires an evaluation of acute and therapeutic services, guaranteed comprehensive care without per-visit financial thresholds, out-of-area coverage, full-time access, preventive services, and annual reviews of benefits per cost.

2. *Lack of facilities:* Requires an evaluation of access to all necessary facilities.

3. *Lack of providers of care:* Requires an evaluation of regular hours, removal of nonprofessional administrative functions from physicians, and adequate pay scales to ensure effective specialty practice (primary, secondary, and tertiary care).

---

[1] U.S. Department of Health and Human Services, Health Care Financing Administration, Office of Health Maintenance Organizations. *Guide to Development of Health Maintenance Organizations.* Rockville, Md., DHHS, 1982. DHHS Publication No. (PHS) 82-50178

TABLE 9-1   Phases in the Creation of an HMO with Selected Characteristics

PHASES	ISSUES	ACTIVITIES	DECISIONS
I. Feasibility 1. Objectives: state of readiness	• Organizational structure • Long-range goals • Objectives	• Initial planning • Funding for feasibility study	Whether to proceed to a formal feasibility study
2. Feasibility Study	• Legal climate • Marketing potential • Provider relationships • Financial capabilities • Need/demand identification	• Management of feasibility study • Data analysis and display of results • Review of analysis by sponsors and funding sources	Whether to proceed with development of an HMO
II. Planning	Same	• Detailed planning • More complete data • Work plan development	How to proceed to initial development phase
III. Initial Development	Same	• Establish HMO as legal entity • Begin marketing and enrollment • Employ or contract with physicians • Complete arrangements for facilities • Complete any insurance contracts	How to proceed to operational phase
IV. Initial Operation 1. Start-up	Same	• Delivery of care to enrollees • Processing of claims • Continue marketing effort • Balance needed services with delivery capability	• Day-to-day policy decisions • Personnel decisions • Whether HMO is self-supporting financially
2. Normal Operations	Same	Same (Also continue evaluation of level of care and services)	• Normal operation decisions • Whether to increase size of HMO, add facilities, increase benefits

4. *Lack of appropriate financing mechanisms:* Requires an evaluation of all financing mechanisms, including private third-party coverage (service plans and indemnity companies, employer- and union-sponsored payment mechanisms, and governmental programs).

The feasibility phase culminates with the completion of the reviews and evaluations of need, identification of appropriate organizational structures and management arrangements, legal climate, marketing potential, health services delivery and provider relationships, and financial capabilities. Depending on the availability of initial funding and the interest and commitment of the planners and their capabilities, this phase may be completed in as little as four months. Generally, however, it may take one year, and sometimes up to two years, to complete feasibility activities.

Costs of the feasibility stage vary, depending on whether the work is done by in-house staff or whether a consultant is used, the availability of community data, the availability of funds to complete the study, and so on. Some experts have suggested that these costs could be as low as $50,000 or as high as $500,000.

A quick review of the major issues that must be considered in the first stage follows. Each must be thoroughly evaluated.

FEASIBILITY CHECKLIST

1. Health plan mission statement, goals, and objectives have been identified and clearly stated. The goals and objectives of expansionary activities are well defined and understood by the health plan board, management, and physicians.

2. A plan of developmental activities or a work plan has been detailed (network programming using techniques such as Program Evaluation and Review Technique [PERT] or Harvard Software's "Project Manager").

3. The management team has all of the requisite resources (time, money, expertise, experience) to develop or expand the HMO.

4. Funds for feasibility, planning, development, and start-up or expansion are available or are forthcoming.

5. The legal review indicates no national or local statutory barriers to the formulation or expansion of the HMO (e.g., blue laws, corporate practice of medicine, certificate of need, advertising, tax status).

6. A workable, legal organizational structure has been, or can be, created.

7. There is an unmet need/demand in the catchment area.

8. There is a broad base of support in the community from which enrollment can be drawn.

9. There will be a sufficient level of initial and break-even enrollment (specify level).

10. The prevailing health insurance premiums and benefits are at a level that permits the HMO to be competitive.

11. The demographic, socioeconomic, and epidemiological data necessary to complete underwriting activities are available.

12. The income (or purchasing power) of the target population is high enough to purchase the benefits package.

13. There is provider support in the numbers required to deliver care (including hospitalization).

14. Capitated payment to providers, physicians, and hospitals is acceptable.

15. The preliminary demand, capacity, and funds flow analyses appear to suggest break-even within an acceptable time period.

PLANNING PHASE

The planning stage essentially expands on the activities started during the feasibility study. At the completion of the feasibility study, the planner should briefly evaluate the information collected and decide whether to continue. During the planning phase, the question of how to proceed through development is clearly addressed: the data base for the major developmental issues listed in Figure 9-1 is expanded and refined; the decisions that must be addressed prior to actual development are clearly defined; a detailed work plan that describes the tasks to be accomplished and the time sequence for performing each task is completed; and sources of funding, including governmental and private sources, are identified.

Because of the substantial studies that are accomplished during the feasibility phase, the planning stage needs only to be a refinement of the data and plans for development or expansion. The time period allowed for these activities should be short—several months at most. Many HMO planners, however, find that the early stages are critical for identifying development or expansion funds and will extend the planning phase, because the search for funds is a slow process and may indicate a general unwillingness of the community to support the HMO; these early fiscal problems should indicate whether or not the newly developing HMO will be successful in becoming operational. The planning phase is complete when all activities and plans for development or expansion have been delineated and when sufficient funds to continue have been identified and obtained. In addition to the items on the feasibility checklist, the following elements also should be a part of the development plan at the completion of the planning phase.

PLANNING CHECKLIST

1. For a new plan, the organizational structure has been developed and is an independent legal entity; for the expansion of an existing plan, the organizational structure has been modified to accommodate the expansion.

2. Community support and acceptance is neither neutral nor negative; physician and target population attitudes are positive.

3. Highly skilled individuals for top managerial and developmental positions are employed by the new or existing HMO entity (executive director, medical director, marketing manager, and finance manager).

4. A marketing strategy (membership objectives, marketing and enrollment procedures) for each target population is in draft form.

5. The benefits packages and other structures have been generally described.

6. A guaranteed commitment from providers has been obtained.

7. Guaranteed commitments from groups of enrollees have been obtained.

8. Facility planning is completed.

INITIAL DEVELOPMENT PHASE

Plans formulated during the previous phase now become operational. Actual implementation of the work plan will involve the selection and training of staff, a functional organizational entity, and a facility. According to federal executives involved with monitoring HMO development and operations, seven major project areas are identified in the initial development phase. Each of these tasks is shown in Figure 9-3 and is discussed in the following sections.

Organization and Board Development: If the organization's selection of a board of trustees and its institutionalization as a legal entity have not been completed during planning, these matters should be finalized at this time. Likewise, if expansion demands that board composition be changed, the plan should undertake these modifications.

Marketing: Activities in this area include the development of benefits packages to match the demands of target populations; creation of a sales strategy; assembly of literature and other sales materials; finalization of dual-choice agreements with employees, unions, and governmental agencies; and enrollment of members.

Provision of Care: This encompasses all activities necessary to arrange for delivery of care. Thus, a medical care program at the health plan's center must be designed and implemented. Services of outside providers also must be arranged; contracts with providers for services that the health plan itself cannot provide economically or physically may include medical specialists,

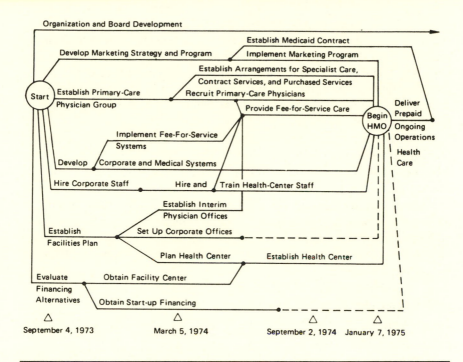

FIGURE 9-3   **HMO development plan.**

pharmacies, hospitals, therapists, and others. Referral relationships also must be facilitated.

Corporate and Medical Systems: These systems include information systems, accounting systems, appointment systems, and personnel management systems, as well as those activities that are necessary to support, evaluate, and control the quality of medical care delivered to members. Medical systems are internal to the corporation; they support the delivery of care. Examples include evaluation of the quality of care, creation and maintenance of medical records, and procedures to handle member complaints regarding the quality of care.

Personnel: New organizations will require the formulation of hiring, censure, recognition, and termination procedures; these procedures should be used in developing a staff that will perform at a level of productivity required by the organization. This is a major managerial task and requires close coordination with all other developmental activities.

In the initial development phase, the HMO should include a plan administrator, medical director, nursing director, marketing manager, and financial manager. Each should be hired when their tasks first appear in the development plan. The administrator and medical director should be the first to be hired by the new organization's board of trustees and, generally, will have been active during the feasibility and planning stages, even though they may not have been formally employed by the plan.

Because the most common reason for early HMO failure is the lack of management expertise, the choice of an administrator and medical director is most important. In studies of federally funded HMOs, it has been found that placing the initial HMO planner/advocate in the position of administrator of the formal organization has not been a wise choice. This position requires an individual with organizational, financing, marketing, and control skills, while the initial HMO planner generally is a lobbyist, negotiator, or politician who helps forge and strengthen the relationships between the health plan, its providers, employers, unions, and the population in the service area. Both individuals are essential to the development of the HMO, but they have separate and very distinct tasks to perform. The administrator may come from a sponsoring organization or may be recruited from another health or insurance plan. Additional staffing might follow the ratios provided in Chapter 6.

Administration: Because administration is a continuous function, it is discussed here to emphasize that good management throughout the process of creating the HMO is necessary for its success. The process of management—planning, organizing, directing, staffing, controlling—is the cement that holds all of the organization's activities together so that services can be delivered effectively and efficiently. The administrator must be able to view the entire program's activities from the lowest common denominators—service and the dollar. Evaluating financial alternatives, obtaining required funds for development and start-up, and budgeting are very important activities of this developmental function and are described in detail in Chapter 11.

Facility Development: This project area provides for the development of necessary facilities in which to carry out the corporation's activities. Included are all problems associated with site selection, leasing, construction, and furnishing and equipping the offices and medical service facilities to be operated by the HMO. Activities in this project area might include setting up corporate offices, establishing facilities for temporary services, and building and occupying a permanent health center.

Generally, facilities for the administrative and delivery functions need to be addressed. Administrative office requirements may be quickly met through the lease of retail or office space in office buildings, although the plan may eventually find that office facilities dedicated to health plan administrative

TABLE 9-2   Outline of Delivery Site Developmental Activities

A. Prearchitectural Planning (15 months)

   1. Long-range Planning

      a. Service area analysis
      b. Ambulatory care program analysis
      c. Financial analysis
      d. Facility analysis master plan
      e. Alternatives/solutions
      f. Program selection/approval

   2. Development of External Team (architects, consultants, others)
   3. Financial Feasibility/Financing/Budget Control
   4. Regulatory Submission/Approval

B. Facility Implementation

   1. Simple Projects (15 months)

      a. Establish program
      b. Establish budget
      c. Develop building concept
      d. Bid/award contracts
      e. Construction
      f. Activate
      g. Monitor/evaluate

   2. Complex Projects (32 months)

      a. Establish budget/program
      b. Develop functional program
      c. Prepare block drawings
      d. Prepare schematic drawings
      e. Prepare developmental drawings
      f. Prepare working drawings
      g. Bid/award contracts
      h. Construction
      i. Activate
      j. Monitor/evaluate

functions only are desired. The planning, design, and construction of an ambulatory care facility is more complex; it involves five distinct stages and may take from 30 to 47 months to complete, depending on the project's complexity and size. As outlined in Table 9-2, the facility development stages occur in the major project phases of prearchitectural planning and facility implementation.

About half the time is devoted to the prearchitectural planning phase. During this phase, critical tasks are accomplished and decisions made; for example, creating a patient demand model, clearly defining and documenting the required ambulatory care program, projecting staffing and utilization patterns, and devising a plan to use ancillary services. Other considerations are examined and courses of action forged regarding the health plan's governance and management structure, capital finance sources, marketplace positioning, and consumer behavior regarding products and services, prices, and location, as noted previously.

Construction costs vary according to whether the facility is new, a renovation of existing space, or a renovation of a nonmedical structure. If hospital space is being used, renovation runs 60 to 75 percent of the cost of new construction; however, where added basic construction costs accrue due to specialized units such as radiology, this figure can go to 85 to 90 percent. Early 1990 construction costs of a new freestanding ambulatory center, including built-in equipment, ran from $100 to $240 per square foot. Total project costs—including financial, legal, design fees, and equipment—usually run approximately twice the general construction costs.

The following is a checklist for facility development.

FACILITY CHECKLIST

1. Establish facilities plan
2. Establish interim physician offices
3. Set up corporate offices
4. Plan health center
5. Establish health center

Since most of the developmental process to this point has concerned the organizational program design and implementation, careful attention must be given to the activities on the righthand side of Figure 9-1, relating to facility development; the initial cost of a facility has an important and dramatic impact on the operation of the program.

INITIAL OPERATION PHASE

When all developmental activities have been completed, the HMO is ready for the delivery of care to enrollees. Start-up activities should have been well orchestrated prior to the operation phase—with all staff members totally familiar with their duties. During the operation phase, therefore, the HMO manager's major responsibilities are to ensure an even day-to-day operation of the organization and to collect and analyze data to evaluate the level of care being delivered, consumer and provider satisfaction, growth in the organization, and financial and operational stability of the new HMO. This phase ends when the program "breaks even," that is, when the membership grows to a level where the cumulative cash flow no longer shows a deficit.

Ordinarily, it takes several years for a new or expanded HMO to reach this stage.

Developmental Guidelines

Three additional issues may be helpful to the HMO developer—rules of thumb, the critical areas in development, and the major problem areas. In the following two sections of this chapter, "critical" and "problem" areas are presented. The list that follows is intended to provide the HMO developer with the experience gleaned from the field regarding the rules of thumb generally accepted by HMO managers. These provide a starting point in the development of assumptions, *but are not intended to be used without modification and caution.* Rules of thumb are merely indicators, guides, and approximations and should not be considered as fact. Several of the categories are discussed in detail in other chapters of this text, and the reader should refer to those discussions before applying any of them. Bearing this in mind, rules of thumb are provided for several HMO activity areas.

HMO PLANNING RULES OF THUMB AND ASSUMPTIONS

Population and Service Area

1. There should be a minimum of 250,000 to 500,000 people in the general population (service area) and the possibility of obtaining at least 1,000 enrollees per physician.

2. A penetration rate of at least 10 percent of the total population (250,000) at the break-even point should be possible.

3. The size of the initial, eligible target population to be enrolled should be at least 5,000 and likely to reach 20,000 in two to three years (i.e., 5,000 to 6,000 families).

4. At least 80 percent of the service area population should be below age 65.

5. Target population family income should be $20,000 per annum or above.

6. At least 70 percent of the projected service area population must live within a 30-minute drive of the facility.

7. No more than 80 to 85 percent of the general population (250,000) should be covered by present insuring mechanisms.

8. The service area population should be at least 20 times the target population that is eligible to be enrolled.

9. The most important population characteristics are age and sex distribution, family size, income level, urban/rural mix, ethnic makeup, and geographic location.

10. Population segmentation may be as follows: by age and sex; by employer or union affiliation; by residency within particular geographic boundaries; by third-party payer representations; or by ethnic, racial, or language characteristics.

Employers and Other Payers

1. Large businesses (more than 1,000 employees each) should be a part of the local service area; these large employers should have experience with managed care health plans and be willing to offer the new or expanded HMO or other managed care packages to their employees.

2. Employers should generally express satisfaction with HMO health plans. For HMO development, employers should not prefer to offer PPOs exclusively.

3. Employers should feel that the HMO benefits packages are better than those of competing plans, that the HMO's premiums are lower than those of competing plans, that increases in HMO premiums are not as large as those of the competition, and that the HMO is the better buy for the employer and his employees and dependents.

4. Employers are interested in hybrid packages that provide for cost savings; the managed care organization should provide options for selection by employers, such as point-of-service, less than comprehensive benefits, and larger copays by employees.

5. Employers offer managed care programs because of cost savings; clearly show how and where cost savings occur.

6. Some employers have observed that healthier employees and dependents have chosen HMO coverage, while employees and dependents in poorer health (higher risk) have chosen traditional plans like the Blues. This adverse selection tends to raise the total health insurance premiums paid by the employer. The new or expanding HMO's strategy with employers should address this issue in a straightforward manner, and premiums should reflect the actual risks of enrollees.

7. Efforts to educate employers concerning the quality of HMO physicians is of high priority during the planning and developmental stages. This is important because employers still have the perception that the traditional system has superior doctors, even though research shows very few differences between doctors in the traditonal and HMO systems.

Providers

1. The project begins with at least five full-time-equivalent physicians in the following specialties: general medicine, general practice, family practice or internal medicine, obstetrics and gynecology, pediatrics, and general surgery.

2. Physicians in these specialties will provide 70 to 80 percent of all health services needed.

3. Other specialists will be provided on a referral basis by affiliated or out-of-plan physicians.

4. Each full-time physician will provide 30 to 35 hours of ambulatory office care and 10 to 15 hours of in-hospital care.

5. Staffing will be according to the following ratios (Please refer to the discussion on physician staffing in Chapter 6):

Internal medicine	35 physicians per 100,000 enrollees or 1 physician per 2,850 enrollees
General medicine	10 physicians per 100,000 enrollees or 1 physician per 10,000 enrollees
Pediatrics	15 physicians per 100,000 enrollees or 1 physician per 6,650 enrollees
Obstetrics/gynecology	10 physicians per 100,000 enrollees or 1 physician per 10,000 enrollees
General surgeons	5 to 8 physicians per 100,000 enrollees or 1 physician per 12,500 to 20,000 enrollees

6. Paramedical staffing (Please refer to the discussion regarding nonphysician staffing in Chapter 6):

5.3 FTE staff per physician, or 3 paramedical personnel per 1,000 enrollees

1.35 FTE business and clerical staff per physician

3.53 FTE paramedical staff (excluding radiology and laboratory) per physician

0.13 FTE physician assistants per physician

0.50 FTE registered nurses per physician

1.10 FTE non-RN nursing personnel per physician

0.17 FTE maintenance personnel per physician

7. As an example, based on 16 full-time-equivalent physicians, the following personnel are required:

0.5 to 1.25 FTE laboratory and X-ray technicians

0.5 to 3.0 FTE all other health delivery personnel

1.0 to 5.0 FTE business and clerical personnel

8. Project 1 physician per 1,000 to 1,200 enrollees.

9. Inpatient hospital beds—1.5 to 2.0 beds per 1,000 enrollees.

Marketing and Enrollment

1. If purchasers (employers, unions, associations, government) do not offer multiple-choice health plans to beneficiaries, attempt to have such a practice instituted. Include the managed care option as one of these plans.

2. Provide open enrollment at least annually.

3. There must be a potential market of several good-sized (more than 100 employees) nonnational firms, unions, associations, and so on.

4. The HMO should attract at least 25 to 50 enrollees per group, except where the account may grow or has the potential to critically influence other groups.

5. Plan on community rating, but use loading and experience rating for special groups if and when required.

6. Assess the HMO's ability to receive either a Medicare or Medicaid contract (or both) and to provide services to these recipients using risk contracts.

7. If contract marketing is used, a commission rate may be as low as one-tenth of one percent of premiums.

8. To achieve an enrollment rate of 10,000 members, 4 to 8 marketing people will be needed initially; however, maintenance marketing after start-up and plan stability may demand 3 to 4 marketing employees regardless of enrollment in the plan.

9. Do not depend on one group for more than 10 percent of health plan income (except during initial operation). An acceptable initial market penetration for an HMO is the enrollment of 10 percent of one group.

10. Attempt to enroll a population mix that approximates the characteristics of the total community population (balanced enrollment).

11. In groups, for those given a true dual choice, the expectation of a 5 to 10 percent initial enrollment rate may be appropriate.

12. Penetration-rate studies should be completed by payment mechanism, employer group, age and sex, and so on.

13. An increased deduction of from $10 to $15 per month from an employee's paycheck is the maximum acceptable increase over the present health plan deduction. Stated somewhat differently, there should be no more than a 10 percent differential between the HMO and the other health insurance plans in the community.

Benefits Package and Utilization of Services

The items listed below are a sample of morbidity rates that might be used during planning and development; please refer to Chapter 11 for a more complete discussion of morbidity rates and rate tables.

1. Plan 400 days per 1,000 commercial members per year for inpatient care, 2,000 days per 1,000 Medicare members per year, and 475 days per 1,000 Medicaid members per year.

2. Plan 83 hospital admissions per 1,000 commercial members per year, 270 hospital admissions per 1,000 Medicare members per year, and 120 hospital admissions per 1,000 Medicaid members per year.

3. Plan psychiatric services (if provided) at 15 to 20 visits per member per year, plus 30 to 45 days of hospital treatment.

4. If extended care is included in the benefits package, plan at least 100 days per benefit period for each member in need of extended care facilities.

5. When most financial barriers are removed, approximately 25 to 30 percent of persons entitled to service make no visits during the year.

6. Plan 3.7 physician visits per commercial member per year, 6.0 physician visits per Medicare member per year, and 4.0 physician visits per Medicaid member per year.

7. Plan 3.7 nonphysician visits per commercial member per year, and 5.7 nonphysician visits per Medicare member per year.

8. Plan 4.89 prescriptions per member per year (all members); 2.56 prescriptions per commercial member per year, and 6.16 prescriptions per Medicare member per year.

9. Plan 1 radiology session for each commercial and Medicaid member per year, and 3 radiology sessions per Medicare member per year.

10. Plan 1.6 lab tests for each commercial and Medicaid member per year, and 4.8 lab tests per Medicare member per year.

11. Plan 1 immunization for each commercial and Medicaid member per year, and 3 immunizations per Medicare member per year.

12. Plan 0.2 emergency room visit per member per year.

13. Plan 0.2 day (outpatient) surgery per member per year.

14. Plan 0.01 ambulance trip per member per year.

15. Approximately 20 to 30 percent of all care received by members will be from out-of-plan services (excluding out-of-area coverage reimbursed by the plan), that is, 20 to 30 percent leakage.

Financing and Facilities

Please review the financial data provided in Chapter 11.

1. Plan approximately 1,500 square feet per physician in the HMO's health delivery center.

2. Plan a construction cost for the health services delivery center at $100 per physician for a new facility and $75 for a renovation.

3. Feasibility, planning, and developmental costs: $100,000 to $500,000.

4. Start-up costs: $75,000 to $1,000,000.

5. Add approximately 1.5 percent to these costs for each month that construction, planning, start-up, and operation is delayed.

6. Project a 1- to 2-year planning and developmental stage prior to operation.

7. Plan not to break even or to make a surplus within the first three years after becoming operational; return on investment may then average 6 to 8 percent per year.

8. Plan on bearing up to $30,000 for costs of care per member per year prior to reinsurance (stop-loss coverage) taking over.

9. Use the financial ratios and value ranges that are shown in Chapter 11. (Example: current ratio [measure of liquidity] = total sources/total uses.)

10. As a percent of total gross revenues, the sources of revenue for the plan may be from the following:

	% of Total Gross Revenues
Premiums	0.65
Fees-for-service	5–10
Copayment	5–10
Pharmacy and other sales	4– 8
Coordination of benefits (COB)	2–15
Reinsurance recovery	1– 5
Other income	8–13

11. Member costs might be reduced $0.15 to $0.20 per month per group member each time 2,000 group members are added as enrollees.

12. Average costs of insurance may be:

	% of Total Expenses
Nonphysician employee insurance cost (health, disability, life)	0.65
Physician insurance cost (health, disability, life)	0.75
Professional liability insurance premiums	1.1
Other liability insurance premiums	0.25
Reinsurance premiums (stop-loss insurance)	1.0
Total	3.75

13. Distribution of expenses may be as follows:

	% of Total Expenses
Physician services	35–45
Hospital inpatient services	25–35
Administrative services	12–15
Other medical and hospital expenses	10–15

In addition, funds may also be used for reserves required by insurance regulations, retained earnings, or dividends. These funds may be 0–25 percent of premiums.

14. Services contracted with insurance companies (including administrative services—collection of premiums; checking enrollment cards; paying commissions, if used; and so on) may account for 1.5 percent of the premium dollar.

15. The lag time between enrollment and time of premium payment is 45 days.

16. Include in any projected financial plans an inflationary factor based on the *Medical Service Index* for the United States. As an example, the index has shown the following changes from year to year: 6.37 percent in 1986, 6.64 percent in 1987, and 7.53 percent in 1988. The change from 1989 to 1990 was 8.3 percent, and 6.3 percent between 1990 and 1991.

CRITICAL AREAS OF DEVELOPMENT

It is helpful to understand which areas in the development and expansion process are considered most critical and to be aware of the problems that occur most frequently. In studies of 10 HMO federal grantees, the areas and issues that are discussed below were considered to be the most critical to development.

Financing

The funding of HMO development, expansion, and operation was considered a major area of concern by managers in the field. Financing in this context includes debt and equity capital for facilities, underwriting of risks, research and development or expansion of programs, start-up costs, and prebreak-even operational costs. Although some financial support for these areas is usually available during the developmental or expansionary period, the funds may be either insufficient or, for many HMOs, the period for break-even extends past that for which the HMO budgeted.

Most developing health plans describe their almost futile efforts to obtain outside financing, especially for risk underwriting or for covering initial operating losses prior to breaking even. Like other health care organizations, HMO resources and operations do not provide an acceptable form of collateral for obtaining the usual forms of financing. In most situations, therefore, developmental or expansion funding is provided through equity financing from surpluses of the business or debt arrangements with outside financial institutions using the existing business as collateral. With the recent bankruptcy filing of the MaxiCare health plan and its reorganization plan under

Chapter 11, however, financial institutions are now more cautious in financing managed care programs.

In interviews with HMO administrators and DHHS's Office of Prepaid Health Care officials, they were asked to suggest a management approach to indicate financial progress during development (i.e., a financial indicator). Foremost was the measurement of whether or not present or proposed sources of funding were sufficient to support operation until the break-even point is reached. An indicator may be an inventory of sources and uses of funds and acceptable financial ratios. These might include actual total income as a percentage of actual total expenses (which should be above 100 percent), net worth, operating margin, return on sales, return on equity, return on total assets, the current ratio (current assets/current liabilities), the debt to equity ratio, and the profit margin of the health plan. The very existence and use of a financial plan and a financial management information system, however, is a strong indication that the plan is managing its finances and has them under control.

Big Brother

Many new plans are backed by organizations that provide much of the fledgling MCO's support. The "big brother" might be defined as an organization or individual that supports the developing MCO. The support is either formal or informal and can be in the form of experience, knowledge of capitated medical delivery, or essential resources. Obviously, for plans that are expanding their programs and service area, the structure and systems of the existing health plan are vital to and provide the necessary support for newly developing health plans, taking the place of a big brother.

Establishing relationships with a big brother substantially increases successful progress in development. This is especially true if the big brother organization is a power base in the community and can help arrange initial marketing contacts with major employers, trade associations, business coalitions, federal and state agencies, and union representatives. If, on the other hand, the MCO has not established a big brother relationship, it must look elsewhere for its resources—technical assistance, influence in the community, and status may be obtained by using consultants and becoming involved with local business coalitions, DHHS regional and national offices, other local MCOs, and state agencies such as the state Medicaid programs.

Providers

Health plan directors state that both hospital and physician relationships with the plan are critical to successful progess in development; the formation of a physician group or panel is the primary concern, and a source for inpatient care is a close second. The first issue in development or expansion is how service delivery can be guaranteed to members. This may require creating a new multispecialty group practice or contracting with an existing one, or it may mean that the plan should help sponsor the development of an individual practice association (IPA). If neither of these methods are acceptable, the health plan may want to actually hire physicians (staff model) to guarantee that physician services are available. On the other hand, hospital arrangements usually are not difficult to achieve; hospital working arrangements with the plan can include actual ownership and/or operation of an inpatient facility, contracts with local hospitals for beds, or merely staff-admitting privileges for HMO physicians. Moreover, the hospital may actually be the sponsor of the HMO.

The services of physicians are the most difficult to obtain, according to seasoned executive directors. To complicate this issue, based on changing enrollment projections and practice patterns, physician needs change. Physician attitudes, which also affect physician participation, are difficult to measure and can quickly change during the development or expansionary period. Thus, the plan must generate physician interest and a firm, contractual commitment during development. Eliciting the leadership of a well-known and accepted physician is one of the techniques that helps build physician interest.

Monitoring formal physician-plan contracts may be an acceptable indicator of provider acceptance and commitment in this critical area. Letters of intent, although of limited use, are the first stage in building a solid physician commitment. Formal contracts usually are signed one to two months before operations begin. Contracts, however, should not be signed prior to completion of the delivery components of the system (i.e., before financial arrangements, marketing, and enrollment are well under way).

Legal

Plan directors agree that the legal area very often becomes a major stumbling block to MCO progress. Numerous legal restrictions and regulations are mentioned, so it is necessary to identify all legal impediments to development and expansion as well as possible alternative legal courses of action. The assistance of a lawyer specializing in managed care may facilitate identification of potential legal problems and their resolution. An inventory of legal problems may be useful to the HMO manager to clearly define such problems and their potential solutions. This inventory might include the following:

1. Federal laws and regulations describing participation in federally funded programs such as Medicare, Medicaid, Federal Employees Health Benefit Programs, and IRS classifications concerning profit and nonprofit status.

2. State laws and regulations that may govern professional associations and corporations (Medical Practice acts), HMO-enabling legislation, insurance (commissioner) regulations and state attorney general restrictions, liability for negligence and malpractice, health care service corporation acts (blue laws), corporate practice of medicine problems, and so on.

3. Local jurisdictional regulations and laws, including zoning and health planning regulations, local income tax laws, and property tax laws.

4. Medical society policies concerning advertising, practice ethics, and so on.

The general availability of legal council may be a good indication that the plan is able to cope with most legal restrictions and problems.

Advocacy

Plan managers describe the need for support from a community-minded individual to act as the plan's advocate (the person who is the main supporter of the MCO development), one who can lead others to accept the idea and concept of an HMO or PPO. Advocates can be either physicians or laymen but usually are not the plan manager or project director. They are important during all phases of activity but especially during the inception stage when the health plan is attempting to obtain private financing and support from community leaders. Moreover, one of the advocate's most important skills must be the ability to negotiate—the ability to arrange for outside support through loans, employer-employee recognition, and support from organized medicine, if possible. The advocate's standing in the community, personality, drive and tenacity, charm, ability to build relationships, and charisma are some other characteristics that are necessary and important.

Attitude

The attitudes of consumers, providers, and third-party payers is critical to successful development or expansion. Negative attitudes toward the HMO must be identified and resolved during the early stages, because such problems can severely limit development. On the other hand, positive attitudes enhance the progress of the developing and expanding HMO. Positive patient-physician relationships under the fee-for-service system suggest that the development of a prepaid, closed-panel group practice may be difficult.

The developing or expanding health plan must determine its image in the community, the ties patients have with physicians, and the overall consumer-employer-physician attitude toward the MCO. Measurements that may be used as indicators in this area include the plan's success in attracting physician cooperation and participation and the rate of consumer enrollment. Actual physician participation and consumer enrollment can then be compared with projected levels of physician staffing and subscription. It also may be helpful to perform an informal survey to identify either positive or negative attitudes toward the plan.

Some plans reported that the good reputation of established HMOs in their geographical areas contributed to positive attitudes and, thus, to easier development or expansion. If established HMOs do not adequately meet their contractual relationships or oversell themselves and do not fulfill all of their promises, the newly developing or expanding HMO will experience difficulties with consumer and physician attitudes.

Timing

Another critical issue identified by all plans was the timetable for expansion or developmental activities. Timing was one of the basic areas in which many HMO federal grantees in the 1970s and early 1980s failed in their development attempts, obviously a symptom of other major problems that were encountered by the HMO. Naturally, the time frame must be tailor-made for each plan and must be flexible enough to compensate for blocks in progress. This suggests the invaluable use of milestone, Gantt, or PERT charts to describe the tasks and the time required to accomplish each task.

The management guides suggested by plan administrators include an evaluation to determine whether HMO management has available and is using a timetable. Major emphasis should be placed on frequent updating and explanations of deviations from the timetable. When deviations exist, the plan director should initiate action to correct time sequencing and perhaps to obtain assistance from outside sources.

Management

Generally, it was agreed that the successful development of an HMO depends, to a large degree, on the managerial ability of the plan's executive director and his/her assistants. Management includes the basic administrative abilities of planning, organizing, leading, directing, controlling, coordinating, and decision making. It also includes the following specific areas: knowledge of the HMO plan objectives, negotiating skills, knowledge of the HMO concepts (i.e., prepayment, capitation, insurance, direct service), knowledge of the community characteristics, relationships with community members, marketing, and financing. Executive directors stress the need for flexibility and adaptability by the HMO and its management. The ability to cope with changes is recognized as vital to successful development.

MAJOR PROBLEM AREAS

It is interesting to note that approximately 15 years ago, in June 1976, the Department of Health, Education, and Welfare identified several of the critical issues heretofore reviewed as being key factors in the failure of 23 federally funded HMO feasibility projects. In all but one, the lack of management skills and expertise and strong commitment to the development of the HMO were identified as reasons for the failure of the projects. The DHEW study suggested that greater efforts should be made to more fully develop the management skills of HMO administrators and staff. Recognizing the lack of well-qualified managers, graduate programs in health administration have begun to offer courses in the management of HMOs and other managed care plans. Several include a residency or fellowship in an HMO setting. Table 9-3 lists the reasons identified by the DHEW study for the 23 failures.

Joint Ventures and Other Linkages

One method by which managed care organizations have developed and expanded into new markets has included linking with existing providers and/or health plans. As discussed in detail in Chapter 4, HMOs, for example, have expanded through multiorganizational, multistate arrangements and have been included in both horizontally and vertically integrated systems. An example of such systems includes the nonprofit Kaiser Health Foundation and its affiliated Permanente Clinics, and the Bess Kaiser Hospitals and their health plans in at least 10 states. Arrangements like the Kaiser/Permanente clinics have developed through buyouts and acquisitions, mergers, joint ventures, and management contracts and agreements. Managed care developers and those involved in the expansion of existing health plans may wish to use joint ventures and other linkage arrangements to accomplish their objectives. Such actions require extreme care but may provide for successfully achieving the developer's objectives. These may include the expansion of capital, the creation of a marketing advantage through linkages with successful plans, and the improvement of management by tieing the new health plan to well-run existing organizations with substantial expertise and experience in the new service area.

Health plan managers first must clearly define their objectives for such an arrangement. Then, the process of identifying and evaluating a suitable "partner" is initiated. A request for proposal (RFP) may be used to solicit responses from likely national venture partners for certain activities or involvement. For example, a business coalition may wish to sponsor the development of a new HMO or PPO that will contract with local employers; a management contract with a national HMO firm may be desired because the new HMO or PPO

TABLE 9-3 Frequency of Reasons Why 23 Feasibility Projects Did Not Proceed Under HMO Law

Sponsorship	No.	Insufficient Sponsor Commitment	Lack of Understanding of Goals and Objectives of P.L. 93-222	Provider Opposition	Lack of Providers	Failed to Supply Marketing/Financial Feasibility Outputs
Consumer Groups	6	3	6	1	4	6
Hospitals	8	4	7	1	5	7
Physician Groups	8	4	8	2	6	8
Private Organizations	1	—	1	—	1	1
Totals	23	11	22	4	16	22

Source: Karen A. Hunt, ed. *Health Services Information,* 3(25):2, June 28, 1976.

will require managerial expertise that can be found only in existing, successful health plans located in other states. The RFP approach could be used to describe the desire of the new HMO to consummate a management agreement with a national HMO and to solicit bids. In other situations, the partner may be a natural ally that exists in the local service area, such as a hospital and its medical staff; the staff and the hospital may choose to develop a joint venture to create an HMO or to become a preferred or exclusive provider for local employers. Or, a Blue Cross/Blue Shield organization and a local multispecialty group practice may develop a new joint venture health plan that will offer an HMO package to local employers.

Both partners to these arrangements may desire substantial information about the other. A group practice, for example, that would like to enter into a joint venture for the expansion of an existing HMO would collect and analyze the HMO's financial status, its marketing philosophy, its relationships with purchasers and other providers of service, and other related issues. Initial communications with potential MCO partners may include a request for the financial, utilization, membership, and other general information listed below.

DATA TO BE REQUESTED FROM POTENTIAL JOINT VENTURE HMO PARTNERS*

Financial:
Audited financial statements
Income and expenses per member per month
Health plan administration expense as a percent of total expenses
Actual surplus or deficit per member per month

Utilization:
Annualized incurred patient days per 1,000 members
Annualized physician encounters per member
Annualized total encounters per member

Membership:
Membership growth and level
Medicare and Medicaid members
CMP activities
Average percent change in net membership/month
Average net change in membership/month

Model and General Information
Type of health plan that parent firm operates/owns
Location and size of each affiliated health plan
Date of affiliation(s)
Accreditation, certifications, and qualification reports

*These data should be provided for the parent firm and each affiliate.

With this information, the medical group will be able to make more informed decisions about becoming involved with the HMO. Table 9-4 provides a summary of the data elements that may be useful in analyzing potential HMO or other partners. The HMO may first be requested to supply much of these data in written form and then through face-to-face interviews with the top candidate HMO firms. Rating scales may be applied to the data elements, with weighted values applied, as noted in Table 9-4. A final decision regarding which HMO firm to associate with would be based on the total scores of each candidate firm, as well as overall impressions gleaned from the interviews.

The following scenario exemplifies the venture relationships that are currently developing. A 460-bed community general hospital wishes to strengthen its relationship with its medical staff; the administration understands that by developing closer ties with its staff, it may be able to keep its occupancy higher and more adequately control its market share. Conversely, the medical staff is composed of 80 solo physicians and a few small, single-specialty medical groups. The physicians have noticed a slow but steady attrition of their patient population, mainly to an HMO that uses another hospital in the area. None of the physicians are provider members of the HMO, and only a few hold joint staff privileges with the other, competing hospital. The administration of the 460-bed hospital suggests to the medical staff that they sponsor and develop an individual practice association, the stock of which will be available for purchase by all members of the medical staff. An IPA is developed and a majority of the staff do buy shares in the new corporation at $100 par value.

Negotiations between the board of the IPA and the hospital culminate in the development of a venture firm, 50 percent of which is owned by the hospital and the other 50 percent by the IPA. The objectives of the new venture firm are (1) to develop a new HMO or bring into the service area an existing HMO to compete with the other HMO in town, (2) to serve as a preferred provider for employers who wish to sign discounted fee-for-service contracts, (3) to negotiate risk contracts with the Health Care Financing Administration, DHHS, to serve Medicare recipients, and (4) to negotiate capitated contracts with the state Medicaid agency to serve Medicaid recipients. The new venture company negotiates provider contracts with the hospital, individual and small groups of physicians on the medical staff, pharmacies, radiology groups, and other providers. It is then in a position to negotiate contracts with HCFA, employers, and the local Medicaid agency. In addition, the venture firm sends an RFP to seven national HMO firms requesting that they develop an HMO business in the local area. Five firms respond with proposals, and the venture firm elects to interview representatives of three of them. One is finally chosen to develop a satellite HMO operation in town. This new (or expanded) HMO operation is created as a joint venture (limited partnership) between the venture company and the national HMO, with the HMO becoming the managing partner and the

TABLE 9-4 HMO Affiliation Data Elements and Rating Form

Data Element	Company 1	Company 2	Company 3

GENERAL INFORMATION:

1. Name
2. Corporate headquarters
3. Primary locations
4. Date established
5. Sponsoring organization
6. For profit/not-for-profit
7. Primary lines of business
8. Other lines of business
9. Organizational structure

RATING ISSUES:

10. Form of affiliation
11. Management contract available
12. Involved with other joint ventures
13. Ownership level desired
14. Familiarity with our organizational model
15. General track record
16. Provider friendly
17. Financial resources
18. Commitment to our service area
19. Knowledge of our community
20. Share of our insurance market
21. Proposed share of market
22. Depth and breadth of management talent
23. Marketing strengths
24. Long-term viability
25. Willingness to invest in our project
26. Management information system and capability with our programs
27. Extent of current license
28. Ownership of new license, if required
29. Assurance of on-site managers
30. Medicare experiences
31. Medicaid experiences
32. Board composition
33. Level of board control
34. Quality assurance and utilization control
35. Adverse risk management program
36. Ability to arrange liability insurance
37. Projected break-even level
38. Stability of company
39. If HMO/CMP, federally qualified
40. Accredited by whom
41. Return on investment
42. Current physician relationships
43. Current hospital relationships
44. Marketing strengths
45. Name recognition
46. Grievance procedures for consumers/providers
47. Liability/credentialing of providers
48. Directors' and officers' insurance
49. Sharing of risks
50. Sharing of actuarial assumptions
51. Growth rate
52. Quality of presentation

venture company acting as a limited partner. After several years of operating both the venture corporation and the limited HMO partnership, the physicians realize that they have stabilized and, in some cases, even improved their share of the market, the hospital has experienced a 20 percent increase in bed use, and the new HMO has broken even and has successfully attracted 30 percent of the health insurance market in the local area. The IPA has been able to avoid major taxes by passing its "surplus" from operation to the hospital and individual physicians through increased (yet discounted) fee-for-service. All objectives have been achieved! Real life may not go as smoothly, but such convoluted linkages are developing frequently to take advantage of market conditions. Obviously, there could be major pitfalls, such as the possibility of antitrust and restraint of trade suits. These issues are discussed in the following section.

ANTITRUST[2]

One of the most difficult current issues affecting managed care systems is the possibility of antitrust suits. This is especially important during the development of HMOs and PPOs and the creation of their medical group provider contracts. In the following paragraphs, some of the most pressing issues are described. This discussion is introductory in nature, and it is critical that the planner obtain legal services to resolve any antitrust concerns.

HMOs and PPOs have become extremely antitrust-sensitive. The activities of both HMOs and PPOs may be governed by the Sherman, Clayton, and Federal Trade Commission acts regarding restraint of trade, prohibitions against monopolies, attempts to conspire or combine to monopolize, and unfair methods of competition or deceptive acts or practices in or affecting commerce.[3] The following issues are the most important.

Implied Congressional Exemption: Generally, antitrust laws are considered by courts to be important statements regarding national policy; however, there may be an implied exemption from the application of these laws when Congess creates federal legislation with the express intent to do just that. No congressional desire either way is available regarding PPOs, since there is no federal PPO statute that regulates or controls their activities (although there are at least 14 states that have enacted PPO-enabling legislation or modified insurance laws to allow preferred provider arrangements). Unlike

---

[2] Adapted from Robert G. Shouldice, "Antitrust and HMOs," *Medical Group Management Journal,* 35(4):12, 13, and 33, July/August 1988.

[3] Bernard T. Ferrari and Thomas H. Sponsler. "Health Maintenance Organizations and the Specter of Antitrust Law." *Loyola Law Review, 31*(4):797–824, Winter 1986.

PPOs, Congress, through the 1973 HMO Act and amendments, authorized the concept of the HMO for the provision of economical medical care and thus removed many antitrust challenges to HMO activities; however, particular actions and practices of the HMO may still be under scrutiny.

Exemption Based on the Business of Insurance: In some states where PPOs and HMOs are governed by state laws that identify the PPO's or HMO's activities as the "business of insurance," the McCarran-Ferguson Act exempts them from antitrust law when the business of insurance is regulated by the state. Generally, PPOs cannot meet the insurance test and thus meet this exemption; for example, they do not transfer or spread the policyholder's risk. HMOs do, however, perform insurance functions by spreading and underwriting substantial health illness risks for their enrollees. But, medical groups as contractors with HMOs may *not* be protected by the McCarran-Ferguson Act because the business of insurance relates to the contract between the insurer and the insured and the medical services agreement may be outside the definition of insurance activity.

Note, however, that if the state HMO-enabling law classifies HMOs as *outside* the business of insurance, then the HMO loses the protection it might otherwise have under the McCarran-Ferguson Act.

Price Fixing: When HMOs contract with providers in IPA, group, or network models (rather than staff models), greater antitrust concern is created. This is especially relevant for PPOs whose physician members agree to establish maximum fees that they will accept as payment in full for services they provide to policyholders of specific insurance plans. In *Arizona v. Maricopa County Medical Society* (1982), the court found that price agreements between insurers and providers were essential in this type of health insurance business and were not illegal; however, when physicians as a group (such as a medical group or an IPA) set fees for individual services rendered, then the practice is illegal. In effect, the physicians as competitors were coming together for the purpose of fixing prices. A *per se* violation of the antitrust laws occurs anytime two or more competitors agree to charge a certain price for services, whether or not that price is above or below the market price. Thus, when several medical groups that otherwise compete with each other agree to and establish fees to be charged (or discounted fees to be accepted from) an HMO, they may be price fixing. The best advice in this area is for the medical group to think of itself as a "seller" of health services and to think of patients (or the HMO or PPO acting on behalf of its enrollees) as buyers of services; hard bargaining should be observed and expected between buyer and seller.

Agreements among physicians are not always *per se* illegal, however. Physicians or groups of physicians who join together to form a new entity such as a joint venture IPA, PPO, or HMO and agree to share the economic risk that there might be gains or losses from this new business are not creating antitrust problems. The pricing agreements between the joint venture and member physicians also are within the law.

On March 14, 1988, a U.S. District Court found against ChoiceCare, a nonprofit IPA model HMO, in a class action suit representing current and former HMO physicians.[4] Finding that the health plan, its president, and executive director were in violation of federal antitrust, securities, and racketeering laws, the court found that the HMO conspired to set prices at anticompetitively low rates, and interpreted the pricing decisions of ChoiceCare's physician-run board as price fixing. In effect, it appears that proper attention was not given to physician involvement in the setting of the fees (prices) to be paid them by the health plan. During the trial, 1,800 physicians in greater Cincinnati alleged that the plan conspired to set anticompetitive low rates. The HMO maintained that it merely contracted with participating physicians for their services and did not impose restrictions on the amount a physician could charge. The jury found that the plaintiff physicians suffered damages in the amount of $34 million; because antitrust laws provide for "treble damages"; the damages assessed against the HMO and other defendants totalled $102 million. This decision (and others with similar outcomes) has major implications for the more than 370 IPA model HMOs nationwide.

Monopoly: Monopolization is described in the Sherman Act as a willful acquisition or maintenance of monopoly power as distinguished from growth or development as a consequence of a superior product, business acumen, or historic accident. Monopoly power is further defined as the power to *control price or exclude competition*. Courts would view the HMO's or PPO's relevant market share, its products (benefits packages as well as provider arrangements), the level of competition, barriers to entry into the market by others, and the health plan's conduct and performance in its trading area. Within this context, the Federal Trade Commission (FTC) and courts would apply a rule-of-reason approach in evaluating the extent to which the HMO or PPO controls the market and prices.

The PPO's size and creation of exclusiveness signals potential antitrust concerns. A PPO network that involves a large number of providers representing more than 20 percent of the provider market may be deemed anticompetitive. In Stanislaus County, California, a physician-sponsored PPO accused of antitrust voluntarily dissolved rather than go through a long court battle. For PPOs

---

[4] Group Health Association of America. *HMO Managers Letter,* 5(6):1–2, March 28, 1988. For further information regarding the settlement between ChoiceCare and its plan physicians, please see "ChoiceCare and Docs Settle," *HMO Managers Letter,* 5(21):2, November 21, 1988; and William J. Kopit, Robert J. Moses, and M. Kathleen Kenyon, "Through the Looking Glass and Back: Sherman Act Claims by Health Care Providers Demanding Higher Fees from Health Insuring Organizations," *St. Louis University Law Review,* 34(5):241–275, Winter 1990.

exceeding the 20 percent rule, the Department of Justice will consider the PPO's competitive effects and the size of the physician panel needed to adequately service PPO enrollees, as well as the extent to which member physicians are willing to participate with other PPOs.[5]

Regarding physician-controlled HMOs, FTC addressed the issue of the HMO's size and exclusiveness.[6] Their 1981 statement defined merged and partially integrated health plans and found that where physicians have fully integrated their practice with the HMO (usually a medical group or staff model), antitrust will not likely occur if the physician membership represents less than 30 percent of the area physicians. In effect, the merged physicians have lost their individual business identities and the group has become a single business entity. On the other hand, partially integrated plans are evaluated on the basis of the group's share of the provider market, and the issue of the HMO's control of the physicians as the "agent of the competitors" is of concern.[7] Obviously, the partially integrated arrangement is a more difficult judgment call, and thus may be more fraught with antitrust danger.

Hospitals and a medical group practice (or the hospital's medical staff) may join together to create a new venture with the express purpose of offering PPO and HMO services. This new venture firm may be guilty of monopolization if it possesses the requisite power to prevent competition by excluding competitors, and by excluding other HMOs from entering the market or limiting the ability of other PPO arrangements from forming. For example, the venture firm may include exclusive clauses in its provider contracts with the hospital and physicians that may limit their ability to become providers with other HMOs attempting to enter the market. And because of the new venture's capital position, it may be able to set its prices (premiums) and PPO-discounted fees at levels that might be termed predatory. These predatory prices may effectively block the entrance and success of competing HMOs.

As HMO and managed care linkage arrangements continue to develop and as medical groups become more involved with alternative delivery systems, the question of potential antitrust issues needs to be evaluated, with careful planning as the method of avoiding such surprises. This discussion is intended to inform the reader about the possibility of such antitrust implications; it is not intended as legal advice and should not be used to solve legal problems. Legal counsel should be consulted early in the negotiation process between medical

---

[5] Clearinghouse on Business Coalitions for Health Action. *What Employers Should Know about PPOs*. Washington, D.C., U.S. Chamber of Commerce Coalition Clearinghouse, June 1986, p. 52.

[6] Ferrari and Sponsler. "Health Maintenance Organizations and the Specter of Antitrust Law," p. 812.

[7] Ibid., p. 813.

groups, HMOs, employers, and hospitals before the new venture relationship is consummated.

Summary

Activities in the development or expansion process of an HMO can be defined by reviewing the various phases or stages involved. The HMO developer should identify the critical areas where major problems may occur. According to federal regulations, development consists of four phases—feasibility, planning, initial development, and initial operation. The feasibility phase is characterized by the completion of a feasibility study that provides the developer or manager with data and a rationale for deciding whether to continue or to terminate development or expansion activities. Tasks to be completed during this phase, in addition to the feasibility study, include locating funds to complete the study, organizing a development team, composing a set of HMO objectives, and establishing a general framework for the new organization.

Development or expansion of the HMO includes several activities—setting objectives, planning, programming, initial operation, and implementation. It is important to note that all developing health plans do not follow a rigorous step-by-step approach to development, but that preexisting conditions constrain the process; each developmental activity must be completed but, because the process is circular and iterative, tasks may be completed concurrently and may affect other developmental activities. Feedback is an important aspect of successful development. All developmental activities must, however, be completed before operation of the plan can begin.

The feasibility study requires the completion of five tasks—development of a management program to control the study, and determination of the plan's legal feasibility, market feasibility, provider-relations feasibility, and financial feasibility. The Department of Health and Human Services's *Guide to Development of Health Maintenance Organizations* provides a good method for a complete study. A study issue that is critical to an adequate analysis of the feasibility of development or expansion is the evaluation of health care need/demand in the service area. High unmet need/demand is justification for additional health care providers and financing mechanisms. Evaluation of the five tasks included in the study provides evidence for a "go" or "no go" decision to be made by the developer and manager.

The next phase, planning, is essentially an expansion of the activities started during the feasibility study and, thus, should include a more complete review of the developmental activities. This phase is concluded when all activities and plans for development or expansion have been delineated and when sufficient funds to continue development have been identified.

Plans developed during the planning phase become operational during the initial development period. Initial developmental activities include the organization of the health plan legal entity, appointment of the board of trustees, marketing, arrangements for the provision of care, corporate medical system development, personnel administration, the process of general administration, and facility development. With the completion of these developmental activities, the plan is ready to "start up," to provide services to its members. This initial operation phase provides a period when the program demonstrates its ability to succeed. During this period, management assesses the health plan's strength in the areas of level of care delivered, consumer and provider satisfaction, organizational growth, and financial and operational stability. Initial operation ends, usually after several years, at the "break-even" point, when a cumulative surplus begins to replace a cash flow deficit.

To assist the MCO manager, sample guidelines, rules of thumb, and assumptions are available, as well as an evaluation of critical areas in development and expansion. Rules of thumb, although crude, can be used with caution and are available in the areas of population, employers and other payers, providers, marketing and enrollment, benefits packages, utilization of services, and financing and facilities. Critical areas in development include financing, "big brother" support, providers, legal advocacy, attitudes, and management. Lack of adequate management capability appears to be the key factor in the failure of new HMOs. An evaluation mechanism is available to assist developers in gauging their progress toward a successful, operational HMO.

Expansion of HMOs and other managed care organizations is frequently facilitated through the use of a joint venture or other linkage arrangement. These new organizational structures are described in detail in Chapter 4; they offer the developer of an expanding MCO many options to ownership, control, financing, and management of market share. Their flexibility in organization adds substantial strength to the relationships among providers and health plans, but these arrangements may open the venture organizations to possible antitrust, price-fixing, and monopoly charges. Caution is required in their formulation.

References

Arthur Young and Company. *HMO Feasibility Study Guide*. Rockville, Md., Bureau of Community Health Services, Health Services Administration, U.S. Department of Health, Education, and Welfare, 1974. DHEW Publ. No. (HSA) 74-13020

Bierig, Jack R., and James C. Dechene. "Antitrust Issues for Preferred Provider Organizations." *The Health Lawyer*, 2(3):8–12, Fall 1984.

Elden, Douglas L., and Richard A. Hinden. "Legal Issues in Networking with Alternative Delivery Systems." *Journal of Ambulatory Care Management, 10*(2):51–78, May 1987.

Enders, Robert J. "Hospital-Physician Collaboration and Competition: The Antitrust Connection." *Healthcare Financial Management, 40*(4):60–68, April 1986.

Ferrari, Bernard T., and Thomas H. Sponsler. "Health Maintenance Organizations and the Specter of Antitrust Law." *Loyola Law Review, 31*(4):797–824, Winter 1986.

Holoweiko, Mark. "Watch Out for These New Liability Risks." *Medical Economics, 65*(8):66–87, April 18, 1988.

Joffe, Mark S. "Potential HMO and Physician Liability Arising from Physician Incentive Arrangements." *HealthSpan, The Report of Health Business and Law, 5*(11):9–14, November 1988.

Martinsons, Jane. "HMO Lawsuits Are Sparking Liability Concerns." *Trustee, 42*(5):10–11, May 1989.

U.S. Department of Health and Human Services, Health Care Financing Administration, Office of Health Maintenance Organizations. *Guide to Development of Health Maintenance Organizations.* Rockville, Md., DHHS, 1982. DHHS Publication No. (PHS) 82-50178

U.S. Department of Health, Education, and Welfare, Health Services Administration, Bureau of Community Health Services. *The Health Maintenance Organization Facility Development Handbook,* Rockville, Md., DHEW, 1975. DHEW Publication No. (HSA) 75-13025

Waxman, J. Mark, and Robert J. Enders. "HMO's, Antitrust and the Changing Health Care Marketplace." In: *HMOs and the Law: Legal Issues for HMO Lawyers and Managers. Proceedings of the Group Health Foundation and the National Health Lawyers Association Conference, Los Angeles, California, September 8–10, 1982.* Washington D.C., Group Health Association of America, 1982, pp. 1–42.

10

MARKETING

Historically, medical services planning involved the development of health care facilities and programs without any consideration for matching services to people's needs. With the advent of Titles XVIII (Medicare) and XIX (Medicaid) of the Social Security Act in 1965, individuals previously unable to afford medical services flocked to providers; their care was financed in large part by the Federal Government. The immediate outcome was a tremendous demand on the medical care system, contributing to the inflationary spiral in health care costs and escalating total expenditures by the Federal Government. Several pieces of legislation that were enacted in response to this situation involved the allocation of and planning for health services facilities; if demand was expanding because Medicare was paying the bills, then one way to control the cost was to control the supply of services available to Medicare recipients.

Health planning laws, although not as effective as originally intended, introduced a more rational method of viewing the need and demand for medical services, as well as sophisticated methods to allocate resources using advanced planning. The industry moved from little or no planning for medical services on an areawide basis to planning for such services in regional areas. This process included studies of population needs and analyses of what providers viewed as acceptable levels of care. Drawing from the experience of other industries, medical care institutions then began to perform individual planning activities by measuring need/demand, evaluating provider attitudes, and creating programs and facilities based on these studies. During the last decade, however, medical services administrators have been forced by increasing costs, feast-or-famine utilization, and governmental regulations to base their planning for medical services on population needs; managers are now studying the long-range or strategic demand for such services and are building programs to meet that demand. Currently, programs exist for and because of consumers rather than in spite of them.

Marketing Defined

This logic is extended even further in managed care organizations, especially HMOs. The HMO seeks members by creating consumer satisfaction through an integrated marketing program.[1] In an HMO, marketing is defined as the performance of a wide range of activities, including market surveys, the design of benefits packages, pricing, promotion and selling, and enrollment. It includes any activity that affects the flow of health services, the enrollment of members, and ongoing account maintenance; in fact, almost all activities performed by the HMO can be considered marketing activities. This is not to say that the concepts and goals of quality care are degraded or mitigated but, rather, that they are enhanced by improving customer satisfaction and expanding the definition of quality of care to include marketing activities. An understanding, therefore, of the patient's perspective of satisfaction with the services, benefits, physician's office manner, and congeniality of the staff is a major part of the marketing process.

Marketing results are a measure of the program's success—its validity as a concept and its ability to educate the public, meet the needs of its members, meet its financial obligations, and so on. More than in any other health services delivery mechanism, consumers, through their decisions on whether to purchase HMO services, voice their acceptance or rejection of the HMO. It is not an overstatement to suggest that successful marketing is the key to a successful HMO and managed care program.

Marketing should also be viewed as a concept and a process. The concept is understanding the needs and desires of members, while the process is creating and delivering services that satisfy patients' desires and meet both quality and financial goals.

The marketing schema illustrated in Figure 10-1 provides a visual depiction of the marketing process; it outlines the flow of funds, beginning with premiums generated by HMO members (or their employers) and ending with expenditures for services to these plan members. Premium income is used to

---

[1] Philip Kotler has been most instrumental in conceptualizing and defining the use of marketing concepts in the medical services industry. His concepts of marketing are provided in the following publications: Philip Kotler and Roberta Clark, *Marketing for Health Care Organizations,* Englewood Cliffs, N.J., Prentice Hall, 1987; Philip Kotler, *Social Marketing,* Englewood Cliffs, N.J., Prentice Hall, 1990; and Philip Kotler and Gary Armstrong, *Marketing,* Englewood Cliffs, N.J., Prentice Hall, 1991.

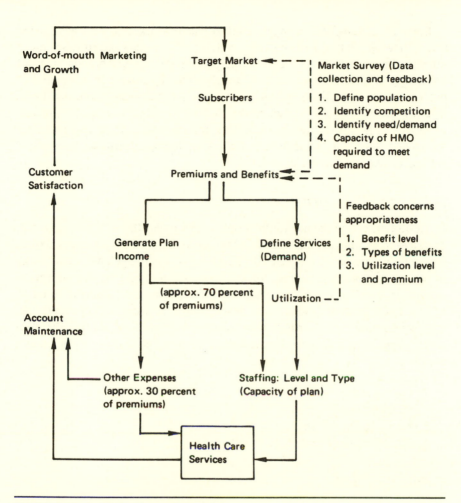

FIGURE 10-1   Marketing schema.

provide services included in the benefits package. The growth and success of the HMO is affected by the free market system, where members' attitudes and beliefs are important to marketing success. Note that Figure 10-1 assumes that once the initial marketing activities are completed, account maintenance by HMO employees and further marketing through word-of-mouth by members are required. Marketing is a continuous, nonstatic process. In this schema, the orientation of the medical care delivery system is toward the market, the purchasers of the program (i.e., employers, the Federal Government, etc.), and the members and potential members instead of toward the products—although service must be competitive or the system will fail.

Some physicians and managers tend to equate marketing with advertising and selling. Marketing includes these activities, but it also encompasses many other issues. Advertising is merely one part of the implementation stage of marketing. It occurs only after a thorough planning process is completed to determine who the clients are, what services the members desire and need, and how their needs will be met by the HMO's providers. Thus, marketing can be described as a two-stage process. The first stage is analysis and planning; the second stage is implementation of plans, including advertising, promotion, selling, education, and evaluation.

MARKETING OBJECTIVES[2]

Philip Kotler, one of the most influential writers on health services marketing, describes marketing as "the analysis, planning and implementation, and control of carefully formulated programs designed to bring about voluntary exchanges of values with target markets for the purpose of achieving organizational objectives. It relies heavily on designing the organization's offering in terms of the target market's needs and desires, and on using effective pricing, communications, and distribution to inform, motivate, and service the markets."[3] Thus, the objectives of marketing involve the following four major areas:

1. Communication
2. Planning and forecasting
3. Management of demand
4. Management of exchanges of value

Communication

Communication is the social process of educating various publics about the HMO's benefits packages and premiums, its physician and hospital providers, and its facilities and locations. These publics include other providers to whom the HMO's physicians refer patients, hospitals where members are admitted, governments that regulate affairs and contract for services of the health plan, and potential managed care members. To each of these audiences, the health

---

[2] This discussion and the next, Positioning, is based, in part, on Robert G. Shouldice, *Marketing Management in the Fee-for-Service/Prepaid Medical Group*, Denver, Colo., Center for Research in Ambulatory Care Administration, 1987, pp. 2–6, with permission of the Center for Research in Ambulatory Care Administration.

[3] Philip Kotler. *Marketing for Nonprofit Organizations*. Englewood Cliffs, N.J., Prentice-Hall, 1975, p. 5.

plan will communicate its needs, describe its services, review its activities, arrange relationships, and so on. Ultimately, the HMO will communicate the ability of the health plan and its providers to meet the needs of members in its service area. Above all, marketing is communication between the physicians and the HMO and its existing and potential markets.

Planning and Forecasting

Marketing also includes planning for the availability and delivery of medical services. A part of the planning process is forecasting the need/demand for services by segments of the population in the service area. Planning is the process of describing the future environment in which the health plan will operate; it includes both assessing the future and providing for it. Planning includes data collection, research, forecasting, data analysis, and the drawing of inferences from the data. It is making management decisions today concerning future activities of the HMO. As a part of marketing, planning represents market research activities; it is necessary in identifying target populations, determining their needs, identifying competition, and then developing services to meet the needs of existing and potential members.

Management of Demand

The management of demand is a technical process of identifying a service population, determining the level of need (and risk to the health plan), and developing marketing strategies to capture that portion of the market. The HMO, therefore, identifies the management of demand as a major marketing activity. Administrators of traditional delivery systems manage finances, personnel, buildings, and so on. They rarely become involved in managing the categories and types of people who require medical services. Some attempts at managing demand by using the traditional delivery system take the form of appointment or scheduling systems, development of waiting lists, and staffing (or availability) of certain services at certain times. Through the use of marketing, the process of managing demand is extended to the prospective identification of consumers who may wish to become prepaid enrollees. Through an analysis of demographic characteristics and the application of actuarial and underwriting methods, the HMO determines the need for care, that is, the demand for services and the risks the HMO will assume are determined before prospective members are given the option of enrolling. A decision is then made as to whether the HMO, through its provider panels and groups, wishes to accept the risk of providing services to groups of enrollees for whom the level of service to be demanded is known in advance.

Management of demand emphasizes a serious concern of the HMO manager, that is, choosing providers who are willing to work with the HMO using modified practice patterns and hospital admitting behavior. As described in previous chapters, HMOs try to control the use of hospital services by emphasizing ambulatory services. These changes in practice patterns (e.g., reductions in hospital days with slight increases in ambulatory visits) are accomplished by providing financial and professional incentives to the participating physicians to change from hospital-intensive to physician office-intensive practices. Health plan managers, both physician and nonphysician, provide strong control over the utilization of physician services. Management of demand, therefore, is enhanced by control over the practice behavior of physicians.

Management of Exchanges of Value

Voluntary exchanges of something of value occur continually between two parties. Each party gives up something of value for something that will fulfill a specific need or want. The parties are motivated to make these exchanges when they feel that what they are getting is at least equal to what they are giving up. Marketing, then, simply includes managing, in a rational way, the exchanges that constantly occur in the HMO so that organizational goals and objectives are accomplished. Because many exchanges occur (e.g., in planning, health services delivery, and referrals), the use of the concept of management of exchanges is another tool for planning and accomplishing goals and objectives.

The three basic values or categories of items exchanged are: services, goods, and money. For the HMO member and patient, money (a premium) is paid by subscribing employer groups for a health benefits package. In exchange, services are made available to the enrollee when a health need arises. These prepaid services are described in the HMO's benefits packages. Once these packages are offered and accepted by the subscriber and a consideration is provided (i.e., payment of the premium), the health plan, through its affiliated panel of physicians and medical groups, has a contract to provide services. Each element in this process is a marketing event. Development of the benefits package that meets the needs and wants of a population is one element. A second element is a pricing strategy to ensure that the premium will be attractive and competitive with the premiums of other health programs. Third, communication of the availability of the health plan and its packages is part of the marketing process. The culmination of the exchange system is the enrollment of employer groups and their employees; delivery of services and feedback about the satisfaction level of members complete the marketing loop. All of the activities shown in Figure 10-1 can be considered part of the exchange system.

The exchange system is not limited to the HMO's delivery activities or to the members' relationship with physician providers. The HMO and its provider groups exchange goods, services, and money with a variety of constituencies, including other subspecialty physicians in the community, companies that provide equipment and supplies, local hospitals, nursing facilities, and the like. There are also exchanges with governmental agencies, such as insurance and planning agencies, in states where certificate-of-need (CON) legislation still requires HMOs and other providers to obtain certification of new facilities and equipment. Thus, the exchange system is used to balance the internal activities of the HMO and its providers with the external environment. Marketing techniques as a tool of management help keep all exchanges, as a total system, in equilibrium.

POSITIONING

Another way of viewing marketing is to examine the current position of the HMO in the medical marketplace. A mature health plan will be considered by members, physicians both in and outside the system, and the community to hold a certain status, image, and position. Indeed, it will have attracted a level of membership and will experience a fairly predictable amount of enrollment, disenrollment, and reenrollment each open season. As a successful health plan in a competitive environment, the HMO will have attracted a comfortable share of both the health insurance business and the medical services delivery market; this share can be easily described by studying the demographic characteristics of the HMO's members and the employers who offer its benefits packages. One can identify the HMO's service area by describing its geographic location, membership size, types and demographic characteristics of members attracted to the plan, the kinds of hospitals used by the plan, and even the referral patterns to and from the HMO's physician providers. These data will identify the HMO's current position in the marketplace.

A market analysis (described in the next section) may identify the need to reposition or redefine the HMO's goals and objectives and to develop a strategy to attract new and different types of employer groups and members. Data collected may identify the health plan's loss of market share and its vulnerability to further loss of current members to competing HMOs and other managed care programs. An analysis may also identify opportunities for expanding and/or improving the plan's position within the community. For example, expanding the service area through contracts with new medical groups can help reposition the health plan and can also boost an existing fee-for-service medical group that needs to reposition itself in an increasingly competitive market. For the new medical group just joining the HMO, the health plan can be considered a marketing device that emphasizes the need for a more competitive strategy and organizational renewal. It allows the group to more fully develop its services and service capacity, or to use existing unused capacity to its fullest. Ultimately, marketing through a managed care system places the medical group in a more competitive position to take command of the marketplace rather than follow in the wake of others.

Repositioning acknowledges the existence of a competitive environment among several quality health plans and their affiliated providers. From the members' perspective, all providers appear to have high-quality clinical services, but the satisfaction derived from a visit to one particular provider may be higher because of certain conditions or events that occurred before, during, or after the visit. Thus, repositioning suggests that even though a competitor's services are of high quality, the HMO and its medical group can develop a marketing strategy that will cause the competitor's members to change their minds about satisfaction with their current health plan's benefits packages and services, including hours of operation, service availability, usefulness in meeting the patient's needs, and so on.

Ultimately, a repositioning strategy should provide the HMO a more acceptable or preferred market share, that is, a membership whose characteristics, number, and level of health risk match the goals set by the health plan. The health plan repositions itself by determining where it is now, where it would like to be, and how it can bring about the desired change. The current position may be viewed as the HMO's niche in the market. Through the efforts described in the next section, the HMO attempts to change its niche and reposition itself to attract and capture a larger or different market share.

Marketing Strategy and Plan

Marketing HMOs and other managed care programs requires both careful planning and developing a strategy that is tailored to the target population. Strategy development demands that funds be available and that experienced marketing personnel be employed for the strategy to be effective. It is the responsibility of the marketing director to develop the marketing strategy, which is a part of the HMO's overall strategic plan.

The creation of a marketing strategy is grounded on the HMO's mission and objectives. The major objective is to identify and select the target populations. The second objective is to develop a "marketing mix," that is, to select the marketing elements that the HMO intends to bring together to meet the needs of the target population. The ultimate goal, however, is to ensure that the HMO is successful in attracting a particular level and type of membership and making available high-quality health services so that members are satisfied with the health plan. The creation of the marketing strategy is a multistep process. As

TABLE 10-1   Steps in the Market Strategy and Plan

Step 1   *Collect data and set initial goals*
   a.   Primary data sources (market surveys, interviews, observations, etc.)
   b.   Secondary data sources (existing data from reports, studies, market analyses performed by other researchers, etc.)

Step 2   *Conduct a market analysis*
   a.   Environmental analysis of the target service area
      (1)   Geographic characteristics
      (2)   Demographic characteristics of the employers and socioeconomic characteristics of potential members
      (3)   Epidemiological data: morbidity, mortality, and disability
   b.   Analysis of the competition
      (1)   Insurance competition
         (a)   Analysis of competing HMOs and managed care programs
         (b)   Analysis of competing indemnity and Blue Cross/Blue Shield programs
      (2)   Provider competition
         (a)   Analysis of nonparticipating physicians, hospitals, pharmacies
   c.   Analysis of consumer opinions, that is, employers/employees and providers

Step 3   *Decide on target markets and set final goals*
   a.   Segment the market and analyze penetration rates
      (1)   Segment by employer, geographic location, payment mechanism, and current coverage
      (2)   Compare segments using cross tabulations
      (3)   Select segments to include in current marketing campaign
      (4)   Prepare justification for inclusions
   b.   Select the target markets and goals; obtain agreement of board and all managers

Step 4   *Design a marketing mix for target markets*
   a.   Review need/demand statements
   b.   Review actuarial and underwriting studies
   c.   Create marketing mix elements
      (1)   Medical services and products (benefits packages)
      (2)   Place (location and availability of services)
      (3)   Price benefits packages (premiums, copayments, deductibles)
      (4)   Promote plan (education, selling, advertising, communication with publics)

Step 5   *Forecast enrollment (and identify break-even point for a developing or expanding HMO)*
   a.   Identify variables that affect enrollment
   b.   Estimate disenrollment and reenrollment levels
   c.   Estimate enrollment in future periods
   d.   Create strategic (long-term) marketing plan

Step 6   *Make choices available*
   a.   Active marketing and enrollment
   b.   Account maintenance and growth

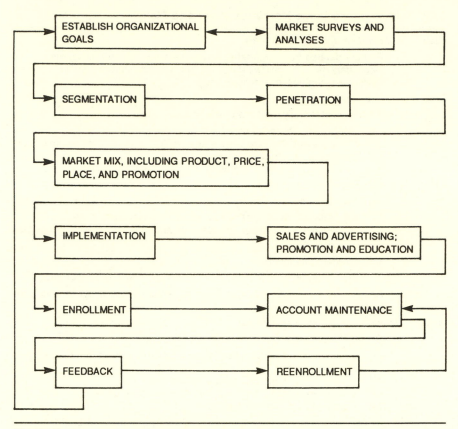

FIGURE 10-2 The HMO marketing process.

shown in Table 10-1, and described in the sections that follow, the marketing strategy and plan involve six steps that are a part of the complete marketing process identified in Figure 10-2.

STEP 1: COLLECTING DATA AND SETTING INITIAL GOALS

Health plans developing or expanding their service areas will accumulate data to help set initial goals and objectives. As the plan takes shape and begins operation, additional data from actual experience will provide the basis for subsequent analyses and for modification of the plan's objectives and direction. Thus, the collection and analysis of information is an ongoing process; even though data collection and marketing analysis are discussed separately, they occur concurrently. Both primary and secondary sources of data are used and are described later in this discussion. In addition, specific types of data are addressed.

Most HMO planners will have a stated set of objectives that will be accepted or modified by the HMO's board throughout the planning and development process. Based on the definition of marketing provided earlier in this chapter, most of these objectives will concern marketing goals. For example, one objective may be the development of a 15-physician, multispecialty group that will provide, on a self-supporting basis, comprehensive health care services to 20,000 members drawn from a population base of 700,000. Although broad, this objective limits the character of the marketing study the HMO administrator should undertake. When the results of the survey are available, a comparison of the population data with the objectives may reveal the need to modify the goals to make them realistic and operative. Many HMOs set unrealistic marketing objectives that are never modified, resulting in impossible marketing goals on which staffing is based and financial projections are made. Modifying the HMO's objectives after the market feasibility study cannot be overemphasized.

Data collection activities, also described as market surveys, provide information concerning the general population—the total population residing in the geographic area to be served—and the target population—those segments of the total population to which benefits packages are to be marketed. The service or beneficiary population is that portion of the target population that is actually enrolled in the health plan. To describe the general population of the catchment area, the market survey identifies broad socioeconomic levels, available insurers, and providers of care. These three areas can be considered as the first cut in the market analysis. Examples of minimum market conditions concerning these three areas are presented in Table 10-2.

The market survey also provides information that allows HMO planners to continue refining the general population to the point where target populations surface. The target populations are of more immediate concern than the general population, because they more fully describe the demand that the HMO must meet; these are the populations to which the market analysis is directly addressed and for whom the marketing strategies are developed. During the operational phase, the administrator's primary consideration is the service population, since all operational decisions are made because of and for this enrolled group.

Secondary Data Sources

The majority of data collected at this point will be from secondary sources, that is, data collected and analyzed by others in the community. The task, then, is to locate, review, interpret, and draw inferences from these data. Much of the information deals with the population of the area and its demography;

TABLE 10-2 Minimum Market Conditions

Level	Condition
Socioeconomic	
(1) Income	(1) Above $30,000 per family per year
(2) Social	(2) Ability to develop a "balanced" population mix; adequate group structure; accessibility and limited travel times
Insurer	
(1) Market share	(1) 10 to 30 percent of the population
(2) Type of insurer	(2) Existing pathfinder HMO
(3) General premium levels	(3) Cost of the benefits package similar to existing programs
(4) Coverage	(4) Benefits packages equal to or more comprehensive than existing plans
Purchasers	
(1) Number	(1) Several large, over 100 employee firms
(2) Contribution	(2) Firm picks up most or all or the premium
(3) Multiple choice	(3) Employers willing to offer one or more managed care products
Providers	
(1) Facilities	(1) Existing, modern, and attractive facilities
(2) Existing services	(2) Evidence of need/demand
(3) Attitudes	(3) Supportive and willing to sign provider contracts

Table 10-3 provides a list of the data elements that are useful in analyzing the population. These data, together with socioeconomic and epidemiological categories, should be known and understood for the reasons listed in the table.

Although the task of collecting the data listed in Table 10-3 may appear awesome, the sources are almost limitless, not only for demographic information but also for socioeconomic and epidemiological data. Sources include the Bureau of the Census of the U.S. Department of Commerce; local, county, and state health departments; local and state chambers of commerce; county economic planning commissions and economic development authorities; business coalitions; tax lists; school enrollments; newspapers; state agencies relating to industry, employment, and trade; voter registration rolls; the U.S. Department of Labor's *Digest of Health and Insurance Plans;* Blue Cross and Blue Shield plans; Medicare and Medicaid agencies; union representatives; other HMOs; and local hospitals. State offices may provide substantial regional data, especially regarding the development and level of commerce in the state; the planning office of the state government may be the place to start. For selected regions, *Sales and Marketing Management* magazine publishes

TABLE 10-3 Data Requirements in Market Analysis

Factors or Characteristics	Relevance
(1) Size of target population	Population size affects the relative ease in marketing and the nature and size of health resources required
(2) Distribution and density	Location and distance of health facilities influence choice and transportation requirements
(3) Age, sex, race, and so on*	Direct influence on epidemiological characteristics of the population that affect the desired need for various services (e.g., the health needs of an over age 65 population differ substantially from an under age 10 category)
(4) Birth rates	Pediatric and obstetric sources
(5) Death rates	Age-specific diseases and conditions
(6) Mobility information*	Turnover of subscribers
(7) Family status*	Benefits package development and number of programs offered; family size influences overall plan utilization and, therefore, staffing, utilization, and costs
(8) Income*	Ability to pay or contribute toward premium or eligibility for welfare programs; income is also a measure of the potential for episodic illness and expected bad debt, as well as an indicator of the effort required to bring population to an acceptable level of health maintenance
(9) Employment*	Group enrollment and the possibility that the employer will contribute toward premiums
(10) Educational level	Direct relation to usage rate
(11) Ethnic make-up	Potential for treatment of special diseases that are prevalent in certain population segments
(12) Housing	Reflects the sociological characteristics of the population, approximate level of income and affluence; housing unit information may indicate individual versus family information
(13) Disease incidence	Required for actuarial and underwriting tasks

*These factors are also important because of consumer-held beliefs and behaviors. For a discussion of these issues, see Chapter 7.

a survey of regional buying power twice a year. Innovative sources might include studies and reports that were completed for other purposes but which are applicable to HMO market analyses. These might include the area transit authority and school districts, local utilities (electricity, telephone, gas, and water), planning departments, health planning agencies, and local and central labor councils. Financial data may be available through Dun and Bradstreet listings and special reports completed by the financial analysis and rating departments of brokerage firms. Finally, special reports and studies may be available from local providers, including annual reports and planning studies for local hospital and medical group practices.

Primary Data Sources

To help complete the picture of the service area, primary source "market surveys" may be conducted. These surveys address the collection of specific information that is not available from secondary sources nor from published reports. HMOs collect data from local employers and their unions, as well as from competing health systems such as hospitals and group practices. Insurers, especially local Blue Cross/Blue Shield plans, may have useful information, although it may be proprietary or competitive. Another source of local insurance activity may be the annual reports completed by insurers and submitted to the state insurance commissioner or the state attorney general's office; these documents are usually in the public domain but are only available from the state capitols. The HMO's providers, other physicians, and even the potential members themselves may be queried. But, because most of the marketing activities will be with employers and their employees and unions, they are the most important data sources and should be surveyed first.

Surveys and questionnaires should be prepared only after the researcher identifies the output desired from such instruments. Some of the useful data elements that will be collected are included on the forms, charts, and tables provided in the following discussion. Overall, these data should help identify the population segments that the HMO will want to enroll, and the survey data will be used to develop a marketing mix of services and selling activities that will be directed at each target segment chosen. Much of the information gathered will be used to classify employers, unions, and associations by segment, size, industry, and so on. A format provided in Table 10-4 may provide a useful method for organizing and recording data.

Emphasis is placed on the larger employers and unions, those willing to offer the HMO benefits packages, and other organizations that may have a previous affiliation with the health plan. These potential groups provide the greatest membership return for the least cost per member enrolled. Each of the employers selected for study becomes the target for intensive analysis.

TABLE 10-4   Classes of Employers by Size and Segment

		Number of Firms	*Number of Employees*
Employer groups	Over 1,000 500–999 250–499 100–249 25– 99 Under 25		
Union trust funds	Over 1,000 500–999 250–499 100–249 25– 99 Under 25		
Federal employees	Over 1,000 500–999 250–499 100–249 25– 99 Under 25		
Public employees	Over 1,000 500–999 250–499 100–249 25– 99 Under 25		
Self-employed			

Questionnaires and interview guides may be used for obtaining information from employers and employees, as well as for obtaining the required data regarding the employer or union, composition of the work force, health status of potential members, employer/employee attitudes regarding HMOs, and the present health benefits package being offered. It is important to determine the anniversary date of each competing health plan being offered by employers, because this date defines the HMO's time frame for contacting employers to obtain their agreement to offer a new plan. It also identifies the open enrollment season, the period when employees can change health plans. Table 10-5 provides an outline of the data that are collected through this process. The marketing researcher will also want to complete a benefits comparison of the several plans currently being offered with the benefits package being proposed by the HMO. Major differences should be noted and consideration given to modifying the HMO's offerings so as to meet the competition. Such

TABLE 10-5   Segment and Account-Specific Data

Obtain and analyze the following data for each employer, association, federal or state contract, union contract, and so on.

1. Employer Name
2. Employees
   a. Total employees: union and nonunion
   b. Eligible employees: union and nonunion
   c. Employees in the HMO's service area: union and nonunion
3. Dependents:
   a. Total dependents
   b. Eligible dependents
   c. Dependents in the HMO's service area
4. Current plan(s)
   a. Name of plan(s)
   b. Category (indemnity, BC/BS, HMO, PPO, etc.)
   c. Benefit level
   d. Anniversary dates and open enrollment seasons
   e. Percent penetration
   f. Loss ratio (plan expenses for claims/total premiums)
5. Premium structure
   a. Contract type
   b. Percent of employees and dependents
   c. Total premiums
   d. Employer contribution
   e. Employee contribution
   f. Out-of-pocket differential; HMO vs. current plan(s)
6. Management of the health plan
   a. Decision making: local or national
   b. Union decision or employer/management decision
   c. Receptivity level
7. Enrollment projections
   a. Percent penetration
   b. Projected contracts
   c. Projected members
   d. Projected total contract and member months
   e. Projected year-to-date contracts and members
   f. Projected year-to-date contracts and member months

decision making regarding the populations and employers to be targeted, benefits packages, premiums, and so on, occurs during the next step in the marketing process, the market analysis.

Epidemiological Data

Statistics on the incidence and prevalence of disease are categorized as epidemiological data. This information is imperative for the completion of the actuarial and underwriting tasks—the calculation of risks and the process by which the HMO determines the basis on which it will accept a group from the target population as members of the health plan. These data are used to generate the statement of demand for services and thus affect the benefits package and premium-level development, as well as the level and category of physician and paramedical staffing that will be required to meet the projected demand. Sources of epidemiological data for small communities may not exist. Limited information about infectious diseases will be available on a regional basis because of its reportable nature. Other major sources may be the records of services provided by local hospitals and outpatient providers such as clinics, group practices, other HMOs, insurers, and solo practitioners. Also, actuarial firms have collected rates of HMO service use over many years and have completed special studies for use in their actuarial work for HMO clients.

National statistics, prepared by the Scientific and Technical Information Branch of the National Center for Health Statistics, are available through the National Ambulatory Medical Care Survey. The databases managed by the Office of Prepaid Health Care (Health Care Financing Administration, Department of Health and Human Services) and data provided by firms like Jurgovan and Blair in Rockville, Maryland may also be of some assistance. Care must be exercised in the use of national statistics, because they may not reflect accurate local medical practice and usage rates; thus, these national statistics must be used in tandem with available local information.

Another important source of actuarial information, and typically the most difficult source from which to obtain information, is current local insurers. Incidence rates for disease, accident, and injury are maintained by indemnity companies, local Blue Cross/Blue Shield plans, HMOs, and other health insurers. By obtaining such local information, the health plan could reduce considerably the expense of underwriting activity and may be able to more accurately predict utilization levels.

Data on Existing Delivery Systems

Identifying and collecting data on existing medical services programs and insuring organizations provide the basis for understanding the level of competition. All existing providers within the health plan's catchment area need to be identified by type of provider, location, and market share. This information is easily obtained from community medical societies, professional society registers, community health departments, local hospital associations, other professional associations, and the local health planning agency. Telephone yellow pages provide an excellent source of physicians and other providers and their locations.

Health program insurers, although they can be identified, are more difficult to describe by market share. One rough method of identifying an insurer's market share is through the "payment source" studies completed by most hospitals. Although the data relate to payment for inpatient care, the studies, together with information on benefits packages offered by insurers, provide a general indication of the market share of each insurer. In addition, benefits package and premium-level information is necessary in the development of a competitive HMO package. Some HMO managers have even suggested that a newly developing HMO may assume that the existing insurance benefits packages have been specifically constructed to meet the particular needs of the community and, consequently, an HMO package with comparable benefits will meet the demand of the members; the HMO manager, by using other insurers' benefits packages, might save considerable effort. This is a risky business practice, because many existing programs are dated, are not based on a market analysis, or are not tailored to the specific target populations to which the HMO will market. Moreover, the HMO will be providing outpatient coverage as its prime benefit and will emphasize preventive medicine; the state of the art in the "Blues" and indemnity programs provides few, if any, benefits in the outpatient and preventive areas.

Information about insurers' market shares and their major accounts is vital to an HMO that plans to use a dual- and multiple-choice enrollment practice; dual/multiple choice suggests that a competitive selection process is operational. As described in Chapter 7, dual/multiple choice is an important marketing device that permits the HMO to break into other insurers' accounts and to competitively attract some of their customers. Indeed, if the market has been almost totally consumed by the existing insurers, dual/multiple choice is critical to the HMO's marketing strategy and future success. It is also suggested that, because the members under dual/multiple choice make up a "noncaptive" membership, those joining are apt to be more satisfied; there is a great deal of intellectual and practical appeal to the dual/multiple-choice arrangement. If the health plan is not viewed as a superior system, however, dual/multiple choice can operate to the detriment of the HMO. Loss in membership is an indication that changes need to be made in the HMO.

STEP 2: CONDUCTING A MARKET ANALYSIS

The information gathered during the first phase of market activities sets the base for the second step, that of market analysis. This stage involves three major areas: analysis of the environment, the competition, and the opinions of consumers, including employers, employees, and providers.

Data in these three areas are analyzed to determine what the consumer demand will be so that HMO services and activities can be adjusted to successfully serve this market. The ultimate objective of such an analysis, then, is to provide the HMO with information concerning its competitors and the demographic, socioeconomic, and epidemiological characteristics of the area to guide the decision-making process. Data collected should enable the manager to develop a marketing strategy and, ultimately, to determine if the HMO's goals and objectives are feasible, that is, whether there are enough qualified buyers to support the HMO activity. This analysis leads to the other steps in the marketing process, including development of dual/multiple-choice arrangements, active marketing, and continuing market/subscriber relations.

It is important to realize that market analyses do not end when the initial planning feasibility decision is made. Market study is a continuous process throughout the life of the health plan. Data are required to make decisions concerning new target populations and modifications to marketing strategies for current subscriber groups. Marketing HMOs is a dynamic process that requires continuous feedback of data. It is imperative that the HMO develop a management information system that will generate a continuous flow of purchaser and member data without major market analysis studies. When the decision is made to expand the health plan, current member information will be readily available, to which information concerning new groups may be added. Through this method, better marketing strategies can be designed.

Environmental Analysis

The first step in market analysis, an environmental analysis of the service area, is used to identify the geographic, demographic, and socioeconomic characteristics of the service area and the epidemiology of the target populations. As most health planners know, analysis of the geographic area in which services are planned is basic to understanding the potential targets. Some planners refer to this process as geocoding and geoplotting—locating potential employer groups according to their geographic position in the service area. Employees' residences are also plotted by location, since the health plan will want to assure health service access to employees at home. Geographic characteristics define the plan's ability to assure availability, accessibility, and convenience of services. The availability of this information will allow plan managers to locate medical service sites or health centers. Some of the issues regarding sites are provided in Table 10-6.

The boundaries of the service area are defined by using ZIP codes, census tracts, the planning area, or other methods of determining geographic subdivision. Health plans currently operating will use maps of the service area and members' ZIP codes to plot the location of current members and enrolled groups. Local employers can supply the ZIP codes of target employees; these, too, can then be added to the analysis. The number of proposed and existing health centers will round out this analysis.

TABLE 10-6   Site Location Factors

1. Distribution and density of the population (current and projected)
2. Sites available
3. Demand for HMO services in the areas selected for study
4. Reputation of the health plan and other plans
5. Travel times, distances, and patterns
6. Topology
7. Available buildings or building sites
8. Costs of renovation or construction (using build, lease, or buy evaluations)
9. Health plan physicians' location preferences
10. Community acceptance and strength of consumer loyalty
11. Marketing advantages/disadvantages
12. Zoning constraints and regulations
13. Building use and code restrictions
14. Plan and nonplan physicians—numbers, types, practice locations, and patients
15. Long-range plans for the area
16. Proposed changes in the transportation system
17. Real estate values
18. Image of the location and other social factors
19. Security and safety of the area
20. Parking and public transportation
21. Recommendations of current medical and paraprofessional staff regarding proposed sites
22. Congestion in site location
23. Competition for sites and marketing efforts of others

Boundary decisions must consider the following issues:

1. The service area should include a large number of employers with more than 100 employees each.

2. Health center locations should be within 30 minutes of the service area boundary in suburban areas, and 15 minutes in urban areas.

3. Future growth beyond the original service area should be physically possible and financially viable.

4. The boundary of the service area can be clearly defined and communicated to prospective health plan members so that they can understand accessibility limits and avoid disappointments.

5. The location issues listed in Table 10-6 should be seriously considered in the location decisions.

The second element of the environmental analysis is an assessment of demographic and social characteristics. Demography is the study of vital statistics and, thus, a demographic study is a review and analysis of the characteristics of the people who live in the service area. Information is collected and analyzed regarding the population—its size, density, and distribution. Additional information regarding age and sex, race and ethnic distribution, educational levels, type of employment (or occupation), average and median family income, and family size should be considered. Health issues, including health status, current health insurance coverage, and morbidity, mortality, and disability, may concern the health plan. The rate of population growth and the degree of transiency (emigration-immigration patterns) are especially important to this analysis since new residents are more likely to become potential members of the HMO. Similarly, high-growth areas of middle- to upper-middle-income families are good prospects, and persons with high levels of educational attainment are more likely to enroll in the plan than those with lower levels of attainment. If large ethnic or racial concentrations are identified, they require a marketing strategy and mix uniquely structured for them. Finally, income levels play an important role in determining whether prospective members will be able to afford the premiums not covered by their employers, out-of-pocket expenses, and copayments.

As part of the demographic review, the health plan manager must prepare general and target population projections for the service area. These projections of growth during the next few years should include density and geographic dispersion. Various methodologies that are used to complete forecasts are available from several sources. The method or methods chosen for a given population projection are based on estimates of the availability of data, the type of data that is required by each projection technique, and the various estimates that are desired. To develop satisfactory forecasts, the health plan manager must prepare a description of the requirement for a forecast and the specific situation to be projected, and explain how the current situation will evolve into the forecast state.[4] With a clear understanding of the forecast requirements, the manager can choose a forecasting technique. Five approaches to population projections that are germane to HMOs are reported in detail by Reeves and Coile:[5]

1. Extrapolation
2. Ratio method
3. Correlation method
4. Component method
5. Cohort survival method

---

[4] Philip N. Reeves and Russell C. Coile, Jr. *Introduction to Health Planning*. 4th Edition. Arlington, Va., Information Resources Press, 1990, p. 280.

[5] Ibid., pp. 298–302.

Of the five methods, Reeves and Coile suggest that the last approach appears to provide the most accurate projections. They suggest that the following steps be used in the cohort survival method.

a. The population should be broken down into appropriate subgroups. The interval covered by each of the age groups should be equal to the periods of projection; for example, for 5-, 10-, or 20-year projections, use 5-year age groups (10–14, 45–49, etc.).

b. Multiply each subgroup by the appropriate survival rate. The survival rate is the complement of the death rate for the cohort.[6] If the death rate is 10 per 10,000, the survival rate will be 9,990 per 10,000.

c. Multiply female groups (in the 15 to 44 age group) by appropriate birthrates to get the number of births.

d. Multiply the total number of births by the proportion of male births and the proportion of female births to get the number of male and female births.*

e. Multiply male and female births by the apppropriate survival rates.

f. Add surviving births to the youngest cohorts.

g. Adjust each group for the net migration.

h. Adjust each cohort for the percent who will advance to the next cohort due to age increase during the year.[7]

---

*Aggregate natality rates should be readily available from vital statistics departments. In the event the state data do not provide a breakdown by sex, one can apply the national proportion of male to female births to determine how the births should be distributed in the 0 to 14 cohort.

Examples of the use of the cohort survival method are provided by Reeves and Coile.[8]

The third environmental factor is a description and analysis of the economic characteristics of the area population. These data, collectively known as the economic and socioeconomic dimensions of the population, are concerned with income and the distribution of income, the employment patterns of the population, labor-force characteristics, and the economic expansion potential of the community; they are important elements in deciding which groups will make up the target populations. The data sources referred to in the second environmental element, demography, will be generally helpful in obtaining these data although the HMO manager may find it difficult to obtain access to certain socioeconomic information and, therefore, will need to be more resourceful in this collection effort. Nonconventional and normally

---

[6] A cohort is a group of people with similar characteristics born in the same time period. All white women between 15 and 20 years of age is an example of a race-sex cohort.

[7] Reeves and Coile. *Introduction to Health Planning*, pp. 301–302.

[8] Ibid., pp. 302–304.

nonaccessible sources may include union and employer employment records, professional association records, state unemployment insurance records, Social Security Administration records for Medicare and Medicaid recipients, local tax records, land developers' projections, and department store and local credit card programs, among others. Generally, these data should provide the marketing director with an overall view of the local society and its level of affluence.

The use of charts, maps, and tables to display this information will be helpful for analysis. Data to be analyzed include:

1. The size and growth of the civilian labor force during the past five years and for the next five years
   2. Unemployment/employment levels and trends for the same 10-year period
   3. Future industrial outlook
   4. Major employers, noting national versus local
   5. Commuting patterns of the work force
   6. Industrial breakdown by industry category and size of employer
   7. Unionization of the labor force
   8. Number of Medicare and Medicaid recipients
   9. Number of self-employed and unemployed persons

This information will assist health plan management in identifying and evaluating employees in high-health-risk industries, such as heavy equipment, toxic waste, mining, construction, and so on. In the process, those companies, (electronics companies, educational institutions, banks, and merchandising firms) whose employees have low or different types of health risks also will be identified. The health plan will be particularly interested in identifying those employers whose work force is stable, that is, without seasonal or cyclical variations or high turnover rates and where the health plan can have a high level of penetration and enrollment, such as federal and state governments, utilities, and service industries.

Three special groups are worthy of further consideration: self-employed persons, persons who are between jobs, and Medicare and Medicaid recipients. Self-employed persons and individuals between jobs usually are responsible for their own health insurance coverage. The HMO may find that offering an "individual" group package is advantageous, but such a decision must be based on an analysis of the collective risks of these individuals and the ability to attract enough members to spread the risks. Finally, Medicare and Medicaid risk contracting may also be of interest to the HMO. Specific federal regulations have been developed for health plans to enter into capitation arrangements with the Health Care Financing Administration to serve Medicare members; likewise, each state has its own set of contracting standards for use in developing HMO/state Medicaid arrangements. Both of these groups are discussed in detail in Chapter 5.

A final area of environmental analysis is the assessment of epidemiological data, that is, morbidity, mortality, and disability information. These data are used to determine disease incidence rates among the target populations. The results of the actuarial studies and underwriting efforts help identify for the financial manager the price or premium to charge the target populations. Setting the premium level for each target group, then, is a joint effort of top management, including the marketing manager.

Analysis of the Competition

One of the most critical steps during the market analysis phase is a complete review of competing health care plans, HMOs, and PPOs. During this phase, the data collected in Step 1 are scrutinized for an understanding of the kind and level of competition and the HMO's position in the market. Data to be collected and reviewed include the following:

- Type of health plans (if an HMO, is it qualified?)
- Estimate of market position
- Years in operation and service areas
- Current enrollment and changes in enrollment over the last five years, and projected growth over the next five years
- Categorization of marketing strategies
- Plans for expansion of market areas, facilities, benefits, programs, etc.
- Market segments and groups (especially employers) enrolled
- Benefits packages, premiums, copayments, and deductibles
- Inpatient and outpatient (health center) locations
- Number of physicians, names, specialties, and board certifications, and an estimate of the physicians' reputations
- Estimate of the consumers' and employers' loyalty to and the reputation of the health plans
- Employers currently offering an HMO and PPO
- Penetration of competitive HMOs of major employers
- Marketing management strategy of the competing plans (e.g., use of brokers, in-house sales force, straight salary or commissions, territory of marketing representatives, etc.)

The strength and nature of unions and the likelihood of gaining union support should be assessed. Most importantly, dominant employers, because of their size, geographic location, industry, and the like, must be evaluated to determine if their support and involvement in the health plan can be assured.

In all cases, the plan will need to have data regarding the coverage now in place and the loss ratios experienced by those enrolled in the incumbent plans. Finally, many employers have become self-insured; that is, they bank the funds that represent health plan premiums for their employees and their dependents. A health benefits package is offered to employees, and as services are used, the employer pays for these services from this bank account. Self-insured employers feel that they can effectively monitor the use of services and have more control over the cost of the health benefits package. Because of these employer arrangements, the HMO may have a difficult time entering the self-insured employer market.

The health plan's management can estimate the saturation point for the HMO market by completing the following steps. First, sum the projected enrollment for all HMOs in the area for five years hence. Modify that total enrollment, based on the HMO's ability to achieve only one-third of the planned enrollment. Add the proposed HMO's five-year enrollment estimate to the existing HMO's modified planned enrollment. Finally, divide the total by the population of the service area as projected for five years forward. The results should be between 6 and 10 percent; this saturation percentage rate estimate will determine whether there will be a sufficiently large market to allow the successful marketing of another HMO or to expand the activities of an existing one. The rate of 6 to 10 percent is only a rule of thumb and should be modified as local conditions warrant. In certain areas of the United States, as much as 50 percent of the population receives its care through an HMO, while in other areas there are few or no HMOs.

As mentioned previously, HMOs compete at two levels—selling the health benefits package (insurance) and providing health services (delivery). Regarding the insurance issue, the HMO manager analyzes the market to determine the level of penetration and market share of competing health plans. These include Blue Cross and Blue Shield; private insurance companies; government-sponsored plans (Medicare and Medicaid); other HMOs and CMPs; self-insured employers, including PPO and EPO arrangements; and the uninsured. A sample list of market share by insurance vehicle is provided in Table 10-7. Note that BC/BS has a 40 percent share, which might be considered the dominant position. A newly developing, expanding, or competing HMO might have difficulty entering the market with such a dominant player, although there appears to be a level of fragmentation among the remaining 60 percent of insurers to allow for the entrance of a new HMO.

The benefits and premium patterns also need to be analyzed. They should be arranged by employer, describing the benefits as either low, medium, high, HMO high, or high-enhanced (with drugs, vision, dental, and other unique services included). Each benefit level, by employer, may be characterized by the number of employers and employees (or members) included in the offering at that

TABLE 10-7   Market Share and Position Held by Competitors

Payment Source/Insurer	Market Share/Position %
Blue Cross/Blue Shield	40
Private insurance company "X"	5
Private insurance company "Y"	8
Government-sponsored federal employees health benefits program	2
Government-sponsored Medicare	8
Government-sponsored Medicaid	5
Government-sponsored CHAMPUS (military dependents)	2
Self-insured employers	4
Uninsured	10
HMO "V"	8
HMO "W"	8
Total	100

level; the data should allow the market researcher to describe the percent of the market at each benefit level. The premium charged, along with copayments and deductibles, can be added to the table. The results of such an analysis should clearly identify the kinds of packages currently in existence and the benefits that appear to be preferred, by insurer and employer. The analysis might suggest where the newly developing or expanding HMO can create a market for itself. For example, the analysis might identify the opportunity to develop a point-of-service program or a high-enhanced package that is not now available. Conversely, if current benefits are relatively low, the analysis might suggest that a comprehensive benefits package might not be competitive, since its price may be high when compared with current programs.

Community and Physician Opinion and Support

The support of community employers, potential members, and physicians will dramatically affect the success or failure of the marketing process. Major opposition should be identified and considered. For example, if it is found that local physicians will not participate with an expanding HMO, the health plan may want to develop a staff model with salaried physicians in the expanding service area. But, the plan may encounter stiff resistance to such a development, and local nonplan physicians may be unwilling to engage in referral patterns with the health plan's physician staff. Attitudes of employers, likewise, may enhance or limit the health plan; some employers are very supportive of managed care programs; however, the employers may wish to limit the number of health plans offered to the exclusion of the HMO, or the employers may prefer PPOs to other forms of managed care. Potential members may not understand how managed care programs operate, especially closed-panel HMOs, PPOs, EPOs and CMPs. It may require considerable educational effort to achieve a greater understanding of the managed care concept. The analysis of opinions and attitudes should identify such limitations, which can then be addressed in the strategies that are developed later.

STEP 3: DECIDING ON THE TARGET MARKET AND SETTING FINAL GOALS

The third step in the marketing process is deciding on the target markets and redefining the health plan's goals and objectives—especially the description of the target populations, the level of enrollment, the provider and referral models, and so on.

Figure 10-3 outlines this marketing-financial planning process; it begins with the tasks of population segmentation and estimates of penetration. The process then continues with estimates of demand of the selected target population and, through financial analyses, permits a forecast of the necessary capacity to provide services to meet the demand. The intermediate product of this planning process is the marketing mix—a definition of the product (the benefits packages), place (geographic location, transportation requirements, hours of operation), promotion (advertising and selling techniques), and price (premium structure). The analysis of population and development of the marketing mix allow the administrator to decide on the market feasibility—a decision, made after the marketing-mix plans are established, to offer dual choice and sell the plan's services.

Market Segmentation and Penetration Rate Analysis

Segmenting the population and employers involves analyzing and identifying existing markets and then identifying the potential target markets. The process accomplishes several objectives. First, it makes possible the division of the total population into discrete segments of purchasers, payers, enrollees, and users of health services, and thus allows for greater ease in planning. Second, segmentation allows the manager to define precisely the characteristics of the segments to which the HMO and its affiliated physicians and hospitals will provide services. Hence, it sets the stage for actuarial and underwriting activities that are so important to the success of the entire marketing process. Third, because the grouping of people by demographic, socioeconomic, and epidemiological characteristics is inherent in segmentation, the process of identifying employment groups that might be sources of substantial enrollment

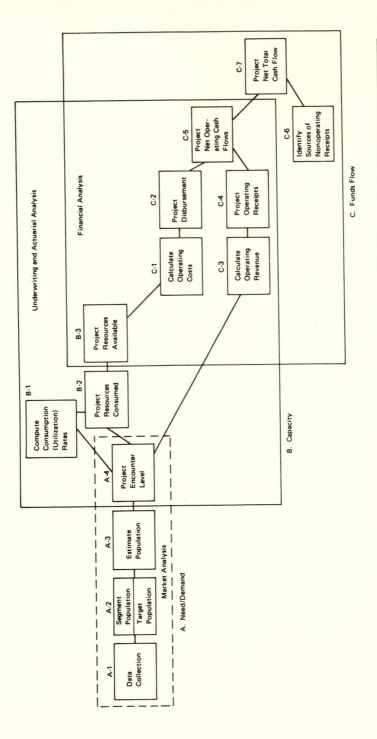

FIGURE 10-3   The marketing/financial planning process.

is enhanced. Finally, a mistake with one segment may not dramatically affect the analysis or hinder success with the total target population.

Marketing objectives, along with the major tasks involved in carrying them out, are included in Figure 10-3, which shows the relationships among the various outputs from the market analysis process, for example, the creation of a need/demand statement; a statement of capacity, which matches the needs of the target population; and a funds flow analysis, which ties all of the marketing and planning activities together. Note that the market analysis leads directly into the actuarial and underwriting activities, and that these actuarial activities create the basis for the financial analysis of the health plan. Thus, these early stages in the marketing process are critical to the ultimate success of the organization. With such issues considered, the board and top management of the health plan can finalize their long-term goals and objectives for the health plan. Goals initially established might be modified upon consideration of the realities of the marketplace, the changing environment and population needs, and financial constraints.

The segmentation process begins by identifying major employer and other groups of 25, 50, 100, 200, 500, 1,000 people, and so on. Certain characteristics of employees, dependents, and others who may become health plan members are important: employer or union affiliation, age, family income, sex, geographic location of employment and residence, third-party payment affiliation, and ethnic or racial characteristics. A review of this information will reveal the most important attributes by which the population should be segmented. More than one attribute of the population should be used to cross-check the validity of the analysis. Examples of cross-tabulations that are useful in analyzing the population include age by employment, residence by income, and employer by insurer. If geographic location appears to be most important because of a rural location, then the population should be segmented not only by geography but also by one or more of the other characteristics, like employment. Finally, the results of each segment analysis should be compared with age, sex, income, and so on, to check for accuracy of demand and capacity forecasts.

It is important to list large- and medium-sized companies, unions, associations, and governmental agencies, since they represent the largest assemblies of potential members. Great effort should be placed on their description and evaluation. Seasoned HMO marketers realize that the employers' or unions' representatives typically control the health insurance programs. These representatives carry substantial weight in the decision regarding which health plans will be offered to employees and union members. It is imperative, therefore, that the health plan's marketing representative work closely with the key representatives responsible for establishing dual/multiple-choice arrangements for employers and unions.

Another important attribute of the population to be studied is the insurance

TABLE 10-8   Segmentation by Payment Mechanism

Health Insurer	Health Care Market by Insurer and Market Share				
	A Current Number of Persons Covered	*B* Insurer (percent of total)	*C* HMO Projected Market Share of Insurer (percentage)	*D* Projected Number of HMO Enrollees (A × C)	*HMO Enrollees (percent of total)*
Blue Cross/Blue Shield	170,000	13.1	1.0	1,700	34.0
Private insurance	700,000	54.1	0.4	2,800	56.0
Health Maintenance Organization	95,000	7.3	—	—	—
Medicare	150,000	11.6	0.08	120	2.4
Medicaid	80,000	6.2	0.006	5	0.1
Armed forces/other noncivilian	24,000	1.9	—	—	—
Noncovered or self-insured	75,000	5.8	0.5	375	7.5
Total	1,294,000	100.0	1.986	5,000	100.0

coverage/payment mechanism. This includes a description of the current insurance companies' market shares, as shown in Tables 10-8 and 10-9. All insurance and payment sources, whether they are service (Blue Cross and Blue Shield), direct service (HMOs and CMPs), indemnity, self-insured arrangements, or governmental programs, should be listed, together with their subscriber, membership, or recipient levels. Again, it is necessary to determine which third-party segments the marketing effort will be effective in addressing. As many market segmentations as are necessary should be undertaken to completely describe the major characteristics of the population.

The next logical task is completion of a market penetration-rate study—an analysis of the target segments that describe the level of the projected market share of each group in each segment. The objective of the penetration study is to precisely identify to whom the HMO will market and to best estimate the membership level from each segment. Table 10-7 gives a basic review of the percentage share of the market for each payment source, while Table 10-8 provides data for a hypothetical penetration-rate study, by payment mechanism, including the HMO's proposed market share estimates for a city of 1,294,000 people.

Segmentation by Payment Mechanism

Based on the objectives established by the health plan's board of directors or trustees and the data that are available about the community, the initial estimate of market share is made. In Table 10-8, the board set its first-year enrollment level at 5,000 members (see Column D), with the highest number being drawn from private insurance companies and Blue Cross/Blue Shield programs. It appears that little hope was given to attracting any members from existing

TABLE 10-9   Segmentation by Employment Group

	A	B	C	D	E	F
			Health Care Market by Employment			
Company by Type	Number of Employees	Percent Eligible	Carrier	Projected Market Share of Total (percentage)	Projected Number of HMO Enrollees (A × B × D)	HMO Enrollees (percent of total)
Local Government A						
Professional	15,000	100	BC/BS	10.0	1,500	30.0
Blue Collar	7,000	100	BC/BS	10.0	700	14.0
Electronics M	1,020	100	Western Life	—	—	
Hotel/Motel	4,300	20	Metropolitan Life	—	—	
Electronics N	2,400	100	BC/BS	25.0	600	12.0
Service X	3,000	100	HMO	—	—	
Publisher	1,200	65	Self-insured	6.0	47	0.9
Construction	1,500	90	BC/BS	—	—	
Research and Development	600	100	Travelers	—	—	
Engineering	1,100	100	—	—	—	
Association	500	100	Travelers	20.0	100	2.0
Service Y	1,200	90	Lincoln National	80.0	864	17.3
Manufacturing	7,000	100	BC/BS	10.0	700	14.0
Light Industrial	2,300	93	Conn. General	17.0	364	7.3
Local Government B	6,000	100	Equitable Life	—	—	
Printer	600	100	Conn. General	—	—	
Unemployed (7 percent of population)	90,580	20	Medicare/Medicaid	0.69	125	2.5
Totals	145,300				5,000	100.0

HMO plans. On the other hand, the figure suggests that the board does have a commitment to provide care to recipients of Medicare and Medicaid programs. In the latter case, the HMO will need to negotiate a Medicaid risk contract with the state in order to serve these individuals. Because the priority appears to be low—five members—and extensive effort is necessary to consummate a state contract, it might be wise to defer activities in the Medicaid area until the HMO is more established. Most state Medicaid programs require a successful track record before contracts are awarded; therefore, in all likelihood, this would not be a successful effort by the HMO at the present time.

Segmentation by Employment/Purchaser Group

In Table 10-9, the same hypothetical market is segmented by employment or purchaser (of the health benefits package) group. Initially, only large employers are included; note that in this example the assumption is made that the HMO will be marketing to employees only and not their families. Again, the marketing manager follows the objectives established by the board, but is also guided by the reality of the current employment situation—the current carriers, the ability for dual choice, the existence of union contracts, the length of time the present health plans have been in effect, and the like.

Comparison of Payment Mechanism and Employment Group Segments

A cross-classification of segments by payment mechanism (Table 10-8) with employment groups (Table 10-9) identifies some contradictory projections, apparent in Table 10-10. Although the segmentation and projections by payment mechanism suggest that 34 percent of the members will come from the present BC/BS programs and 56 percent from private insurance companies, the segmentation by employment suggests that 70 percent of enrollment will be from employers now covering their employees by BC/BS and only 26.6 percent from private insurance companies. Estimates of Medicare and Medicaid by both methods, however, are very close. The marketing manager must continue to study these analyses until an acceptable and realistic penetration projection is agreed upon.

A decision must be based on the projected market share estimates in both Tables 10-8 (Column C) and 10-9 (Column D). Market share estimates must be compatible with the organization's objectives, but they also must be in the realm of reality, based on data collected and alliances formed with community groups—employers, unions, associations, and so on. They are critical projections that must be based on solid information and assurance from key community group leaders. The inability to make these estimates and, thus, realistic decisions suggests incomplete information and lack of understanding

TABLE 10-10 Comparison of Payment Mechanisms and Employment Group Segmentations

Company	BC/BS	Private Insurer	Medicare and Medicaid	Noncovered or Self-insured
Local Government A	2,200			
Electronics	600			
Publisher				47
Association		100		
Service Y		864		
Manufacturing	700			
Light Industrial		364		
Unemployed			125	
Company Total (Table 10-9)	3,500 (70%)	1,328 (26.6%)	125 (2.5%)	(0.9%)
Insurer Total (Table 10-8)	1,700 (34%)	2,800 (56.0%)	125 (2.5%)	(7.5%)

of the community and its social and economic order. It indicates that more work will be required before the discrepancies among the several penetration-rate studies can be resolved.

Deciding on Potential Members

These in-house studies will help to accurately project the service or beneficiary population. This is a critical step that must be completed prior to the development of benefits packages and premium (price) formulation. But, even though all of these activities are completed with care and are reasonable, the marketing manager may bungle the marketing program if personal contact is not established with key individuals who control the health benefits in the large employer groups and unions. The manager should initiate meetings with employment group leaders early in the marketing development process. Key business leaders should be asked to participate in the development of benefits packages; their assistance should be requested in other plan activities; and their personal commitment to the health plan, especially as plan members, should be obtained. Naturally, close alliances will be easier to achieve if the plan administrator, medical director, and marketing manager are long-standing members of the community and are well known and liked. In other instances, contacts will be on a purely professional level; key group leaders will ask for a cost-and-benefit proposal from the health plan. The plan administrator should be prepared to brief community leaders, representatives of employers, and the press on the goals and objectives of the HMO, its potential ability to contain costs, and possible benefits packages and premium schedules. Every effort should be made to sell the capitated concept as well as the health plan's benefits package.

The final products of the segmentation and penetration studies are a list of membership sources and a projection of the level of members from each source. Each source can then be completely described and a marketing mix prepared. Descriptions of employer, union, and association groups and governmental agencies should include the following 15 elements:

1. Name of organization and size of membership group
2. Absolute and relative size of eligible population in membership group
3. Average wage or family income
4. Residence (geographical distribution)
5. Male/female categorization
6. Current insurance carrier and coverage
7. Decision about insurance coverage—local or national control
8. Date of last insurance carrier, benefit, or premium change
9. Premium and contribution of individual member (copayments)
10. Existence of dual choice
11. Family size (distribution)
12. Experience rating or community rating
13. Competition in each segment and in the market as a whole; for example, if a competing HMO concentrates on large national employers, the proposed HMO might heavily target medium and small employers
14. Stability of the revenue flow from each segment
15. Cost-effectiveness of marketing to potential consumers in each segment (e.g., large group presentations versus individual meetings)

Additional data elements will be required for actuarial activities.

The health plan management is now able to decide to which of the potential groups to market. In effect, this decision is the first part of the market feasibility decision—there are sufficient groups from which enough members can be enrolled to meet the health plan's membership-size objective.

Segmentation by Market Share and Premiums

Major market segments should also be described by levels of existing or current premiums (e.g., the premiums now charged, classified by employer, union, amd association groups) and by rate structure (e.g., single enrollment, two-person or double enrollment, parent and child, and over-three or family enrollment). Again, a chart or tabular presentation of these data will assist in drawing inferences. The analysis might suggest that due to the widespread presence of low premiums with limited benefits, the market may be apprehensive about accepting comprehensive, expensive health plan packages. Conversely, high premiums with many benefits may mean that the new HMO will experience difficulty in differentiating its products or services from the competition.

Selection of Target Markets

After studying market segments and analyzing penetration rates, the next step is to determine which market segments should become target markets. All data collected may be displayed so that a specific description of each target employer, for example, will evolve. The market segmentation and penetration-rate studies previously described will be very useful in the decision-making process, especially if cross-tabulations have been completed (e.g., geographic location by insurance coverage, age by geography, etc.) Each target segment should be described according to the 15 data elements listed on page 398. With these data available, decisions can be made as to which segments will become the health plan's target markets.

The process used might be to rate each of the 15 elements for each potential target employer, union, association, and so on, whereby each potential member is compared and rated relative to all others for each of the elements. For example, a maximum rating of 10 points could be assigned for each of the 15 elements, making a possible total score of 150 points. The first element, name of the organization and size of the member group, will be rated for each target group. A larger size group will receive a higher rating than a small one, perhaps eight points for a large organization versus three for a small one. If only 10 groups out of 30 are to be chosen as target markets, the 10 with the highest total ratings will become the plan's targets. Each target market may now be considered an "account." Some marketing managers will plot the target groups on a map to confirm the rationale for their choice. Does the target market make sense as a whole? Can a consolidated/coordinated marketing effort be applied to all target market segments chosen? Decisions about target groups should be viewed in the context of the health plan's entire business activities and, conceptually, with regard to the medical care delivery and need/demand for services for the entire community. Further, the target groups should fulfill the goals and objectives established for the health plan. Remember that the targets chosen will be those that allow for the greatest financial and enrollment success of the program with the lowest risks. But also remember that these targets must undergo further review in the next marketing steps—designing the marketing mix and forecasting enrollment. Thus, opportunities to reconsider the decisions made at this stage occur later, but before the actual implementation of the marketing plans.

Process/Activity	Product/Output

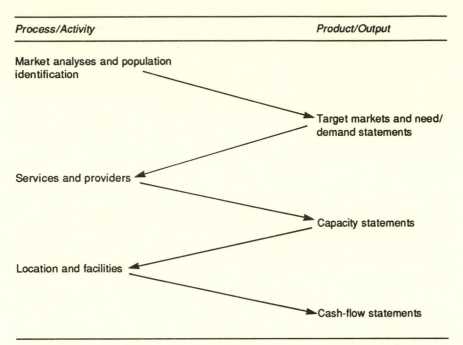

FIGURE 10-4   The marketing/financial planning process by products.

Products of the Marketing Process

At this point it might be useful to consider the results, or outputs, of the marketing process. The output of the first phase (Steps 1 to 3) of the marketing strategy—population and target market identification—is statements of groups to be marketed. For others in the health plan, especially the finance officer, actuary, and medical director, these groups are also considered as having a level of need or demand for medical services; the product of the first three steps for them may be a "need/demand statement." Figure 10-4 outlines this dual output of the population analysis. Following the flow of activities and products listed in Figure 10-4, the demand levels help to determine the size of the organization (facility and staff) needed; the product of this analysis is a statement of capacity or size of the service delivery unit. These two products are finally evaluated through a cash flow study; descriptions of financial needs for the year can then be completed. The following section deals with demand statements.

STEP 4: DESIGNING A MARKETING MIX FOR TARGET MARKETS

The fourth step in the the marketing plan and strategy development is the design of a marketing mix. This consists of four major elements:

- *Medical services and products* (benefits packages) to be delivered as part of the health plan
- *Pricing* of medical services and products (the prices or premiums, deductibles, and copayments of the benefits packages)
- *Place or location* of delivery of medical services
- *Promotion* of the health plan

Each target population (e.g., groups of employees, union members, Medicaid and Medicare recipients) may require a separate marketing mix, which is developed around these four basic variables: product, price, place, and promotion. In effect, the process of marketing mix development concerns the matching or tailoring of the benefits and premiums offered by the health plan to each target segment chosen. This activity is represented by Figure 10-5. Data collected during the market analysis phase are used to decide which markets will become the health plan's targets; the figure suggests that these include Markets A, B, C to N, and Individuals. A marketing mix that meets the needs and objectives of each separate target market, as well as the objectives of the health plan, is then created for each target market. Obviously, as part of this process, the HMO's financial officer will prepare cash flow analyses to determine if premiums and costs of benefits allow for successful financial operation of the plan; if not, it may be necessary to revise premiums and benefits to bring revenues and costs into alignment.

Marketing Mix and the Demand Statement

The process of marketing mix development began with an analysis of the target markets' characteristics. The demand statement is used to help describe the services/providers required to fulfill the needs of the members. Demand is that quantity of health services "wanted" by a patient constrained by limited financial resources. Patients will demand only that amount of service that is economically rational for them to buy. But, in medical care delivery, the level of demand also is related to the type of service demanded. The demand for acute or emergency services is largely inelastic with regard to price (i.e., consumers do not consider the long-term economic loss from receiving such services now, because they want immediate attention). Preventive and cosmetic services, on the other hand, are relatively elastic with regard to price (i.e., consumers will not demand these services if the price is higher than they can easily afford).

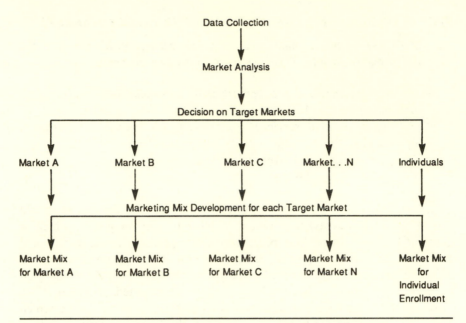

FIGURE 10-5   Choosing target markets and marketing mix.

Another portion of total demand is called derived demand—services ordered by physicians, such as laboratory and radiology examinations or additional office visits.

Demand is generally described from the patient's viewpoint, while *need* is a physician-oriented concept. Need is the quantity of health services prescribed by "expert medical opinion" as necessary to keep a given population healthy over a period of time. While need estimates are based solely on the amount of services experts feel are necessary for health maintenance, demand estimates are based not only on need but also on other factors, including out-of-pocket costs of care and consumer perceptions of need. Consequently, it is easy to envision several problems in demand identification—individuals may not agree with professionals concerning what their needs might be; professionals do not normally consider economic factors in their need statements; and the limited supply of services may not be sufficient to meet the demand level of care, even without considering need.

How, then, shall the health plan prepare a statement of need/demand that will be appropriate for the target populations? The process requires estimates of both demand and need, as well as adjustments of the combined estimates based on the HMO objectives described by the governing board and the medical staff. First, demand estimates are developed, based on estimates of use; it is here that data on ambulatory visits and hospital days per 1,000 population become useful. This method uses a standard visit-to-population ratio and hospital days-to-population ratio. Second, estimates of need are based primarily on studies of epidemiological, morbidity, and mortality data. The need approach is considered to be within the realm of the actuary and the underwriter. Statements using both methods should be developed as a check on the accuracy of the projections.

The results of need/demand studies provide a forecast of the type and number of services (encounters or visits and hospital days) that will be demanded by the target populations. Thus, through the process of projecting demand, the first element of the mix is developed—medical services and products, or the benefits packages. A second element of the mix—estimated price—also is addressed, but final pricing is deferred until cash flow analyses are completed. Moreover, the stage is set for the development of a capacity statement—the size of the HMO and its panel of physicians, and the facilities needed to meet the need/demand. The third and fourth marketing mix elements are place or location of the medical facilities and promotion of the health plan. These four elements are discussed in the sections that follow.

Marketing Mix Element: Medical Services and Products (Benefits Packages)

The needs of the target population are translated into services that might be included in the benefits packages for each target population. Based on the philosophy of the HMO and its participating physicians, one standard benefits package may be developed to meet the needs of most of the target segments, or tailor-made benefits packages may be developed for each target group if needs are substantially different from one group to another. Benefits packages also may be based on the capacity or ability of the provider panel to provide the services. For example, the market and demand analyses may show a need for psychiatric services; however, the physician panel may not include a psychiatrist, the health plan may have no plans to include one, and may be unwilling to refer patients to psychiatrists in the general community. In other words, the benefits package should generally meet the need/demands of the target groups, constrained by the ability of the provider panel to provide or arrange for these services. Remember that the marketing philosophy is that activities are undertaken and services are provided to create satisfied consumers and patients.

At the begining of this chapter, the concept of positioning was discussed; that is, the development of a niche in the market, or the medical group's or HMO's market share. Market position is accomplished by creating an image and reputation for a certain kind of service and developing satisfied and loyal customers. In effect, the health plan has differentiated itself from other providers in the marketplace, and the better differentiated the services from the competition, the more successful the marketing effort. When the HMO and its affiliated physicians develop and market a health plan, they will differentiate themselves in two areas—the medical services that have been customarily provided and the benefits package/premium for the plan. These two areas represent two different but coordinated marketing and service efforts.

The health plan should be able to describe how each service it offers differs from and is better than the competition's. First, the plan's administrators should list all the health plan benefits, medical and nonmedical services, and products that are offered. Then, the unique attributes and features of each should be identified. Likewise, management should be able to identify the benefits of or satisfaction derived from each service or product. Finally, if they are not unique or better than the competition's, the health plan's administrators should identify and determine how the products and services can be differentiated from the competing plans and health services providers. This exercise assists in identifying the distinctive aspects of each service and in determining what benefits and levels of satisfaction are derived. If there are no advantages for consumers, the plan should attempt to differentiate the service by changing it. The plan has a need for a differential advantage, and may want to reposition itself through this process.

A second area in which the health plan must consider differentiation is in the development of the benefits package and premium structure. Benefits packages must meet consumers' perceived needs and demands and must be comparable with other available health insurance benefits packages. Again, the health plan's management, using a similar process to that described above, should question how its packages differ from those offered by the competition.

Traditional HMO benefits packages have been fairly comprehensive, although current practice is to develop products that mimic traditional Blue Cross/Blue Shield, hybrid products, point-of-service offerings, and other innovations. The comprehensive packages usually include so-called first-dollar, first-day coverage for hospital care and physician care provided in a hospital and the physician's office. Additionally, HMO packages include major medical or catastrophic coverage. All together, the service units are provided in three areas: (1) ambulatory services (that may also include preventive services), (2) inpatient hospital and long-term care services, and (3) other services and products such as eyeglasses, prostheses, blood products, and so on. In designing the benefits package, the health plan should consider the following issues:

- Federal and state regulatory requirements (basic and supplemental benefits packages are described in Chapter 2)

- Feasibility of matching major benefits in existing competitive programs and medical care programs
- Possibility of differentiating the health plan by adding supplemental benefits (e.g., prescription drugs, vision, or dental services) or by offering alternative options (e.g., different benefit levels, copayments, and premiums)
- Ability of the health plan to reposition itself in the market by improving its customary services and products
- Cost of each benefit and implications for the total premium
- Provisions for converting a member's contract in cases of employment termination, retirement, movement outside the service area, or change in status
- Arrangements for out-of-area coverage
- Willingness of participating physicians to provide each benefit, and attitudes about each benefit
- Availability of facilities (e.g., hours of operation) and their distribution throughout the service area
- Prevailing physician compensation in the service area, and the level of capitation payments, discounts, or salaries
- Negotiation of per diem rates at affiliated hospitals

Consumer satisfaction can be heightened by increasing the attractiveness of benefits packages. This may be accomplished in several ways. First, there must be a commitment to respond to consumer needs. This includes 24-hour emergency care, a grievance procedure, consumer representation on the HMO board, and a continuing program of member communications. Second, there should be a concern with keeping members healthy, as demonstrated through the use of health education classes, sports medicine clinics, diet and nutrition workshops, and so on. Finally, the member should experience a feeling of personal care and attention; this might be amplified through the ambience of the facility, the quality of the medical devices used, the level of technology available, and the attitudes of physicians and support staff.

Marketing Mix Element: Pricing of Medical Services and Products

Rate making and premium development of each benefits package and benefits level (e.g., low and high option) are carried out by the HMO's financial manager in association with a consulting actuary and the entire management team and board. Price development must also be a coordinated effort with the physician and hospital providers, since adequate payment to these providers must be reflected in the premium charged payers. Prices and premiums that are developed must be such that revenues from premiums plus other revenues, including profit, exceed the costs of operating the health plan. From a marketing perspective, premiums are set so that they are competitive with similar benefits packages offered by other HMOs and health insurance plans. As discussed early in this chapter, the value exchange system describes the rationale for consumer purchases—something of value (medical services) is exchanged for something else of value (premiums). The HMO will probably use price compensation as a major part of its overall marketing strategy.

Economists suggest that a free market can operate effectively only when the purchaser has adequate information on competing products to make a purchase decision. Therefore, it is imperative that a comparison of competing benefits packages and prices be made and communicated to potential subscribers and members. It is almost impossible, however, to make accurate comparisons, although most HMOs do provide comparative information. Comparison of HMO packages is difficult because the products are different and somewhat unequal. Comparisons are further complicated because there are usually differences in out-of-pocket expenses to the member—expenses such as copayments and deductibles that are not covered by the benefits package.

It is important to understand what role employers, unions, or associations play in contributing to the member's premium. A *noncontributory* plan is a health insurance program in which the premiums for the insurance are paid entirely by the employer. A *contributory* plan is one in which the employee or union/association member pays a certain amount. When the employee or union/association member pays the entire premium, the plan is designated *fully contributory.* If health insurance is a noncontributory fringe benefit offered by the employer, price considerations are solely the employer's. Regardless of whether the plan is contributory or not, the key employer contact or union/association representative will be reviewing price very closely to determine what the health care fringe benefits will cost. The experience of some HMOs suggests that employees will not purchase a contributory option if its price is more than $10 higher per month (deducted from their paycheck) than their current health plan. With fully contributory plans, members' attitudes about prices are very sensitive; to be competitive, the HMO's price should be about the same as that of competing health pla.is. If prices are higher than the competition, the following rules of thumb should apply:

- The HMO's prices should be no higher than $10 to $15 above the prevailing single premium rate
- Prices should be no higher than $15 to $20 above the prevailing double premium rates
- Prices should be no higher than $20 to $25 above the prevailing family premium rates

Premium levels have an impact on which individuals in the target groups select the health plan. Low rates and underpricing may result in adverse selection—the selection of the HMO by individuals with abnormally high health risks, resulting in unfavorable utilization patterns. Lower than competitive prices may encourage enrollment at a very fast pace, faster perhaps than the health plan's providers are able to properly serve the members. Recent data suggest that young HMOs enrolling new groups experience higher than normal utilization; use rates among the new groups seem to stabilize at lower, more normal rates after the first year.

Marketing Mix Element: Place or Location of Medical Facilities

Considered during the planning and development of the marketing strategy, the geographic location of health plan offices and the HMO's providers affects the attractiveness of the health plan to potential members. Generally, it is believed that at least 65 percent of the target groups should live within a 30-minute commute of the facility. For urban areas, the facility should be able to adequately serve an area within a 10-mile radius. Together, travel time and distance are described as the "travel function"—an aggravation index that includes distance, travel time, congestion, normal travel patterns, parking, safety, and so on. The travel function and the attractiveness of the service sites create important marketing conditions. Hours of operation and types of emergency coverage also will be important to continued account maintenance. Large HMOs have realized that satellite facilities are useful in providing accessible services to members living in suburban areas.

Marketing Mix Element: Promotion

The final element of the marketing mix is promotion—communicating information about the health plan to the target groups and educating the potential members about their health service needs. Planning activities and the development of staff, equipment, and facilities are of no significance if the availability of the health services cannot be communicated to the target groups, yet somewhat archaic attitudes about advertising and selling persist in the medical community, and it is essential to discuss their use.

The health plan should choose its ad copy carefully and should have a clear and specific understanding about how promotional literature and selling activities are to be used. The principles of medical ethics state that a physician's name cannot be included in promotional material. In these health plans, the concern is not so much of advertising by physicians themselves but advertising on behalf of the physician by the marketing department.

The difference is between advertising the availability of medical services under a specific system—such as an HMO, PPO, or Blue Cross/Blue Shield—and advertising the individual physicians that work with the system. The American Medical Association's Ethical Relations Committee and Judicial Council provide guidelines that allow physicians greater freedom than in years past to advertise their services and charges. This policy has evolved because HMOs have traditionally advertised; fee-for-service physicians have responded to this competitive pressure with their own marketing efforts. In effect, what HMOs have been encouraging—free choice—is finally being achieved.

The degree of promotional activities can vary from intensive and agressive efforts to very little coordinated procedures. Most plans have a relatively "soft sell" approach that includes public service announcements on radio and television, mailings, ads on buses and subways, and newspaper ads. These efforts attempt to create an image regarding the health plan. This might be of a caring organization, or one that is technically advanced, or one that thoroughly reviews and guarantees the quality of its services and providers. Some plans will want an image of accessibility and convenience along with control of rising medical care costs. Generally, the ads will inform the public about the availability of the plan's health services.

Some of the ads are generally supportive of the entire medical community and suggest only the availability of prepaid health plans as another option for medical care delivery. Somewhat stronger advertisements may describe the uniqueness of the prepaid approach—its emphasis on ambulatory and preventive services and its 24-hour availability. Hard-sell techniques have been used infrequently. Ads might, however, include a description of the programs offered and the major advantages of controlled cost and quality, comprehensive coverage, and easy access when care is needed. The use of comparison charts pointing out the advantages of the HMO over its leading competitors can be very effective. But no matter what technique is used, it is imperative that the health plan's marketing director evaluate the impact of the advertising campaign on the other providers in the community before implementing it. Ugly confrontations that could adversely affect the entire medical community and tarnish the health plan's image should be avoided. In all situations, materials presented must be in good taste and factual—neither overstating or understating the HMO's ability to provide services. Advertising should not only inform but should also educate the public. In a situation where a health plan is completing its first market activities and has enrolled its first year's members, an effective advertisement form is word of mouth; its effectiveness depends on many factors that are all part of the image of the health plan and the medical group—quality care, access, friendliness of personnel, and so on.

Advertising is one of several activities in the promotion effort that build the public image of the health plan. Other promotional activities of the HMO that should be continuous include public relations, actual selling activities, improvement of sales literature, preparation of annual reports, periodic preventive health tips for distribution to members, training and utilization of the sales force to be effective yet courteous and helpful, and a courteous receptionist and telephone operator. As Gumbiner suggests in *HMO: Putting It All Together,* the HMO has a relationship with several publics, all of whom react in various ways to the health plan and its activities. These publics include "the general public, the professional public (other doctors, pharmacists, dentists), its in-house public (its own staff, which should never be forgotten), and the consumer public that it serves. Then there are many subgroups: government agencies, industries, unions, insurance companies, and hospitals."[9]

The willingness of consumers and publics to purchase an HMO option depends on their perceptions of its value to themselves, their companies, and their families. Several impediments, described below, need to be addressed when promotional and ad strategies are being developed.

- The relative advantages of the health plan over the traditional system are not readily perceived by the public. During the enrollment process, the public needs to be educated about the advantages of the prepaid health plan.
- The advent of the HMO requires a substantial change in consumer attitudes regarding health services delivery and financing. When buying health services, most people will tend to be more conservative than when buying other products.
- The health plan's product is complex and difficult to understand, particularly in comparison to a known service or product.
- The health plan cannot be tried easily (i.e., pretested) without a significant perceived risk to the consumer.
- Prepaid benefits are neither readily demonstrated nor easily communicated.

STEP 5: FORECASTING ENROLLMENT AND THE BREAK-EVEN POINT

The fifth step in the marketing process is forecasting HMO enrollment and the break-even point. Current and projected sizes of target groups need to be considered and accurately forecast. Such projections affect staffing requirements, for example, since they are a function of enrollment. These

---

[9] Robert Gumbiner. *HMO: Putting It All Together.* St. Louis, Mo., C.V. Mosby Co., 1975, p. 87.

forecasts are necessary in the development of financial projections and budgets. Likewise, these projections help the health plan's board set goals for the plan. Statements of enrollment levels for each month and the year are prepared. For ease in creating use rates and cost estimates, these projections are described in member-months; 7,000 members would reflect 84,000 member-months (7,000 times 12 months).

Enrollment forecasts are based on the results of segmentation and penetration-rate analyses made earlier. Two steps are then used to forecast enrollment. First, management identifies the variables that affect enrollment levels and, second, the plan estimates the additional members who will enroll in future years. The variables that affect enrollment levels include the size of accounts, employee out-of-pocket costs, the differences between the HMO's benefits package and that of its competitors, the level of receptivity to HMOs by firms and payers, the existence of local versus national companies, and the presence of unions or associations. Each of these variables for each market group should be weighed and inferences drawn regarding the number of members expected from the group under study. When these penetration rates are completed for the current year, the health plan manager should then attempt to project levels of penetration beyond the initial year. Although the same variables are important, assumptions should be made regarding disenrollment, new enrollment, and reenrollment trends. In a conservative approach, the manager should assume that only a small percentage of all employees or members of associations/unions will initially enroll. New members during the first year or two may approximately equal disenrollment. But, if marketing efforts are sustained and current members are satisfied with the plan and its services, future enrollment should increase through yearly reenrollment and new members. This process will be enhanced through word-of-mouth advertising by satisfied members. Target growth rates can be described in several ways: (1) as the total number of new members from each group, (2) as the total of reenrollments plus new members from each employer group, or (3) the total number of enrollees in the health plan without defining their enrollment/reenrollment status.

Monthly enrollment projections might be displayed on charts to help in the analysis and to follow the progress in membership growth. Some of the variables described above may be included, along with the size of the employer group and the number and percent of enrollees from the group. New projections should be made monthly, based on the previous month's enrollment figures. Such estimates should be evaluated to determine where break-even will occur, that is, the time when revenue from premiums and other sources equals the fixed and variable costs of operating the health plan. Enrollment projections must be tied to the break-even objective for new plans; after this point is reached, enrollment projections should be an integral part of setting objectives. Each target group and its enrollment should be evaluated regarding its loss ratio (premium income to expenses for the target group); the plan cannot sustain membership in a target group where losses exceed income.

After forecasts are prepared, long-range promotional plans should be considered and some preliminary proposals drawn up. Because future promotional efforts will usually be an extension of programs, these proposals will provide for continuity of enrollment activities with current accounts and expansion to new accounts. Chances are that new accounts will have formed a good impression of the health plan through word of mouth. This "halo" effect should be considered when additional promotional plans are developed.

STEP 6: MAKING CHOICES AVAILABLE

The final step in the marketing process is making choices of health plans available, also known as active marketing. This is the implementation stage when all the plans and strategies developed to this point are put into operation. The health plan takes its programs to the marketplace and actively sells them to the target populations and groups. The aim of this process is to give employees, union and association members, and individuals the option of choosing the HMO's package from among the various health plan options available. Active marketing, then, includes several activities: promotion and advertising, solicitation strategies, the sales process and closing or making the sale, the enrollment process, and account maintenance. These issues are discussed in the next few paragraphs.

Dual/Multiple Choice

Promotion and selling activity begins by offering dual/multiple choice to those firms, unions, associations, and governmental agencies that have been chosen as the health plan's target groups. Dual/multiple choice has been a traditional HMO strategy for breaking into other insurer's markets, and it may also facilitate the development of true, marketplace-driven, consumer choice among programs. Most employers historically offered only one "mandatory" program; the decision of an employer to offer the HMO option as a second choice will require a change in employer attitudes regarding fringe benefits for employees as well as changes in current operations. For instance, the rationale for current benefits plans may be that the employer has "always provided the XYZ health plan." With the need to control rising benefits costs, employers are now willing to consider alternative approaches, such as offering two, three, or more health plans. HMO account representatives find that negotiations with employer representatives, based on sound logical reasoning, are useful in changing current habits and opinions. They must be skilled in presenting the HMO approach and explaining benefits packages and the range of premiums. Advantages to the employer or union should be well understood and communicated, and a thorough knowledge of potential disadvantages is helpful in presenting an acceptable argument for dual/multiple choice. Both positions are presented in the following lists.

ADVANTAGES OF DUAL AND MULTIPLE CHOICE:

1. Greater employee satisfaction with the fringe benefits package and, thus, with their jobs.

2. The potential over the long run for less employee sick time and, thus, higher productivity as a result of preventive services and the use of the less time-consuming ambulatory mode of delivery.

3. HMOs as a cost-containment approach may save money for the employer who contributes to his employees' health insurance, since the cost of the employer's contribution may not increase as quickly as in other insurance programs.

4. The employees' share of the cost of the package also may be moderated, thus providing greater employee satisfaction with the company.

5. A more comprehensive benefits package may entice desirable potential employees to join the firm and induce current employees to remain with the company.

6. The firm may feel a social responsibility to the community and its employees to make several choices available and, perhaps, more valuable health care programs.

7. The firm may wish to offer dual/multiple choice to enhance its public image.

8. According to law, a firm governed by the Fair Labor Standards Act must offer dual/multiple choice to its employees if federally qualified HMOs using group, staff, and IPA approaches are available. (This provision is scheduled to be phased out in 1995.)

9. The firm may offer dual/multiple choice to meet the competition for employees because other local firms are offering dual/multiple choice.

DISADVANTAGES OF DUAL AND MULTIPLE CHOICE:

1. Costs of HMO benefits packages are customarily slightly higher than the plans in effect; therefore, the HMO option may be viewed as an increase in financial liability for the firm.

2. There are increased costs, both start-up and operational, to the employer in administering two or more plans rather than one (e.g., recordkeeping, collection of premiums).

3. By offering more benefits initially, the employer might envision a possibility of accelerating union/employee demands for more fringe benefits.

4. Employers are reluctant to interrupt production by allowing marketing representatives to solicit employees on the job, although firms generally will arrange meetings with union stewards and second-level management.

5. The possibility of a substantial dollar increase in health insurance deductions from an employee's salary may contribute to the loss of employees.

6. Employees and spouses are being asked to break established physician relationships.

STEPS TO IMPLEMENTING DUAL AND MULTIPLE CHOICE: There can be wide variations in implementation methods for dual/multiple choice. Generally, however, the following steps can be considered basic:

1. Employers, unions, associations, and others are approached by the HMO, and the group representative decides to allow dual/multiple choice.

2. The group decides on the level of benefits and the premium. The general approach is to continue with the current premium level initially, although the HMO benefits package might vary substantially from the incumbent plan(s).

3. The group representative will decide whether to allow the HMO to market directly to group members; ask the HMO to coordinate its efforts through the incumbent plan(s) and let the existing plan(s) market, enroll, and complete all other marketing activities, including collection of premiums; or allow the HMO to market and manage the accounts for itself and the incumbent plan(s). A contract will be consummated describing the arrangement agreed upon.

4. Information describing the benefits of all plans is made available to each of the beneficiaries.

5. The beneficiaries are permitted and encouraged to decide for themselves which plan they desire.

6. Each beneficiary is required to make an affirmative choice of plans.

7. Beneficiaries are then given an opportunity annually to transfer from one plan to another. (Enrollment periods must be coordinated with labor agreements and other health plan anniversary dates.)

8. The insurance plans must agree in advance to accept the beneficiaries who select their plan, without percentage restrictions or other qualifications.

For further discussion concerning consumer choice, please see Chapter 7, regarding purchasers and the consumer perspective.

Active Marketing

How is selling the HMO to targeted groups actually accomplished? The process includes several key activities:

1. A schedule of appointments with key account representatives is developed.

2. Each appointment is held, and actual selling to the employer, union, or association representative is accomplished. The employer agrees to the dual/multiple choice option for the employees.

3. HMO sales representatives then market to employees or union/association members and enroll those who opt for the HMO coverage.

4. Each account is serviced.

5. Reenrollment is provided to the accounts in which disenrollment has occurred.

Appointments are scheduled with the largest groups first, smaller groups (50 to 500) second, individual contracts next, and welfare programs such as Medicaid last. Large-group marketing costs per enrollee are the lowest: the effort to sell to 5,000 employees is not much more expensive than selling to 3,000 employees. There is a somewhat higher per-enrollee cost when selling to smaller groups, and substantially higher per-enrollee costs for individuals. Selling to Medicaid recipients can be very time-consuming, and they may be the last group to be enrolled, although negotiation for a state contract should begin early in the marketing process. Another important reason for beginning the active marketing process with employee groups is that the companies, by preemployment screening, generally have already screened those individuals who were severe health risks as being unacceptable for employment. Therefore, a fairly good cross-section of healthy people is selected, which will help to keep health plan utilization expenses low. Full-coverage or better coverage plans like HMOs have a tendency to attract people requiring above-average medical services. This is natural because the paid-in-full, better coverage program means less money out-of-pocket for the member. Scheduling for selling to and signing on unionized groups can be difficult because they operate with negotiated contracts; many employers will refuse to do anything that is not included in the contract and will defer any action until the contract is renegotiated. Even during the negotiation period, there may be little compromise, with both the union and the employer expecting that their specific demands will be met. In general, the HMO manager must maintain the same control over the solicitation activities as all other marketing and health plan activities; thus, solicitation strategies must be carefully developed and strictly followed by the sales staff. Strategies, staff development, and enrollment of specific groups are discussed in the following sections.

Promotion, Advertising, and Public Relations

Before the outset of marketing activity, the health plan and its affiliated providers have agreed on the goals and objectives for the prepaid system.

Marketing surveys and analyses have been completed. With target groups selected through segmentation and penetration-rate analyses, the stage is set to develop relevant promotional devices.

Promotional activity includes the development of dual or multiple choice arrangements, described previously, and how dual/multiple choice fits within the promotional strategy must be considered. For example, many potential members already may be patients of the HMO's physician providers and may be more easily sold on the idea of enrolling in the HMO. Next, recently arrived service-area residents with no physician who are being offered a choice of health plans may be open to the HMO program. Then, service-area residents with no physician and, finally, service-area residents with existing physician relationships may be approached. As one would expect, people without existing physician relationships are more likely to enroll in an HMO than those with established ties. If a company has relocated a number of people or has many young employees, effective promotional messages could emphasize the complete range of health services that can be found in the health plan's service system.

Another key element in promotion is determining how the HMO's message is to be communicated to target employment groups (i.e., choosing the educational and sales tools). The marketing director chooses a message strategy to fit the descriptions or characteristics that were developed during market research on each target group. Thus, the manager selects combinations of communication and educational activities aimed at relaying desired messages. These tools may include advertising, marketing materials, public relations activities, personal contacts, image creation activities, and pure educational services such as health services messages and meetings/seminars. Table 10-11 provides a list of communication tools that might be used. When printed materials are developed, several precautions should be considered. Even though individuals in the medical care industry are tempted to use a caduceus (a staff with two entwined snakes and two wings at the top, symbolizing the medical profession), it does not sell medical services. The message should be in the headline of the brochure or advertisement, since this may be the only part that potential members will read. If more help is needed in developing promotional strategies, consultants as well as advertising, marketing, and public relations agencies may be useful.

Solicitation strategies should be individualized to each market segment, since selling approaches need to be tailored to the specific needs of each potential member. Usually, the following concepts or ideas form the basis for promotional and selling activities.

1. Members need not be ill to benefit from the health plan; preventive medicine and early disease detection keep the members healthy.

TABLE 10-11   Communication Tools and Considerations in Their Use

Communication Tool	Considerations in Use
ADVERTISING • Radio • Television • Newspaper • Billboard • Direct mail to potential subscribers • Yellow pages advertisements • Medical group and/or HMO logo • Direct mail to employees, unions, and associations • New resident's letter	• Good for creating awareness and knowledge of plan's existence among large numbers of people • Limited usefulness in disseminating complex idea • Expensive (advertising agency, media costs) • Potentially effective during heavy enrollment periods when it may reach most potential members; effectiveness is dependent on quality of copy • Potential for internal conflict between business and medical staff around ethics of medical advertising • Advertisements target highest priority consumer group segments (e.g., young families, spouses, opinion leaders) by selecting media with most appropriate demographics • Advantage of controlled placement within selected media to reach priority targets
DIRECT MARKETING MATERIALS • Brochures • Exhibits • Member handbook • Audiovisual shows • Posters • Staff directories	• Generally more effective in communicating greater amount of information than advertising • Plan image enhanced through graphic design • Required to meet federal full and fair disclosure regulations • Materials targeted to specific target audiences and segments (e.g., union slide shows, employer brochures, posters for particular company) • Possible to update easily • Reasonable cost compared to advertising
PUBLIC RELATIONS • Publicity (TV, newspaper, magazine) • Health fairs and wellness services • Newsletters • Patient education programs • Speakers bureau • T-shirts displaying logo	• Free or less expensive than paid advertising • Establishment of professional image and credibility within the community • Difficult to control • Enhancement of awareness among opinion leaders • Involvement of all HMO staff (medical, clinic, marketing, and board members) • Opportunity to make useful personal contacts with community influentials

- Medical group's name
- Community events
- Sports physician
- Civic association activities (Chamber of Commerce)
- Scholarship to outstanding high school student
- Stickers for telephone and medicine cabinets
- School shows for children

PERSONAL SELLING
- Employer meetings
- Employee meetings
- Open house
- Telephone calls
- Representative desk in group practice facility
- Discounted or free care to civic groups/organizations and the elderly

- Necessary communication tool
- Very effective in communicating large amounts of complex information
- Very expensive labor costs
- Able to customize presentation for segments in each target audience (e.g., focus on segment's self-interest)

IMAGE CREATION
- Quality of materials
- Facility design and parking
- Responsiveness
- Organization personnel
- Behavior and dress
- Physician attitude
- Member grievance procedure
- Waiting time
- Appointment scheduling
- Cash payment discounts
- Extended hours
- Suggestion box

- Professional image projected at all staff levels
- Comfortable, attractive environment to dispel clinic label
- Reputation and enrollment dependent on attention to member satisfaction

2. The individual selects a personal family physician.

3. The member's health care is managed; the health plan provides comprehensive services at one location; and a family physician manages the total health care needs of the family.

4. The health plan offers broader coverage with fewer and smaller copayments. Outpatient care is a normally covered service; health plan patients do not have to be hospitalized to receive covered services.

5. Quality care is assured and enhanced through the use of group practices or organized panels of physicians, high medical staff standards, peer review, and the ready availability of specialists and equipment.

6. Freedom of choice under dual and multiple choice enables individuals to best meet their family requirements and to change plans annually if so desired.

7. HMOs are cost-efficient methods of delivery; premiums do not increase as rapidly as those for Blue Cross/Blue Shield and indemnity plans.

8. Unlike the Blues, access to physicians is enhanced in HMOs, since the HMO member need only call or go to the physician panel to find a physician, while Blue Shield members must find a physician from the community willing to accept them as patients.

9. Health education is a part of the entire program offered by the medical group—education concerning the use of the prepaid program and its services, habits to develop for healthier lives, and use of available preventive programs.

Soliciting and Selling

A solicitation and selling strategy developed by the health plan includes some of the following.

1. *Dual/multiple-choice arrangements*—the first approach to employee and union groups. This approach is used to inform union and management leaders and to open otherwise closed markets to medical groups.

2. *Enrollment of key employment-group leaders*—support through example, which may influence other group members.

3. *Solicitation of other influential individuals*—meetings with as many influential people in the employment group as possible, with enrollment lending credibility to the plan.

4. *Individual employee or union/association member solicitation*—the critical second stage of group solicitation. The strategy used will be tailored to each employment group. Normally, it is preferable to meet with employees or union/association members in small numbers rather than one large group. Large gatherings are very impersonal; one employee radically opposed to the program could affect many potential members. These meetings should be held during work-shift changes or weekends.

5. *Work with existing insurance companies*—some companies rely solely on the advice of their existing carriers. If, in fact, the existing carrier markets the HMO, as is often the case, payment for services may guarantee an acceptable selling job.

6. *Small- to medium-size employers*—consider premium level as the most important issue in offering the HMO. Other subjects considered important are premium rates and copayments, employer administration of dual/multiple-choice benefit plans, health services and benefits of the health plan, and master contract provisions.

7. *Community education*—public service announcements, brochures, and other media advertisements designed to foster acceptance and public awareness of the HMO's physician practice panel or group practice.

8. *Mail communications*—effective in group selling. Letters may be more carefully read than a brochure.

9. *Communication with spouses*—generally, spouses have a strong voice in the decision to give up an existing method of care and to enter into a new system. Information concerning the prepaid choice and its services must, therefore, reach spouses.

10. *Open house at the HMO and the physician group practice*—provides potential enrollees with an opportunity to see the facility and lends credibility to promises made in small group meetings. Open houses, however, usually are not well attended.

11. *Door-to-door selling*—this approach usually is one of the last methods used in dual/multiple-choice selling because, although effective, it is sometimes difficult to contact the decision maker in the family. Because of the need for personalized contact, however, it is one of the most important approaches to selling to individual subscribers who are not under dual-choice arrangements and in enrolling subscribers of government-assisted programs such as Medicaid.

12. *Volunteer activities*—enthusiastic and articulate enrollees may be willing to provide expert assistance in financing, underwriting, public relations, and so on.

13. *Endorsement by sponsors*—rely on the reputation of the sponsoring organization by mailing letters of solicitation on its stationery over the signature of one of its officers. Use of a statement of qualification by the Federal Government may or may not be a useful component of the marketing strategy.

14. *Watch the terminology*—presentations should not include the word "clinic" (which may connote charity care) but should refer to the facility as a "medical" or "health" center. A "physician specializing in internal medicine" is preferable to "internist," to avoid the possibility that physician specialists will be confused with students.

15. *Flyers, payroll envelope stuffers, posters, and other take-home litera-*

ture—all are useful in group selling, but remember that they may not make it home.

16. *Comparisons*—comparing the HMO with other available plans is effective in identifying the prepaid plan as a program that provides more comprehensive services for a similar premium. If possible, all health care costs for a specific period (total expenditures for health) should be used, including premiums and out-of-pocket expenses.

17. *Word-of-mouth*—best promotional mechanism over the long run, after the initial enrollment group has been secured, and the major means of acquiring new members.

An HMO marketing representative should attempt to sell the health plan on a one-to-one basis to the key leader in an employment group. Initially, one-to-one selling begins with an educational phase, when the key leader is informed of the health plan's existence, how an HMO operates, its economies, and the plan's overall advantage. The next phase is actual enrollment. The initial phase may last throughout the development of the health plan and, thus, is a cumulative process. A sample promotional strategy on selling to corporate decision makers might include, for example, an initial assessment period, during which the HMO creates an awareness of the HMO's concepts and advantages. The second step might be considered the development of the account, during which the HMO provides information about the health plan, tries to arouse interest in and instill a desire to offer the HMO, and obtains an "action" commitment from the decision makers to offer the health plan. The final stage is the operational phase, during which the HMO makes good on its commitment to perform.

Another target market comprises individuals who are not associated with large employers, unions, or associations. For example, an existing group practice that signs a contract to service local HMO members may wish to offer the HMO to its current patients. In effect, these individuals become another "group" that should be underwritten like all other groups. Traditionally, because the individual group is normally heterogeneous, it is a higher risk group than employer or union groups. The pricing of the benefits package may result in somewhat higher premiums under the experience rating method. In its underwriting process, the HMO will have established, as marketing objectives, the size limitation on unaffiliated individuals. The choice of a community rating approach may help to reduce the cost of the program to the individual group by spreading some of its potential expenses to other members.

Decision to Buy—A Value Choice

The decision to buy the HMO product is viewed by the consumer as a value choice. The consumer may buy the HMO, a Blue's plan, or indemnity coverage, or may remain a self-paying patient (i.e., not buy at all). The consumer decision is based on how well the perceived value of the HMO's products and services matches his or her own needs and desires. The decision to buy can also be viewed as an exchange of values—that is, the consumer believes that he or she is receiving service equal to or worth more than the charges for the service. What, then, are the product values of an HMO, and how well do they match the general need/demand for services? The following are four basic HMO product values.

1. *Comprehensive care:* Many customers of service and indemnity plans have been disappointed or upset when they find that their "comprehensive" insurance coverage only partially pays for services they have received. As part of the HMO promotional activity, comparisons of the indemnities, the "Blues," and the HMO may assure the potential members that HMO coverage is more comprehensive than that of existing plans. Additional services that emphasize prevention and ambulatory care also may be viewed by the customer as value added.

2. *Accessible care:* The consumer with a fee-for-service, private family physician too often finds that no service is available on weekends, on weekdays when the physician has no office hours, and during evening and nighttime hours. The HMO attempts to provide 24-hour coverage and telephone consultation. Emergency care in HMOs, however, may be provided on a referral basis, through out-of-area coverage, or in a hospital's emergency room. Long waits and impersonal service may be the result for the HMO member.

3. *Quality care:* Although this is a very difficult area to document, consumers value quality care and satisfaction very highly. They consider quality/satisfaction to be the ability to see a physician when one is needed, the degree of respect and sensitivity with which patients are handled, the impression provided by the facility, the degree of choice of physician, the use of the family or managing physician, and the closeness of the consumer's relationship with the personal physician. Consumers cannot easily judge the quality of the medical treatment they receive, but they can and do evaluate the quality and satisfaction of the personal treatment.

4. *Reasonable cost:* The pricing of the benefits package is critical to the success of the marketing strategy. It can only be used as a selling point if it is competitive with the current insurance program's premiums. As mentioned earlier, the employee's monthly payroll deduction for the HMO should be no more than $15 higher than the incumbent plan. When skillfully explained, consumers will understand that although the HMO premium may be higher than their present coverage, they also may be receiving more services for their money in the HMO system.

Enrollment Process

Sales occur over two phases, as described above—obtaining employer or union commitments to offer dual/multiple-choice, and selling to employees or union/association members. Internally, the HMO marketing department should:

1. Determine who in the employer/union group will be responsible for coordinating the enrollment campaign with the HMO marketing representative and which representative will handle the account.

2. Make decisions regarding:

   a. Date of mailing the HMO offering to employees (usually two months before the effective date of the potential contract)
   b. Enrollment period (usually a two-week period beginning approximately six weeks before the effective date)
   c. Eligibility criteria for potential enrollees, such as time with the company or union, full-time versus part-time status, and the like
   d. Conversion and retirement provisions

3. Set up administrative procedures for the organization, such as payroll deductions and selection and enrollment forms.

4. Draft and send a letter to each employee's or union member's home on employer/union stationery announcing the health plan.

5. Prepare an information packet to distribute to all employees; be sure that company approval has been obtained.

6. Discuss how the HMO's representative will obtain access to employees or union members. The greater the access, the more success the plan will have in enrolling members. Access may be by way of presentations to the employee group, display booths, and panel discussions with HMO and other plan representatives.

7. Determine what off-site activities may be used (if access to union employees is prohibited in the workplace). These may include open houses at the health center; articles and announcements in employer newsletters; bulletin boards with posters, brochures, and pamphlets in personnel and union offices; mailings to homes; and the like.

During the enrollment process, the HMO representative will provide information about the prepaid program and ask the customer to buy. Although marketing representatives are trained in selling techniques, the representative must "ask the customer to buy" if a sale is to be made. The act of selling is consummated when the potential purchaser actually signs the enrollment card. Those who do not accept should be asked to sign a nonacceptance statement so that the plan has a record that the offer was made by the HMO. After enrollment is completed by the execution of enrollment forms, the marketing representative should arrange for the new members to visit the medical group's facilities to (1) see the health center and learn how to make appointments and use the services, (2) have a physical examination if it is required for enrollment, and (3) choose a family physician from the primary care practitioners or physician pool.

Requiring the potential members to make a timely decision to purchase makes it easy for the health plan representative to complete the sale and to process the enrollment forms. For individuals not covered by dual or multiple choice, the process requires some additional effort on the part of the marketing representative. In either case, the member's signature on the enrollment card finalizes the selling process. Enrollment cards or forms usually state the benefits in general terms and the amount of the member's contribution to the premium. It is recommended that the member be given a complete description of the benefits package (policy and certificates), including any copayments or deductibles and any other service limitations. This statement should be written in layman's language, and the salesman should thoroughly explain the statement. Over the long run, such a practice will substantially reduce misunderstandings and foster better relations between members and the plan.

Signature cards or enrollment forms provide data about the member, including his/her name and the names of his/her spouse and dependents. The cards or forms also may include insurance classification, dates of birth, occupation, sex, annual earnings, and so on, as well as a statement signed by the employee authorizing payroll deductions for any portion of the cost that the employer has specified must be paid by the employee.

The employer or union is the policyholder and receives a master policy form, the legal instrument that describes the complete agreement between the HMO and the employer or union. Employees or union members who are then classified as beneficiaries will receive an insurance certificate. While these certificates do not legally constitute a contract, they are evidence of the benefits package in force and should reflect the benefits and other provisions of the master policy—the formal contract. Persons who have individual policies with the HMO are both the policyholder and the beneficiary and also should receive a comprehensive statement of the benefits and premiums in force. Because these issues may be governed by law, state government representatives should be contacted concerning specific requirements.

Many states have a cooling-off period, during which the new member can decide not to accept the offer to join the HMO. These periods normally are for 48 hours after enrollment is completed. Generally, if the selling has been honest and all questions have been fully answered, the number of enrollees who choose not to continue with enrollment will be low.

A final issue that may be addressed during enrollment is preexisting conditions. When the application for enrollment is completed, major disease risk categories are reviewed. If the member has such a disease or condition at the time of enrollment, the health plan may require a physical examination and may exclude care for this disease or condition from coverage. (Federally qualified HMOs are not allowed to make an enrollment decision based on preexisting conditions.)

Account Maintenance and Growth

The final phase of the marketing activity concerns continuing member relations and identification of new markets. Once the potential subscriber becomes a member of the HMO, part of the marketing effort should be directed toward keeping that member satisfied with the health care program. The marketing agent who sold the plan would make the best contact point should the member have problems. This may not be possible; but there should be a person who acts as the consumer contact point in the HMO, whether it is a receptionist, a physician, or a consumer ombudsman. These issue are addressed in Chapter 7.

Experience has shown that the quality of member relations has a direct bearing on future enrollment. Good relations foster the best form of ongoing promotion of the health plan. HMO programs are sold by satisfied people who refer their neighbors and friends. Indeed, significant increases in enrollment can be expected after the first or second year of operation, primarily as a result of satisfied customers. This also suggests that HMOs should develop growth objectives. Orderly growth requires good management of present and future accounts and members. It also requires the establishment of growth levels for groups of members and control of the marketing activities to ensure that these levels are met and, also, that they are not exceeded. The situation of overenrollment is, in many ways, as bad as not meeting the minimum enrollment level.

The Marketing Department and Its Management

Marketing departments are created as a formal organizational division or unit for the purpose of carrying out planning, development, and operational functions. HMO marketing functions can be categorized into six areas. These include the functions of market surveys and analyses, planning and control, sales, account service, health plan member services, and advertising and promotion.

To carry out these functions, the HMO will identify and hire a director of marketing and a marketing staff. The types and numbers of marketing staff will be influenced by the anticipated workload; some staffing levels are provided in Chapter 8. The number and types of marketing personnel also will depend on enrollment estimates, anticipated member turnover, and the expected technical and managerial needs of the marketing department. Job descriptions will assist the manager in hiring and directing qualified staff. Staffing arrangements will match the limitations of the HMO's organizational structure and its budgetary constraints. Budget allocations for staff may significantly limit the numbers and quality of the staff.

The marketing director is responsible for carrying out or arranging for all of the market surveys and analyses, and for completing forecasting activities. He/she interfaces with all other staff, especially in developing enrollment projections, developing benefits packages, and pricing and setting premium levels. As noted above, the director is responsible for identifying potential marketing personnel and interviewing and hiring the most capable to become marketing representatives.

The director is responsible for implementing the marketing strategy and plan. Initial contact is made with key employer and union representatives and promotional activities with each group are implemented, including group meetings. On a daily basis, the director manages the daily performance of marketing representatives to ensure that enrollment goals are met. Ultimately, the director is responsible for the maintenance of all accounts.

During initial growth, the ratio of marketing staff to membership is generally high, but the ratio usually drops as membership grows. At this point, the marketing director may become personally involved in contacts with potential groups of members and directly involved in account maintenance, along with account representatives, who are responsible for sales to and enrollment of employees and for continuing account maintenance. Often, specific accounts or a territory are assigned to each marketing representative, who then becomes familiar with and develops a rapport with the accounts, thereby reducing apprehension and increasing member satisfaction. If sales personnel also act as member service representatives, they have the added responsibility of developing new member orientations, handling member grievances, and designing activities to measure and maintain member satisfaction.

The size of the sales staff is based on its combined activities, but generally it is estimated that approximately 90 hours of sales staff time is required to market, enroll, service, and reenroll an account. If 10 accounts are to be managed, some 900 hours of sales staff time may be required. Rules of thumb may help plan the staffing levels; for example, it is estimated that for initial marketing efforts, a ratio of marketing/sales representatives per 1,500 program members is useful. After most accounts have been successfully marketed and enrollment is stabilized at or near projected levels, the ratio may increase to one representative for 2,000 members. Thus, if the initial first-year goal is an average 6,000 members, it is suggested that four sales representatives are needed. After marketing activities settle to a normal pace, the application of the 1:2,000 ratio would result in the need for only one representative for a growth of 2,000 members per year.

STAFF VERSUS CONTRACT MARKETING

Who should be involved in the marketing and selling activities depends on the program's design and sponsorship. If the sponsor is an insurance company, the parent company most likely will manage the marketing activities. For independent organizations, there are essentially three broad organizational approaches:

1. Develop ? marketing staff as an integral part of the HMO organization
2. Contract with an existing organization or with brokers, general insurance agents, and existing carriers to complete marketing activities
3. Use a combination of HMO staff and some contract marketing

Each approach has its own strengths and weaknesses. The decision to choose one program over another is based on several factors. Foremost is the ability or inability to attract a competent and experienced marketing director and a marketing staff. In the past, many federal HMO grantees exhibited major deficiencies in their in-house marketing efforts, primarily because they lacked competent marketing directors. Good directors command substantial salaries. For a newly developing HMO with potential financial problems, this added cost may be higher than it is willing to undertake; hence, it may be more attractive to contract with Blue Cross and Blue Shield, for example, to undertake the marketing activities. It is obvious, however, that if the HMO is unwilling to invest substantial funds in the marketing activity, it will not be successful; the marketing budget for a new HMO should be more liberal than for a mature HMO that is relying on word-of-mouth advertising and account maintenance. Although it may appear that the use of an outside agency is the least expensive method of marketing, this may be misleading. These organizations, of necessity, must have a return on their investment, even if they are nonprofit, just to stay in business. Coupled with the possibility that service- and indemnity-plan sales personnel may be inexperienced in HMO solicitation, the ultimate cost to the HMO, in all likelihood, may be higher than if it hired an in-house marketing staff. Questions of cost, ability to attract experienced staff, and control of the marketing activities must be weighed carefully before the decision is made to use either system.

If an in-house staff is created, control can be strengthened by the organizational structure developed for the marketing staff. Organization may follow one of the following methods. The staff may be divided by:

- Account type—government and manufacturing accounts and banks/ service organizations
- Territory
- Function—account sales, enrollment, account services, and member services
- General sales with no specialization

The marketing director must decide which method or combination of methods will be most useful and successful for the HMO and its target accounts.

SALES FORCE COMPENSATION

Compensation for the sales force may follow the normal salaried approach used for other employees of the health plan. Some suggest, however, that salary may not provide the motivation needed to develop sales aggressivenesss.

A second method might be compensation tied to enrollment quotas; but this could lead to adverse selection, because sales representatives might oversell or not be as selective in their selling efforts. Thus, the commission approach is seldom used by plans today.

A third approach, salary plus incentives, has been used successfully by many HMOs. The issue is how to apply the combined methods and what kinds of incentives should be offered; usually incentives are based on some measure of the representative's performance. Incentives must be fair and understood, and the opportunities for such payments must be equally distributed among the sales force. Moreover, quotas, if used as part of the incentive system, must be attainable. Disincentives develop if quotas are too high, and apathy appears if they are too low. Incentives should add substantially to the base salary if they are to become true motivators.

Finally, at times the entire sales staff will need to work together rather than compete for bonuses or incentives (e.g., when major accounts are being enrolled). Compensation arrangements should provide for these cooperative time periods.

MARKETING CONTROL

Marketing directors must address four major control issues. The first, management of the sales force, is described in detail above. A second issue involves the reporting of enrollments on a periodic basis; such reporting should be facilitated by the HMO's management information system. The other two methods include the development of marketing plans and the budgetary process. Continuous market planning should initially develop short-range plans of a year in length but, ultimately, long-range plans of three to five years are necessary. The objectives of such strategic plans may involve statements regarding enrollment, market share, revenue, contributions per enrollee, satellite outpatient facilities, expansion of market share and service area, expansion of the physician panel, and diversification into affiliated products and services.

The planning and control process requires the development of a marketing budget for the health plan, composed of a series of line items that reflect the expenses and revenues associated with the marketing function discussed in this chapter. The marketing director is responsible for developing projected expenses as well as potential revenues from enrollment estimates, and there should be sufficient detail to justify these projections. In turn, these projections will be incorporated in the overall budget for the HMO. Ten items are included in the marketing budget; they include:

1. Salary, incentives, and fringe benefits
2. Travel and expense accounts
3. Dues and fees
4. Brokerage
5. Professional services
6. Media costs
7. Printing and reproduction
8. Postage
9. Equipment
10. Materials and supplies

Monitoring areas that relate to the marketing budget include:

1. Marketing expenses per member per month
2. Marketing expenses as a percent of revenue
3. Marketing expenses as a percent of administrative or total expenses
4. Enrollment per marketing representative
5. New accounts per marketing representative

Summary

Administrators of health services delivery programs, including HMO managers, have realized that marketing of their programs is a legitimate task of management. Forced by a free market system, where consumer attitudes and beliefs are important to program success, HMOs have developed their programs and marketed them to meet the needs of their members. In HMOs, marketing is defined as the performance of a wide range of activities, including market surveys, benefits design, pricing, promotion and advertising, selling, and enrollment. Marketing is also viewed as both a concept and a process. The concept is to understand the need and desires of members, while the process is to create and deliver services to satisfy patients' desires within the boundaries of the HMO's quality and financial goals.

The objectives of marketing activities include four areas. The first, communication, is the process of educating various groups about the HMO's benefits packages and premiums, facilities, and providers. The second area, planning and forecasting, includes planning for the availability and delivery of medical services as well as collecting data, conducting research, forecasting, analyzing data, and drawing inferences from the data. Management of demand, the third objectives area, includes identification of the need/demand for services and management of the categories and types of people who enroll and then need medical services. The last marketing objective concerns the management of exchanges of value; voluntary exchanges of services, goods, and money (or premiums) are managed so that organizational goals are attained. The exchange system occurs between the HMO and its members, physicians, vendors, hospitals, nursing facilities, and governmental agencies, among others.

Marketing managers consider the current position of the HMO—its image, status, and reputation—in the marketplace. Using market analysis, managers identify the need to reposition or redefine the HMO's goals and objectives and to develop a strategy to attract new and different types of employer groups and members. Data may identify loss of market share to competing managed care programs or opportunities for expansion or improvement of the plan's position. Repositioning suggests that there is a competitive environment in which the HMO operates. Even though a competitor's services are of high quality, the HMO must develop a strategy that will cause the competitor's members to change their minds about satisfaction with their current health plan. In this way, the HMO will develop a more acceptable or preferred market share.

Viewed as an HMO-wide set of activities, marketing is a six-step process: collecting data and setting initial goals, conducting a market analysis, deciding on target markets and setting final goals, designing a marketing mix for target markets, forecasting enrollment, and making choice available and enrolling members. Data collection or market surveys provide information concerning the general and target populations. Demographic, socioeconomic, and epidemiological data are collected, along with information on available insurers, providers of care, and the general competitive situation. This first step allows the HMO to recognize appropriate target populations.

In Step 2, information gathered in the first step facilitates an analysis of the environment, the competition, and the opinions of consumers, including employers, employees, and providers. Step 3, deciding on the target market and setting final goals, is accomplished through population segmentation and estimates of penetration for each segment. The process continues with estimates of demand by selected markets and, through financial analyses, permits a forecast of the capacity necessary for providing services to meet demand. The intermediate product of this planning process is the marketing mix— a definition of the product (benefits packages), place (geographic location), promotion (advertising and selling techniques), and price (premium structure). The final products of the segmentation and penetration studies are a list of membership sources and a projection of the level of members from each source, along with a marketing mix for each source.

Step 4, designing a market mix for target markets, is a continuation of Steps 1 and 3, with particular regard to the development of a marketing mix for each target group. Successfully developed mixes allow the health plan to differentiate itself from other providers and health plans. The better differentiated the services from the competition's, the more successful the marketing effort.

The fifth step is concerned with forecasting enrollment and identifying the break-even point. Projected sizes of target groups must be accurately forecast, since enrollment affects staffing requirements and financial projections. Estimates of enrollment, disenrollment, and reenrollment must be considered, and such projections must be tied to the break-even objectives of the new HMO and an integral part of setting yearly objectives for mature plans.

The final step involves making choice available, for example, giving potential members the option of choosing the HMO's package from among the various health plan options available. A part of this step is the development and implementation of dual/multiple-choice arrangements in firms, unions, associations, and governmental agencies that have been chosen as target population segments. This is a traditional strategy of HMOs for breaking into other insurers' markets and for developing true consumer choice. Advantages to the employer offering dual/multiple choice include greater employee satisfaction, potentially higher productivity because of less sick time, cost containment, and increased competitiveness in attracting desirable potential employees. Disadvantages include the slightly higher costs of the HMO package, increased costs of offering two or more programs rather than one, and possible employee backlash because of increased salary deductions or loss of established physician relationships.

Another phase of Step 6 is the actual selling to groups and individuals identified as the target population. Selling to groups is the primary objective, with the largest groups first, smaller groups second, individual contracts next, and welfare programs last. This order, however, depends on the local situation and must be tailored to the characteristics of the target population; for instance, the patients of established doctors may be considered a "group" of individual contracts that may make up the target population. Solicitation strategies are as varied as the groups to be approached. Some of the methods used include dual/multiple-choice arrangements, enrollment of key group leaders, cooperation with existing insurance companies, community education, marketing of services to spouses, open house of facility, door-to-door selling, comparison of plans, and word-of-mouth promotion.

The final phase concerns continuing member relations and the identification of new markets. It is vital that an employee of the HMO act as the consumer contact point and that he/she be directed to keep the consumer satisfied with the health services program. Experience has shown that the quality of account maintenance has a direct relationship to future enrollment. HMO programs are sold by satisfied people who refer their neighbors and friends.

References

Kotler, Philip. *Marketing for Nonprofit Organizations*. Englewood Cliffs, N.J., Prentice-Hall, 1975.

Malhotra, Neresh. "Health Care Marketing Warfare." *Journal of Health Care Marketing, 8*(1):17–29, March 1988.

Martin, John. "Problem Analysis: Application in the Development of Market Strategies for Health Care Organizations." *Journal of Health Care Marketing, 8*(1):5–16, March 1988.

Porn, Lou, and Martin Manning. "Strategic Pricing: Hitting the Mark with Pricing Strategies." *Healthcare Financial Management*, (1):27–32, January 1988.

Reeves, Philip N., and Russell C. Coile, Jr. *Introduction to Health Planning*. 4th Edition. Arlington, Va., Information Resources Press, 1990.

Shouldice, Robert G. *Marketing Management in the Fee-for-Service/Prepaid Medical Group*. Denver, Colo., Center for Research in Ambulatory Care Administration, 1987.

11

FINANCIAL MANAGEMENT

One of the yardsticks for evaluating the success of a business is its return on investment—its ability to bring into the organization more money than it disperses. In the health services industry, success is measured by an organization's ability to provide high-quality medical services and still remain solvent. The HMO planning activities described in the earlier chapters of this text are drawn together here through a discussion of several financial planning models and completion of the financial planning activities. The development of assumptions and the financial planning models are discussed first. Risk management and the use of underwriting techniques are then described, as well as the actuarial aspects of capitation and premium development. Note that both risk management and underwriting and actuarial techniques are an integral part of the financial planning activities and models. A section regarding health insurance concepts is then provided. The chapter concludes with a discussion of some financial management activities, especially the question of incurred but not reported expense (IBNR), that provide the HMO manager with the tools required for successful delivery of services.

Financial Planning

Marketing strategy was described in Chapter 10 as a two-tier process—the selection of target populations or groups and the development of a marketing mix (those elements that the HMO brings together to meet the target population's needs); also covered were the demographic, socioeconomic, and epidemiological data that are collected and analyzed to allow the manager to fully define market segments of the population and the strategy to be used for each. The final decisions concerning target markets and marketing strategies

433

are a part of the broader issues in the financial planning process; for example, estimates of the level of utilization to be anticipated from a population group reflect what it will cost the HMO to provide needed services and, thus, help to determine a premium that will cover these costs. In essence, a part of the marketing, rating, and underwriting process is an actuarial analysis to determine the extent of risk involved in enrolling targeted populations. The HMO then decides which groups to underwrite—agrees to accept the risks and thus the losses for health services described in the benefits package, given the HMO's underwriting rules.

The following discussion addresses the marketing and financial planning issues—specifically, capacity and funds flow analysis—that were discussed in Chapter 9; these issues were outlined in Figure 10-1, Chapter 10, and are reproduced in Figure 11-1. Throughout this section, several broad issues are discussed that the HMO manager must address regarding financial planning; special attention should be paid to these areas, which include the level of anticipated members, the benefits package composition, staffing levels, size and operation of the facility, out-of-plan utilization, and debt service. Good financial management in these areas will help assure success of the health plan.

GOAL SETTING

The HMO, whether it is a newly developed or long-established organization, periodically evaluates its reason for being, that is, its goals and objectives as a health care provider and financing mechanism. Objectives are established that reflect the desires of the board of trustees or directors and the health plan's physician panel and the needs of the consuming public. Boards are usually interested in service to particular segments of the community and the ability to create a surplus or profit from operations. Physicians desire a challenging yet convenient practice, the ability to continue their education, research and teaching opportunities, and acceptable incomes. The needs and desires of the public are reflected in the construction of benefits packages, location of facilities, staffing patterns, and types of physicians employed. Thus, the major objectives of the HMO may reflect the following:

1. The location and the service area
2. The population segments to be marketed
3. The target population or group size and composition
4. An acceptable return on investment (profit or surplus)
5. The demand and capacity of the organization
6. Physician-related goals

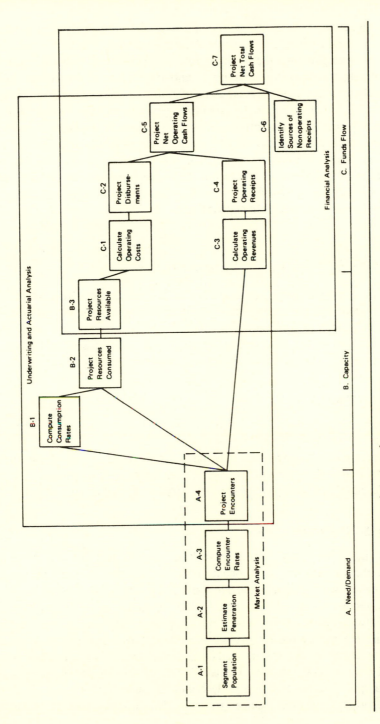

FIGURE 11-1 The marketing/financial planning process.

These objectives help to guide the manager in daily operational decision making as well as financial strategic decision making.

In financial planning, the manager will have available the data described in the planning and marketing chapters (9 and 10). He/she also will be required, especially for a new HMO, to make some planning assumptions to help complete financial planning activities. In establishing programs, operational data may be available that will substantially reduce the guesswork normally found when using assumptions. Such data may be available through outside actuarial firms; good estimates are available from other HMOs in the HMO system, but such guidelines should be used with caution. The areas in which new and expanding HMOs must make some assumptions before their financial plans can be carried out are discussed in the sections that follow.

Financial Planning Assumptions

In the next few paragraphs some examples of financial planning assumptions are provided. After agreement is reached on HMO goals, their creation is one of the first steps in developing the HMO financial strategic plan and budget. These samples should help define the types of assumptions to be made early in the planning process but modified as changes in the plan occur.

STAFFING RATIOS

Physician staffing ranges from 1:1,000 members to as low as 1:1,500 members. The staffing ratios for physicians should be specified by specialty; in addition, paraprofessional staffing ratios must be determined (examples of these ratios are provided in Chapter 6). The issue of whether to use physician assistants must be addressed, and physician ratios adjusted accordingly.

RISK ASSUMPTION

HMOs, like other health insurers, seek to arrange the distribution of risk among the various HMO components and to exert control over the type of risk they are willing to assume. The various incentive and risk-share systems that HMOs use to spread the risk to the physician groups, hospitals, and indemnity insurers were reviewed in Chapter 6. Estimates of the level of risks are created by the actuary—a professional who calculates the risks of enrolling members and arrives at the pure premium. This information is then used by the HMO managers to make decisions concerning the control and type of risk. This second step is described as underwriting—the evaluation of categories of potential member groups to determine the basis on which they will be acceptable to the HMO, taking into consideration legal requirements and other external factors and the HMO's underwriting rules and general philosophy (and objectives). External factors are relatively simple to define: The HMO does or does not fall within the control of the state attorney general or the state insurance commissioner; state laws may regulate the organization and operation of the HMO; federally qualified HMOs must meet the federal regulations. The HMO underwriting rules deal with more elusive issues, especially for the new HMO that has no underwriting experience. These rules must consider several selection factors: type of group; size of group; industry or type of company; composition of group; location of risk; plan of insurance, including eligibility and benefits package; cost sharing; and previous coverage and experience of the group. Assumptions concerning these selection criteria, plus sound data, permit the HMO to predict, within reasonable limits, the probable utilization by and, thus, the cost of each group of members. This process, which is reviewed later in this chapter, is described as rating or rate making. If, based on common sense and past experience, a decision cannot be reached on the level of a particular group, that group should not be enrolled. Underwriting allows for control of the risk by good selection of the groups to be enrolled, defining differential rates for "classes" of risks. These issues are fully discussed in the "Risk Management" section of this chapter.

Another risk category for which planning assumptions must be considered is the possibility of underenrollment. Substantial losses caused by initial enrollment being lower than the projected levels that were used in the planning process create financial risks that may be totally unacceptable to the HMO. Avoidance or minimization of such risks must be a management goal throughout the planning process. Some health plans increase premiums perhaps up to 5 percent above estimated costs to help reduce losses from underenrollment and start-up/expansion costs.

UTILIZATION RATES

Depending on the level of sophistication of the financial planning model used, a variety of utilization rates must be assumed. These include encounter and consumption rates for hospital care, health plan care (doctor and paramedical personnel visits to the health plan), ancillary services (laboratory tests, radiology, prescriptions), emergency services, and out-of-area services. Hospital rates may be in the form of hospital days per 1,000 members per year, admissions per 1,000 members per year, and average length of stay per admission for each group of enrollees, or they may be presented as rates for major specialty areas such as internal medicine, surgery by procedure, obstetrics, pediatrics, and so on. A highly sophisticated system of use projection may require hospitalization rates by disease categories, using the *International*

Classification of Diseases (H-ICDA) specifically "adapted" for use in hospitals, the CPT-4 coding system, or some other classification system. Services of the health plan (ambulatory services) include utilization rates for doctor office visits per member per year for each of the physical, primary, and specialty areas. In addition, laboratory and X-ray service rates, prescription levels per member per year, and out-of-area and emergency service rates also must be estimated. A determination of encounter rates for physician assistants and other personnel also may be necessary.

Local utilization rates for HMOs are seldom available unless a functioning health plan already exists in the same area. If this is not the case, or if sharing of use data is impossible, where would one find such information? Several of the larger, long-established HMOs have consistently collected and analyzed their utilization rates; these data have been reported in the literature over the years and are available to the trained researcher. Some of these data are presented in Chapter 8; other data are provided by HMO actuaries retained by the HMO. Much of this information is available in rate tables and special studies undertaken by members of the Society of Actuaries. In any event the health plan will want to estimate use rates, usually per 1,000 members per year using all sources. Further discussion of rating is provided later in this chapter.

MORBIDITY, MORTALITY, AND DISABILITY RATES

Affiliated with the discussion of utilization rates, underwriting also will require some assumptions concerning the local levels of morbidity, mortality, and disability, which will allow the actuary to perform an

- Analysis of mortality data
- Analysis of morbidity data
- Analysis of disease-specific data
- Estimation of the coverage of the target population by health and related services
- Estimation of the role of extrasectoral factors in the demand on the HMO sector

Other assumptions, broad and specific, are made by the HMO during the development of premium rates and the annual budget. An example of this process is provided later in this chapter.

Models for Financial Planning

All models for financial planning first require the establishment of the organization's objectives, the collection of data concerning the community, and the statement of assumptions in at least the areas discussed above. Some models are simplistic and provide only indications of what might be expected. Others are highly sophisticated, providing more detailed projections, and require extensive data. In the following discussion, several models are presented that may be used to project and analyze the HMO's financial position. The utility of each approach must be weighed carefully in terms of the time, data required, cost, output of the model, and the manager's requirements, and should be cost-effective for the circumstances. Models that provide an analysis of utilization and, thus, cost per member per year may be very time-consuming and costly to prepare and such an analysis may not be useful in a capitated system. On the other hand, such a system may provide the managerial control needed in a highly competitive environment and in an HMO that is heavily in debt and anxious to make the most of every premium dollar. The discussion that follows begins with a review of the elementary approaches used in the field to estimate the need/demand for services, especially ambulatory services; this process might take place while the HMO is creating its financial assumptions. Then the financial planning models in current use are discussed.

SETTING NEED/DEMAND ASSUMPTIONS: SIMPLISTIC MODELS

Ambulatory Facility- and Physician-Focused Approaches

Among the elementary ambulatory health services models that have been used throughout the health care field to estimate the need/demand for medical services are the "facility-focused" and "physician-focused" approaches. In each instance, a ratio is used to project the required facility size or number of physicians. The facility-focused model uses a standard facility-to-population ratio to help establish assumptions about space and staff requirements. This model enables the planner to determine the number of facilities or treatment rooms that will be needed or demanded, either by comparing facility-to-population ratios or by translating projected facility visits into the number of treatment rooms and facilities demanded. Similarly, the physician-focused approach provides a statement of the number of physicians that will be needed by comparing existing physician-to-population ratios to standard ratios. Note that in Chapter 6, physician-to-population ratios are described, with actual ratios listed in Table 6-4, p. 197. The physician-focused approach provides indications of the need/demand for physician manpower but only indirect indications of facility needs. (For group practice and staff models, one might estimate the size of the facility by multiplying the estimated physicians required by 1,200 to 1,500 square feet per physician.) These ratios provide only crude estimates of need/demand, and should be used along with the other financial planning methods described below.

Visit-Focused Approach

The method that provides the basis for setting need/demand assumptions regarding utilization and the treatment of morbidity and mortality data is the visit-focused model. This approach is valuable in that it produces information on the total number of ambulatory visits needed/demanded by comparing the needs of the HMO's members with the historical use of services by members of other HMOs. Assumptions regarding the levels of use of services can be created by applying visit and hospital day use rates to the population, an estimate of the need for care. The product of these use rates, multiplied by the cost per unit of care, becomes the basis for the raw or pure premium.

TRADITIONAL BUDGETARY MODEL

Not unlike other businesses, HMOs use a strategic budgeting process in which costs are developed for several expense areas based on generally recognized operating ratios; these are adjusted for specific and current market conditions and inflation. Premium revenue, together with revenue for copayments, sales of medical equipment and supplies, fees for service, Medicare reimbursement, and the like, are then developed, and a budget and funds-flow analysis are prepared. The following provide the cost areas of this model and the basic computations for a staff model HMO:

A. *Physician Salaries and Fringe Benefits*

 1. The projected number of enrollees *times* the physician-to-population ratio *equals* the number of physicians required.
 2. The number of physicians required *times* the prevailing income for a particular specialty *equals* the total physician-income costs for that specialty.
 3. Compute physician-income costs for each specialty, then total all costs.
 4. The total physician-income costs plus 20 percent of physician-income costs for fringe benefits *equal* the total cost of physician incomes and fringe benefits (note that 20 percent is an example).

B. *Nonphysician Salaries and Fringe Benefits*

 The total nonphysician-salary costs plus 15 percent of nonphysician salary costs *equal* the total cost of nonphysician salaries and fringe benefits (note that 15 percent is an example).

C. *Supplies, both Business and Medical*

Four ambulatory physician services per year *times* the projected number of members *times* the cost of supplies per ambulatory service *equal* the total costs of supplies (again, the figures are examples).

D. *Out-of-Area Benefits*

The unit cost *times* the projected number of members *equals* the total cost of out-of-area benefits per year.

E. *Drugs and Appliances*

The unit cost *times* the projected number of members *equals* the total cost of drugs and appliances per year.

F. *Building and Occupancy*

The projected square footage required *times* the anticipated square-foot rental rates *plus* the cost of utilities *equal* the building and occupancy costs. (As an example, it is estimated that 2.0 square feet per member are required at the 10,000 enrollment population, 1.5 feet at 20,000 enrollment, and 1.0 foot at 30,000 or more.)

G. *Depreciation of Furniture and Equipment*

The number of physicians *times* the cost per physician *equals* the annual total depreciation of furniture and equipment.

H. *Hospitalization*

The projected number of members *times* 400 hospital days per 1,000 enrollees *times* the average daily hospital expense *equal* the total hospitalization costs (again these figures are illustrative only).

I. *Amortization of Start-up Costs*

Costs can be amortized using a variety of methods, but the cost of amortization per member should be maintained at less than 5 percent of the total premiums.

J. *Other*

An estimate of other costs that the HMO will encounter will be included in the budget at this point.

TABLE 11-1   Group Capitation Rate Computation Using the Budgetary Model

	Cost per Member per Month	
Cost Area	Year 1	Year 2
MEDICAL EXPENSES:		
Physician Services	$ 38.00	$ 42.00
Hospital Services	40.00	45.00
Other Medical Services	19.00	21.00
Pharmaceuticals	13.00	17.00
HEALTH PLAN ADMINISTRATION :		
Health Plan Management, Operation, Marketing, Debt Service	15.00	16.00
Reinsurance Premium	3.70	4.20
Reserves	2.00	2.10
Profit/Surplus	1.25	1.40
MEDICAL CENTER OPERATIONS:	0	0
less:		
Reinsurance Recovery	(2.50)	(2.80)
Coordination of Benefits	(2.40)	(2.75)
Copays	(.60)	(.65)
Total Cost Per Member Per Month	$126.45	$142.50

K. *Administrative Reserve*

The total annual plan revenues *times* a percentage designated by the board (such as 2.5 percent) *equals* the total administrative reserve for debt service and possible insurance reserve.

The total of items A through K provides the annual cost of the HMO. Monthly per capita costs are obtained by dividing the total costs by total membership and then by 12 months. But more frequently, the HMO will estimate its total member months for the year (the total number of members enrolled each month) and divide this number into the total costs to arrive at a cost per member per month and the base premium or "capitation rate." Premium rates are built around the product of this computation, with adjustments made for differences in the characteristics of the groups enrolled. A pro forma operating statement and cash flow analyses can then be completed. Usually costs and income will not be equal, and adjustments must be made to the costs—especially staffing levels and premiums. Table 11-1 shows an example of how the per member per month costs for an HMO using this model can be determined. Note that by describing individual cost areas in PMPM values, the total cost PMPM is created.

This approach follows the general formula, where the cost PMPM *equals* the annual utilization rate *times* the unit cost *divided* by 12. For example, if office visits are budgeted at 3.5 per member and each visit costs $30, the cost PMPM would be $3.5 \times \$30 \div 12 = \$8.75$ PMPM. In the example shown in Table 11-1, the total PMPM cost for the first year is $126.45; for the second it is $142.50. These PMPM values will be used in a later example to create the capitation rates.

Caution should be exercised in the use of the term "capitation rate." As noted later, this is the amount of per capita revenue that the health plan must generate to cover its costs; the base rate will then be modified according to the types of contracts the plan sells. Conversely, in previous chapters the term capitation and capitation rate described the base PMPM that was provided to an outside-the-plan contracting medical group; for example, the capitation rate for a medical group might be $32 PMPM, and the total capitation might be $32 *times* 1,000 members served, or a total prospective monthly payment to the physicians of $32,000.

COMPREHENSIVE UNITS-OF-PRODUCTION MODEL

Another, quite unique and rarely used, financial planning model, including both ambulatory care and hospitaliztion, was developed for the National Center for Health Services Research and Development, DHHS. It is included here to emphasize the need for managers to understand the relationships between the demand for services by the membership and the level of resources needed to meet that demand, all tied together using a budget and an analysis of funds flow.

The first objective of the model is to determine demand in terms of encounters with (or visits to) health care delivery personnel both on an outpatient and inpatient basis. The second step in the model is to match the required plant capacity (staff, equipment, facilities) to the demand statement, so that resources will be available to provide adequate services; this step uses "consumption rates" for each resource required to provide services to subscribers. Multiplying the total number of encounters by the consumption rate for each resource consumed provides the total amount of resources needed to meet the projected demand. Because resources are limited, a comparison of total available resources with those resources that are needed identifies possible deficiencies/surpluses in staffing or in other resources. The HMO also may elect not to make available certain resources, thus consciously deciding not to provide selected services (e.g., identifying a need for mental health services but realizing that obtaining the services of a psychiatrist is not feasible). The third step in this approach allows the planners to apply a cost per unit of resources (disbursements) and a revenue per encounter (receipts);

cash budgeting can then be completed. Depending on the results of the cash-flow projections, adjustments to reduce possible operating deficits may be necessary.

The steps necessary to complete this model are presented graphically in Figure 11-1 and are superficially reviewed in the outline that follows.

A. Develop a statement of demand by

1. Segmenting the target population.

2. Estimating the penetration of each segment chosen, following the method provided in Chapter 10.

3. Computing the encounter rates; total encounters are determined by multiplying the projected number of members by the encounter (or visit) rate per person. Encounters by type of service also should be determined by multiplying the encounter rate per service per person by the number of members.

4. Projecting the encounters over a period of time by estimating the number of times per month that members will use services.

B. Determine capacity and resources by

1. Defining the universe of resources necessary to provide the types of services (medical, surgical, obstetric, pediatric) for which there will be encounters (demand). These resources should be compared with the benefits that are listed in the subscribers' benefits packages to ensure that the HMO will have the specific resources necessary to provide each benefit. Some broad resource categories, in addition to medical specialists, may be other personnel; outside services, including a detailed description of types of inpatient services; space and rentals; consumable supplies; equipment; pharmaceuticals; and employee benefits.

2. Computing the consumption rates by determining the average number of units of a resource consumed by *one* encounter. Personnel resource units may be defined in terms of time, facilities in square footage, supplies in numbers of items, and other resources in terms of a proportionate share of their total consumption. To determine the number of units to be consumed for each type of encounter, multiply the total number of each type by the consumption rate for each resource consumed. (Completing for only the variable direct resources simplifies the process; the cost of indirect [fixed] resources can then be added to the total costs in step C5.)

3. Projecting the resources available by identifying the types of resources that are available and describing each in terms of the number of units of service that can be provided by the resource. For instance, a laboratory technician might provide one service every 6 minutes—10 per hour, or 2,000 per month

(200 hours per month times 10 per hour). Multiply the encounters by the service projected per month by the resources' consumption rate. Compare the product of this multiplication with the available resources to determine over- or underutilization of that resource and, thus, whether more or less increments are needed. (This may be completed for only variable direct resources.)

C. The funds flow analysis reduces the resources to a common denominator—dollars—so that disbursements and receipts can be compared; a positive cumulative cash flow over a two- to three-year period must be the outcome. The steps in this process are to

1. Determine the cost per unit of resource, then multiply the unit costs by the units of resource available.

2. Determine the total monthly disbursements according to established personnel policies or contractual agreements.

3. Compare the costs of resources to the disbursement.

4. Determine the charge or revenue per encounter, then multiply by the number of each type of encounter per month. Reduce the total revenue by the percentage that will not be collected. (Uncollectables may amount to 5 percent of the total premium revenue.) At this point, capitation and premium rates can be proposed. For example, the resources needed to provide physician services may be $300,000 for a membership of 1,800 individuals. Physician services may be expressed as $300,000 ÷ 1,800 ÷ 12 months or $13.89 PMPM.

5. Add indirect costs to disbursements if not included in steps B2 and B3. Then compare operating receipts with disbursements. The differences between the two represent the net operating cash flow. Cumulative cash flows can then be presented.

D. Adjustments will likely have to be performed to bring receipts and disbursements into close alignment.

The units-of-production model requires a high level of sophistication and an understanding by the HMO manager of the industrial production function. To use the model successfully, the HMO manager must have available the data to estimate encounters per type of service and consumption rates for resources. Aggregate rates of encounters and consumption are available from several sources, but rates per medical service are much more difficult to obtain. If this major data requirement can be met, the units-of-production model has the capability of providing very useful estimates of demand capacity and funds flow analysis, because it builds on the most elementary units—encounters per service, consumption of resources per encounter, and costs per unit of service. Decisions concerning projected utilization are made at the most basic levels and relate to small segments of the total demand; thus projections of aggregates, such as total visits per 1,000 members, are avoided, which, if erroneous, could create fallacious cost projections of major negative impact.

The model requires that the HMO manager think in terms of units of service and project costs and revenues on a basis similar to that of the manager in commercial and manufacturing sectors. This is a reversal of the commonly used method of relying on aggregates of services and using them as the basis for the development of premium rates for groups of members and capitation arrangements with physician groups. But, because of its sophistication and complexity, the cost of the units-of-production model may outweigh the benefits derived. Thus, the manager should evaluate the time, energy, and expense necessary to use the model and to determine whether this level of detailed financial planning is necessary for his/her HMO. Indeed, the HMO may ultimately use this, along with the comprehensive insurance underwriting model approach, as its sophistication in financial strategic planning improves.

Because the model requires that units of production be identified with the several medical care services of the health plan, the HMO manager may decide to use these projections as the basis for an accountability mechanism as well as a budgeting device. Indeed, since physicians control the provision of services, they can be held accountable for their activities. Accountability can occur only if the physicians are involved in the planning process for establishing production levels and rates, and this model allows for such activity on a monthly basis.

COMPREHENSIVE INSURANCE UNDERWRITING MODEL

Although the budgetary approach may use annual utilization rates for major classes of cost, another approach may be based on detailed analyses of use rates by individual service units. This financial planning model may be built around the activities associated with the insurance functions of underwriting—risk taking, actuarial analyses, incentive/risk-sharing formulas, and establishment of rates and rate setting. In one such model, the HMO management analyzes the service area population by segmenting it and tentatively chooses groups of potential members, much the same as the units-of-production model. Following the methodology provided in Chapter 10, a penetration-rate study is completed, and demographic, epidemiological, and socioeconomic data are collected concerning the target groups. Actuaries are then asked to analyze these populations to determine the types and levels of services required (i.e., the risk that the plan is to underwrite). From these studies, the HMO manager can develop lists of services that the target population will require, as well as estimates of the utilization rate for each service. Categorization approaches from which the lists of services can be developed are the *H-ICDA* and the CPT-

4 coding systems previously discussed or a form of the relative value systems, such as the Resource Based Relative Value Study (RBRVS) newly adopted by Medicare. The latter has the capability of quantifying, in terms of relative value, the degree of effort, education, and training of the providers; complexity of the procedure; and other issues that help describe the "relative" differences of the procedures as compared to all other procedures. At this point, the HMO manager may decide to base the remainder of the financial analysis on one of the comprehensive models previously described or by the following method.

1. Determine, based on knowledge of available health resources, which services will be provided (i.e., describe the benefits packages to be offered).

2. Develop a protocol (or detailed description) for each service to be provided (classified by one of the methods noted above). Protocols basically are decision-logic trees that chart a course of treatment: they allow the physicians to establish practice patterns that ensure quality of care; permit the development of standard courses of treatment that become the basis for outcome studies; and enable the professional staff to determine the level of functioning of various paraprofessional personnel such as physician assistants. The HMO management, in association with the medical director and a group of the HMO physicians, establish these protocols, and then a detailed description of the resources that will be needed to provide care.

3. Determine the cost of the protocols for each service to be provided and multiply this cost by the number of each service category. Normally, only direct costs will be involved in this process; therefore, indirect costs such as heat, light, and amortization of debt should then be added to arrive at total costs or disbursements.

4. The per capita cost (the capitation rate) can be computed by dividing the total costs by the estimated number of members and then by 12 months. Loading and discounting the quotient, if experience rating is chosen, permits the manager to develop premiums.

5. Revenue, including premium income, sales of prescriptions, fees for services, copayments, and so on, are compared to total costs and adjustments are made.

In general, the insurance underwriting model permits the HMO manager to take advantage of the expertise of the underwriters and actuaries whose profession it is to determine the risks involved in insuring populations. Their major tools are the utilization rates or frequencies provided by rate tables and special studies. These rates are expressed in terms of an individual or per 1,000 members (such as 400 hospital days per 1,000 population). Their recommendations normally are conservative but accurate. This model also requires involvement by the physicians in establishing protocols—or, at the least, broad descriptions of medical services—that can be used in financial analyses and physician capitation negotiations and that also can be used in professional review activities. Protocols that precisely describe the activities required of the physicians should also allow for the collection of productivity data to be used in the physician incentive system. Generally, this model does not require the sophisticated encounter and consumption rates of the units-of-production model, but the development of protocols is difficult and time-consuming. There are, however, examples of ambulatory and inpatient protocols currently available; these would provide a place to start the development of a protocol system.

EXPENSES AND INCOME

The following is a summary of the income and expense items mentioned in each of the models described earlier. Expenses fall into four primary categories:

1. *Medical care costs:* These costs include all medical service and supply expenditures for both inpatient and outpatient physician care.

2. *Hospitalization costs:* Included in this category are all hospital-related charges incurred during the delivery of inpatient care.

3. *Administrative costs:* All expenditures incurred by the health plan that are related to the administration and support of either the medical and/or hospital services.

4. *Other costs:* This category includes all other costs associated with the operation of the health plan.

Income items include:

1. *Premiums:* Revenue from membership dues directly related to the level of enrollment.

2. *Fees for service:* Income from services provided on a per-unit-of-service basis to non-HMO members—patients of HMO physicians who, prior to joining the health plan, were in private practice; emergency services to local residents; services provided as a courtesy to residents in close proximity to the health plan; or income derived from planned fee-for-service activity.

3. *Copayments:* Revenues from charges (approximately $1 to $10) levied at the time selected services are provided—for office visits, laboratory tests, radiology, injections, pharmaceuticals, and so on.

4. *Sale of drugs, supplies, and prosthetic devices.*

5. *Federal, state, and local welfare program payments:* Include revenue from the provision of services to recipients of programs such as Medicare, Medicaid, worker's compensation, and local welfare programs.

6. *Loans, grants, and gifts:* Income from outside sources and philanthropy.
7. *Investments and interest income.*

Insurance Concepts

By now the reader will agree that HMOs are organizations that insure groups of individuals against the costs of medical services and also provide those medical services. Thus, knowledge of health insurance principles, especially group health insurance, benefits package development, and premium rate setting, is important. Most HMO contracts are sold to groups of employees; this is termed *group underwriting.* It is a process by which the HMO determines what level of group risk it is willing to accept and the terms on which the group contract will be written. The initial step in group underwriting is to determine the pricing structure, the *premium*—the consideration (money) paid by the employer and employees to the health plan for an insurance contract. Moreover, to provide *insurance* means that a contract is created under which one party— the health plan—undertakes to guarantee health services or payments to the second party for losses due to ill health; such a contract specifies the period of time and the conditions or peril under which the contract will be in force. As noted in Chapter 1, commercial insurance companies *indemnify* against loss; they reimburse or compensate the insurance subscriber for losses or damages incurred due to illness. HMOs, however, do not indemnify against loss; they *assure* that medical services will be available and provided when the member needs them—although the health plan may indemnify itself against catastrophic losses through reinsurance purchased from outside commercial insurance companies.

One of the more important concepts in group underwriting is *rating,* fixing the amount of premium to be charged and the subsidiary issue of identifying *risks.* Both go hand in hand, as the actuary attempts to identify the level and kind of health service needs of the target groups, for example, the risks that they will become ill. These risks are influenced by many issues, but the size of the group is one of the most important. Insurers rely on the *law of large numbers.* This concept suggests that the larger the group enrolled the more widely the group risk can be spread, while the smaller the group, the greater the level of risk per member. The insurer must be able to precisely identify total group risk as stated in rates per 1,000 population. As the enrollment increases, these rates should moderate, because risks can be spread across a greater number of enrollees. It is interesting to note that the member, individually, is not able to accurately describe his/her risks since, without the "support" of the group members, the insurer would consider them to be high and uninsurable.

Insurers thus choose to enroll larger groups first and smaller groups after the health plan has a substantial enrollment base on which to spread the risk.

This brings us to the issue of rating. The process of rating or pricing the benefits packages has become as important to the success of the health plan as the need to operate an effective health services delivery system, and most HMOs now spend considerable effort in rate making. Generally, this includes, first, the development of *base rates* (or capitation rates).[1] This base reflects the organization's budget, as developed, using one of the financial planning models described earlier; it defines the per capita revenue requirement of the health plan. Second, the capitation rate is converted to *premium rates,* a charge, payment, or price that is fixed according to a scale or standard. It is the amount of premium per unit of insurance, where the pricing unit is not the member or person enrolled but rather a contract such as a single person contract, a family contract, a two-person contract, and so on. Thus, the method used by the HMO to set premiums is referred to as its premium rating system, and each HMO has its own unique method of performing this process. Some plans, for instance, may rely on the use of health insurance *rate tables* and *rate books,* the manual of standard rates used by insurers to determine premium rates by class of member, and for different benefits packages. Others may depend more heavily on the use f internal budgeting processes, or actuaries who perform special studies to determine base rates for the HMO's market. Other factors, such as changes in technology and medical devices, the insurance effect on members' use of services, inflation in the medical industry, and increased competition, also affect the premium rating system used by the plan. A further discussion of rate making is provided later in this chapter.

Risk Management[2]

Health maintenance organizations are health delivery mechanisms, but they also have the dual and equally important role of insurer. Many argue that HMOs do not insure but that they provide "assurance" of services, thus attempting to avoid regulation by the state insurance commissioners; this issue concerns every HMO manager who has offered a benefits package to subscribers. Most experts today agree that HMOs indeed use many of the insurance concepts described above. Of concern here are the insurance functions of risk management that must be performed by the HMO to assure the financial

---

[1] Peter R. Kongstvedt. *The Managed Health Care Handbook.* Gaithersburg, Md., Aspen Publishers, Inc., 1989, p. 217.

[2] This discussion is based on Robert G. Shouldice, "How HMOs Control Risks," *Medical Group Management, 34*(3):11–12, May/June 1987.

stability of the organization. The HMO seeks to distribute the risk of providing care to a selected population within a financial budget and, therefore, attempts to control the type of risk that it is willing to assume. How do HMOs control the risk that the premium will not be sufficient to cover all of the health services required by the members according to their contract with the health plan? Are there other risks that the health plan assumes, and how are they managed?

HMOs encounter three categories of risks. These include:

1. Normal business risks similar to other businesses (loss from fire, theft, and poor business decisions, for example)
2. Risk of loss because of professional liability for malpractice by individual physicians
3. Underwriting risks of enrolled populations

Many normal business risks are covered by umbrella insurance policies that include fire, theft, property, casualty, and so on, although the business still faces the prospect of financial instability if it is not managed well; the outcome of this last situation may be voluntary reorganization (Chapter 11) or involuntary dissolution (Chapter 7) bankruptcy.

In the second situation, most malpractice risks are passed along to an indemnity insurance company through purchase of professional liability insurance. In the third situation, several mechanisms are used for managing the underwriting risks of the HMO. These include the following four categories:

1. Benefits package design
2. Actuarial analyses, underwriting, and rate making
3. Risk sharing using capitation payments to and withholds from providers
4. Other management techniques

BENEFITS PACKAGE DESIGN

Control of risk begins with the planning and design of benefits packages. Basic packages are developed to meet the perceived needs of the target groups but are influenced by state and federal regulatory requirements, as well as offerings of competitors. The health plan, by including or excluding benefits, controls access to the related health service without coverage; patients may be reluctant to seek the service, and physicians may be reluctant to provide or even offer the service. An infamous non-HMO example of benefits controlling use of service is Blue Shield's historic unwillingness to offer benefits for physician services that are provided in the physican's office, with resulting inappropriate hospital admissions. Ultimately, under pressure from competing HMOs, the Blue's benefits packages were changed in the 1970s to include physician services both in hospital and in the physician's office.

Even though the HMO may offer a particular benefit, service availability might be limited or a copayment might be required when the member receives services. The copayment reduces risks by supplying additional revenue to cover the costs of service delivery. The health plan might include the benefit and offer the affiliated services, but it may also control access by limiting the number of providers and available appointments.

ACTUARIAL ANALYSES, UNDERWRITING, AND RATE MAKING

Health plans also manage risk by detailed study of the probability that members will use services provided in the benefits package. Based on historical data, actuaries determine the cost to the health plan by describing the rate of service use *times* the cost per service. By adding the costs for all services that might be used, the actuary creates the pure premium or base rates. As underwriters, the health plan's board and administrator then determine if the pure premium should be "loaded" or "discounted" to arrive at the actual contract unit premium rates to be marketed; that is, the board may feel that the populations to be enrolled may have higher or lower risks of service use than described by the actuary and, therefore, may adjust the base rates accordingly. Single contracts, for example, may be the actual base rate derived by the actuary. But, the two-person premium rate would be loaded at 2.5 times the base rate, and a family contract (three or more contract units) may be 3.0 times the base rate, even though the average family size averages 3.5 persons. Eventually, the premium charged will reflect the health plan's (underwriter's or rate maker's) estimate of its risks of enrolling selected populations.

SHARING RISKS

Most health plans try to reduce their risks by sharing them with other organizations. The purchase of reinsurance allows the health plan to share some of its catastrophic losses with indemnity insurance companies; for example, the HMO may purchase stop-loss insurance to cover 80 percent of its costs above $30,000 worth of services provided to a critically ill member. Stop-loss protection may also be extended to its physician groups to help reduce the risks they take by accepting capitation; the physicians pay the HMO for this stop-loss coverage by agreeing to a reduction in their capitation payment. Generally, the HMO's decision regarding risk assumption will fall within the continuum shown in Figure 11-2.

To summarize, the HMO will try to develop capitation arrangements with providers that will allow the HMO to share risk with other organizations. These per capita, prospective payments place medical groups, hospitals, and other

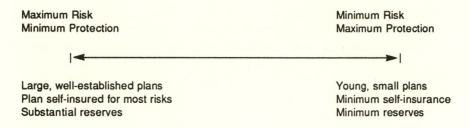

Maximum Risk
Minimum Protection

Minimum Risk
Maximum Protection

Large, well-established plans
Plan self-insured for most risks
Substantial reserves

Young, small plans
Minimum self-insurance
Minimum reserves

FIGURE 11-2 Stop-loss continuum.

providers at risk through contractual limitations on total payments. Similar results are obtained by the health plan when providers are paid fee-for-service and a withhold is applied; the withheld funds are at risk, since payment to the provider is contingent on the provider's acceptable control of members' use of services (usually inpatient care). Other methods that tie provider remuneration to control of service use are also used, such as basing bonuses to salaried physicians on use rates; HMOs even use the term "shared risk pools" to describe the funds that are allocated to risk sharing/incentive arrangements—usually used for hospital inpatient and specialty services. The risk pools are established during the financial budgeting process. Payments for services are drawn from the specific pool; if providers manage utilization appropriately, funds may remain that then may be shared with the providers. But if health care expenses are higher than the risk pool, the losses are shared with the providers, usually by deductions from their capitation payments during the next fiscal period. In fact, some plans have a policy of deducting a certain shared risk percentage from the providers capitation on a monthly basis; these withheld funds are then maintained as part of the shared risk pool and are used to pay for services or returned to the provider at the end of a fiscal period.

OTHER MANAGEMENT TECHNIQUES

In addition to these methods, HMOs use other management techniques that can be equally effective. Many of these are under the direct control of the HMO's manager, medical director, and physicians.

1. Use more outpatient surgery and reduce inpatient admissions for surgery.
2. Require preadmission screening and certification of all hospital admissions.
3. Require concurrent reviews and monitoring of lengths of stay of all hospital patients.

4. As part of the peer review process, require retrospective reviews of all hospitalized patients as a standard procedure.

5. Establish and use a standing quality assurance/utilization review committee.

6. Provide care at home when it is more cost-effective and medically appropriate. Physician extenders may be effective in the delivery of home services.

7. Provide care in an extended care unit and hospices when it is more cost-effective and medically appropriate.

8. Use outpatient services rather than inpatient hospital services.

9. Require ambulatory work-ups and testing before hospital admissions.

10. Use physician extenders where appropriate and paraprofessionals that have skills in several areas.

11. *Ceteris paribus,* choose the lowest cost provider.

12. Use aggressive coodination of benefits (COB) procedures and pay special attention to subrogation procedures.

13. Use aggressive reinsurance recovery procedures.

14. Use the gatekeeper concept to appropriately control access to the system.

15. Use a policy of no self-referrals to specialists and special medical care units.

16. Use physician assistants and other nonphysician personnel as first contact care providers.

17. Use preauthorization for specialty referrals to facilities such as emergency rooms, urgent care centers, surgicenters, centers of excellence, radiology and laboratory services, physical and occupational therapy, and so on.

18. Concentrate on assuring that there are concurrent and retrospective reviews of selected specialty services where risks are high (e.g., adult and pediatric psychiatry and other mental health counseling services, alcoholism and drug treatment services, excessive allergy and dermatology treatment, overmarketing of routine or annual physical examinations, oral surgery).

19. Create a formulary using generic drugs, and require that it be used by providers; exceptions should require preauthorization by the medical director.

20. To help guarantee appropriate use, develop central books for inpatient admissions and for physician appointments, including specialty services and tests.

21. Institute patient education programs that train enrollees regarding appropriate use of the health system, and behavior modification to encourage life-style changes that improve health and encourage cost-effective utilization.

22. Support the development of a strong medical director who approves/disapproves service delivery, recommends medical staff disciplinary action for noncompliance with established policy, recommends standards of care,

evaluates medical staff professional performance in accordance with approved policy, resolves conflicts arising between physicians, coordinates quality assurance/utilization reviews and ethical medical practices, acts as the direct liaison with the HMO regarding physician problems and involvement with the HMO, and so on.

23. Develop and use protocols or clinical algorithms that set standards and describe appropriate and accepted medical practice in the medical group.

24. Institute a provider education program regarding HMO procedures and the need for efficiency, economy, and an understanding of the budget that will set the boundaries and resource constraints of the group practice's operation with HMO enrollees.

25. Control out-of-area occurrences by limiting coverages and costs in the subscriber contract to emergency visits only.

26. Limit, through the use of a ceiling, the amount or cost of rare, unusual, and expensive services that normally are outside the capability of the HMO providers, or illnesses that are very expensive to treat. Another method may be the use of reinsurance for expenses over a selected level, as described above.

27. Exclude or reinsure epidemic occurrences or disasters.

28. Avoid low enrollment levels by performing adequate market analyses and using an appropriate marketing strategy. The lack of underwriting expertise and the setting of unrealistic enrollment goals should be avoided.

Underwriting

Underwriting is the process by which the risk of accepting populations as members is evaluated and determined. It includes the financial responsibility and liability for losses and costs of medical services underwritten in the policy. A part of the underwriting process is the actuarial analysis—the calculation of premium rates for each unit of service (unit of exposure or benefit unit) that is included in the benefits package. Thus, underwriting and its associated actuarial analyses provide a method of rate making for the HMO—a method for determining the types of services to be provided, the level of utilization of services, the risk involved in the provision of such services, and the rates that must be charged to subscribers to cover the cost and the risk involved in the provision of such services.

UNDERWRITING GROUPS

Figure 11-1 outlines the several activities that may be included in underwriting; note that this activity is a part of both the marketing process and the financial planning process, and it includes analyses of need/demand, capacity, and funds flow. There is no step-by-step process to be followed by HMO underwriters, but each group of potential members is evaluated according to several underwriting assumptions, or rules, that are agreed upon by the board of the HMO and that describe the general acceptability of the risks involved. A description of these rules follows.[3]

1. *Types of groups:* The most common type of group is *individual employers,* who insure their employees for health insurance benefits. Consideration should be given to the character of the employer company or firm and its reputation as an employer in the community. A second type is the *union group.* Of major concern in underwriting unions is the source of funds to pay the premiums, since the Taft-Hartley Law prohibits employer contributions to be transferred to a union. Thus, the premium payment for a union member's coverage must come from the individual union members, whether it is from dues or a separate collection. *Multiple employers* (i.e., a number of employers in the same industry) sometimes band together to purchase health insurance as a single group, which can be considered a third type of group. Such an arrangement may be made by using a negotiated trusteeship, as required by the Taft-Hartley Law, for employees covered under a bargaining agreement. Eligibility requirements for benefits should be flexible enough to allow a substantial number of employees to join but still exclude transient employees. Voluntary trade associations also may establish a fund for their members and employees. Other important groups that may not be included in these three categories are jointly administered programs and federal, state, and local governmental groups. Again, the major concern in underwriting such groups is the capability of receiving and maintaining a high level of participation from each employer group.

2. *Size of the group:* Generally, the larger the group enrolled, the greater the degree of accuracy in mathematically predicting the probability of loss. Thus, HMOs attempt to attract large groups in which the expense ratio (ratio of expenses to earned premiums) is relatively low and in which there is a consistency of losses over time. Small groups have higher expense ratios because of their inability to spread the risk and the possibility that there will be wide fluctuations in use and, thus, cost. More rigorous underwriting rules may be applied to smaller groups.

3. *Industry or type of company:* Disability and morbidity rates for certain industries are high because of the physical conditions in which employees must work. If a disability is job-related, it is covered by the worker's compensation

---

[3] This discussion draws upon the Health Insurance Association of America's *Principles of Group Health Insurance I,* Chicago, Ill., HIAA, 1972, Chapter IV.

law (and the cost of care is covered by the state worker's compensation program), but secondary effects on an individual employee's health are not covered. Long-term effects must be carefully evaluated prior to underwriting more hazardous occupations and industries. Historically, the insurance industry has excluded the following industries or has charged high premiums for coverage:

a. HAZARDOUS WORK: Mines, quarries, oil drilling and rigging, logging operations, charter and unscheduled airlines, aviation and pilot-training schools, munitions plans, sanitation businesses, asbestos-related industries, pest control services, and scrap dealers.

b. LOW-PAYING OR SEASONAL WORK: Hotels, motels, restaurants, car washes, laundries, cleaners, entertainment and arts groups, beauty salons, barber shops, bowling alleys, service stations, convenience stores, fishing enterprises, golf clubs, ski resorts, camps, farms, and ranches.

c. HIGHER RATE OF CLAIMS: Doctors, dentists, nurses, chiropractors, and other medical workers.

d. HIGHER ADMINISTRATIVE COSTS: Government-financed nonprofit organizations and municipalities.

4. *Composition of a group:* The risk of underwriting varies with the makeup of a group. Factors such as age, sex, and dependents affect use patterns. Generally, groups of extremely young or old persons tend to have high use patterns. Female employees, according to surveys conducted by the Department of Health and Human Services, have 25 percent more disabilities than male employees and have more short-duration disabilities during their younger years. Dependent coverage presents another set of problems: In organizations with a high percentage of married women, the percentage participation of these employees may be very low, because many of their husbands will have coverage for themselves and their dependents through their own employers. Generally, the objective of the HMO that offers only one benefits package in underwriting groups is to provide a benefits package broad enough to cover all activity at work (that is not included under worker's compensation) and off-the job, full-time employees, and union or association members. Thus, the benefits package should not be directed at any one class of employee or earnings level.

5. *Location of risk:* The ability to adequately provide service and to attend to administrative activities is an important factor in the HMO's selection of a group of potential members. Long travel times or distances will compound the problems of service delivery. Thus, the HMO will select a service area that it can adequately and conveniently cover with physicians and other providers.

6. *Plan of insurance, including eligibility and benefits package:* Eligibility determines who will be included as a potential member. Normally, employee- and union-member eligibility is based on conditions that pertain to employment;

thus, eligibility cannot be determined by age, sex, or race because, by law, these cannot be conditions of employment. Moreover, the coverage provided generally is extended to dependents; size of family and ages of dependents are, therefore, important data in assessing the risks of underwriting the group.

HMOs are recognized for their willingness to develop tailor-made packages for particular groups of employees. Special note should be made of extremely minimal or rich benefits packages; these situations may create underenrollment through lack of employee interest or adverse selection.

7. *Cost sharing:* There are two basic methods for payment of premiums—noncontributory, in which the policyholder (employer, union, association) pays the entire premium, or contributory, in which the enrollee may pay a portion or all (fully contributory) of the cost. Underwriters prefer noncontributory programs because they assure full employee participation, which simplifies marketing and administration. Fully contributory plans have many drawbacks (lack of employer interest, marketing problems, possible loss or lack of participation) and should be used only under special circumstances, such as supplemental packages to other health insurance programs and programs limited to higher salaried employees who generally do not have personal financial difficulties. An example of a noncontributory plan currently being offered by HMOs and CMPs is the supplemental or wrap-around package purchased by those over age 65 to enrich their Medicare coverage, provided by the health plan under contract with HCFA (see Chapter 5).

8. *Previous coverage and experience of the group:* The cost of prior coverage appears to be the main reason that groups shop for new health insurance coverage. Underwriting such groups is based on a review of previous coverage and experience. Information about the group's coverage and use patterns for the three previous years at least is important and may be evaluated as described in the following examples, the first using the traditional indemnity insurance approach, and the second using a capitation unit (HMO) approach:[4]

Indemnity Insurance Approach

a. Review rate and loss experience:

Current Benefits Packages	Number of Insured	Monthly Premium
Employee	115	$ 97 per employee
Dependents	75	$115 per dependent unit

---

[4] Health Insurance Association of America. *Principles of Group Health Insurance I,* pp. 103–105.

Year	Premiums	Utilization Experience
1st policy year	$240,300	$230,500
2nd policy year	260,000	220,000
3rd policy year	262,000	280,000
	$762,300	$730,500

b. Determine the present insurer's expected annual premium:

Employees	115 × $ 97 × 12 months =	$133,860
Dependents	75 × $115 × 12 months =	103,500
Total Premium, 12 months		$237,360

c. Develop ratio of actual premium to premium calculated in step b:

$$\frac{\text{Actual premium 1st year } \$240,300}{\text{Calculated premium } \$237,360} = 101.2\%$$

$$\frac{\text{Actual premium 2nd year } \$260,000}{\text{Calculated premium } \$237,360} = 109.5\%$$

$$\frac{\text{Actual premium 3rd year } \$262,000}{\text{Calculated premium } \$237,360} = 110.4\%$$

d. Determine through actuarial analyses the new rates the HMO must charge:

Employee	115 × $105 × 12 months =	$144,900
Dependents	75 × $130 × 12 months =	117,000
Total premium, 12 months		$261,900

e. Adjust total premiums developed in step d by the factors from step c:

1st policy year	$261,900 × 101.2% =	$265,043
2nd policy year	$261,900 × 109.5% =	286,780
3rd policy year	$261,900 × 110.4% =	289,138
Total		$840,961

f. Determine the loss ratio of the HMO:

$$\frac{\text{Total three-year actual incurred expenses } \$730,500}{\text{Total three-year premium of new HMO rate } \$840,961} = 86.9\% \text{ loss ratio}$$

g. A management decision must be made to determine how high a loss ratio will allow for a surplus or profit when other expenses are added. Assuming a loss ratio of 80 percent in this example, the HMO's premium rates must be *increased* to an amount equal to 108.6 percent (86.9% + 80%) of the HMO's average rates for an equal benefits package (or, if using commercial insurance manuals, 108.6 percent of manual rates).[5] If the acceptable ratio was 90 percent rather than 80 percent, adjustments to manual rates would be a *reduction* of approximately 3.4 percent (86.9% ÷ 90% = 96.6%) to determine the premiums to be charged.

Capitation Unit/HMO Approach

a. Review rate and loss experience:

Current Benefits Packages	Number of Insured	Total Member Months	Monthly Premium
Single	115	1,380	$ 97 per employee
Family	76*	912	395 per family

*20 families at 3.8 individuals per family.

Year	Premiums	Utilization Experience
1st policy year	$240,300	$230,500
2nd policy year	260,000	220,000
3rd policy year	262,000	280,000
	$762,300	$730,500

b. Determine the present insurer's expected annual premium:

Employees	115 × $ 97 × 12 months =	$133,860
Family	20 × $395 × 12 months =	94,800
Total Premium, 12 months		$228,660

c. Develop ratio of actual premium to premium calculated in step b:

$$\frac{\text{Actual premium 1st year } \$240,300}{\text{Calculated premium } \$228,660} = 105.1\%$$

$$\frac{\text{Actual premium 2nd year } \$260,000}{\text{Calculated premium } \$228,660} = 113.7\%$$

$$\frac{\text{Actual premium 3rd year } \$262,000}{\text{Calculated premium } \$228,660} = 114.6\%$$

---

[5] Manual rates are an insurer's standard rate tables, included in its rate manual or underwriter's manual, that are used to develop premium rates. Please see the discussion of rate making later in this chapter.

d. Determine through actuarial analyses the new rates the HMO must charge:

Employee	115 × $105 × 12 months =	$144,900
Family	20 × $400 × 12 months =	96,000
Total premium, 12 months		$240,900

e. Adjust total premiums developed in step d by the factors from step c:

1st policy year	$240,900 × 105.1% =	$253,186
2nd policy year	$240,900 × 103.7% =	249,813
3rd policy year	$240,900 × 114.6% =	276,071
Total	-	$779,070

f. Determine the loss ratio of the HMO:

$$\frac{\text{Total three-year actual incurred expenses } \$730,500}{\text{Total three-year premium of new HMO rate } \$779,070} = 94.5\% \text{ loss ratio}$$

g. A management decision must be made to determine how high a loss ratio will allow for a surplus or profit when other expenses are added. Assuming a loss ratio of 80 percent in this example, the HMO's premium rates must be *increased* to an amount equal to 118.1 percent (94.5% ÷ 80%) of the HMO's average rates for an equal benefits package (or, if using commercial insurance manuals, 118.1 percent of manual rates). If the acceptable ratio was 95 percent rather than 80 percent, adjustments to manual rates would be a *reduction* of approximately half a percent (94.5% ÷ 95% = 99.5%) to determine the premiums to be charged.

To summarize, certain factors are considered in underwriting and enrolling groups of subscribers, including difficulties in administration (especially with small groups), negotiated trusteeships, and groups that are partially or fully contributory. In addition, the law requires that employer groups provide a conversion privilege for employees leaving an employment group. Conversion may not always be to an individual membership in the HMO; or the HMO may offer individual enrollment but with highly restricted benefits. Dual/multiple choice may offer potential underwriting problems if, in fact, it creates an adverse selection mechanism; high users from the group might select the HMO option because of its broader coverage. Overall utilization does not appear to be affected. For those groups that appear to be high risk/high utilizers, rate adjustments with loading factors may be used as described under rate making.

Finally, for federally qualified HMOs, the passage of the Health Maintenance Organization Act of 1988 (P.L. 100-517) allows HMOs to use other than community rating. The HMOs are provided an option to set rates based on adjusted community rating methods; under this approach, HMOs can determine premium rates for employer groups based on the anticipated revenue requirements for that group, and can base rates on the prior costs and utilization experience of that particular group. But note that the rating must be prospective, at the beginning of a season; unlike indemnity insurers, the HMO is prohibited from using experience rating that includes retroactive refunds or dividends for good experience by the group.

UNDERWRITING INDIVIDUALS

There are circumstances under which the HMO may wish to offer individual subscriptions outside the usual group arrangement. This may be provided not only because of the HMO's sense of social responsibility to the community, but also as a marketing technique to attract the patients of physicians who join with the HMO, and others who are moving into the community, are self-employed, or are otherwise not associated with a group. Because the chances for adverse selection and billing difficulties are higher among such potential subscribers, underwritng rules for these individuals may be highly restrictive. In addition to a statement of health, their contracts may include preexisting condition limitations or exclusions (if not limited by federal qualification). Higher premiums because of the greater risk are inevitable for individual subscribers.

Benefits Packages

The benefits packages offered by the HMO are its products and services; as such, they are at the heart of the organization and serve several important functional objectives—to meet the need/demand of the members, to reduce financial deterrents to early care, and to develop a wide range of treatment alternatives that are available to the HMO's providers. In developing benefits packages, the HMO may follow the offerings of traditional Blue Cross/Blue Shield and indemnity programs, as well as of existing HMOs. Because the HMO's packages will be competing with the existing programs, the structure of the packages must be similar to the BC/BS plans—they must be comprehensive and offer first dollar/first day coverage, with few copayments and deductibles.

INCLUSIONS

For federally qualified plans, the Health Maintenance Organization Act and its amendments provide a list of required "basic health services" and a list of supplemental health services that may be provided at the option of the HMO;

TABLE 11-2   Basic and Optional Services Commonly Included in HMO Benefits Packages

Basic Benefits	Optional Benefits
Physician services	Psychiatric treatment
Hospital services	Treatment of alcoholism and drug
Emergency health services	addiction
Home calls	Eye examinations and prescriptions
Diagnostic laboratory services	Ambulance service
Diagnostic and therapeutic radiologic	Visiting nurse service
services	Artificial limbs, eyes, and orthopedic
Specialist care and consultation	braces
Maternity care	Dental services
Well-baby care	Provision of allergens
Treatment of allergies	Prescription drugs
Physical examinations	Loan of crutches, wheelchairs, and so on
Immunizations	Treatment of conditions requiring care in
Anesthesia	other than general hospitals
Educational activities	Home health care
	Extended-care facility services

these appear in Chapter 2, pages 37 and 38. *Basic benefits* are those services that are considered essential to the provision of health care and that are included as benefits in most health care plans. *Optional benefits* are those additional services that are normally selected to meet a unique need of the target population or to increase the market acceptance of the plan. Unlike the BC/BS and indemnity packages, the list of services offered by HMOs is somewhat more comprehensive and places equal emphasis on outpatient and inpatient services and includes some preventive health services as regular basic benefits. Basic health service packages also are defined by both the Medicare and Medicaid programs and may include additional services and more detailed requirements in the contract between the HMO and the responsible government agency. HMOs, however, are most concerned with meeting the level of competition and minimums established by law and, more importantly, with meeting the special needs of target populations. This becomes more complex each year as HMOs and their competition offer hybrid programs, multiple- and triple-option packages, point-of-service programs, and the like (see Chapter 4 for a discussion of these options). The HMO management understands these market forces and forms objectives that become the basis for benefits package development, constrained by cost.

The basic and optional benefits that are commonly included in HMO benefits packages are listed in Table 11-2. These services can be categorized as follows:

1. *Outpatient Services:* Diagnostic services, office visits, physical examinations, medical consultations, and laboratory tests. These services are provided by both primary (internists, general practice, OB/GYN, family practice, and pediatrics) and specialty physicians.

2. *Inpatient Services:* Care provided in hospitals and extended-care facilities, and the ancillary services provided to inpatients.

3. *Out-of-area and emergency care:* Services required in emergency situations within the HMO's service area and services provided for emergencies that occur outside the service area.

4. *Catastrophic illnesses:* Services to meet unique health needs requiring the services of superspecialists; they are usually very costly and service-use intensive.

5. *Drugs and appliances:* Prescription drugs, eyeglasses, and other prosthetic and corrective devices.

6. *Other special care:* Services that might include home health care, therapeutic and rehabilitative care, and health education.

EXCLUSIONS, LIMITATIONS, AND COPAYMENTS

Exclusions to the benefits package and limitations on services that are included in the package may be used for various reasons—to limit or control risk and thus maintain financial solvency, or to prevent inappropriate use of services. Most often such limitations and exclusions include war clauses, coordination of benefits (COB) with other insurers, services covered under worker's compensation or other public programs, physical examinations required for employment or by insurance companies, preexisting conditions beyond a dollar limit of care, intentionally self-inflicted injuries, personal comfort items while hospitalized, and private hospital rooms, unless medically ordered. In many of these circumstances, the liability for the service logically resides with other groups, such as an employer, a life insurance company, and local or federal governments. Antiduplication or coordination of benefits clauses are agreements among insurance companies, using language developed by the National Association of Insurance Commissioners, that describe the responsibility of each insurer involved and the order for primary and secondary responsibility in a subscriber's claim. They are included so other carriers will bear their fair share and prevent double payment for services when a member has coverage from two or more sources. For example, working wives may be covered first by the plan where they work, with the HMO assuming the difference in cost for care. Experts in the field suggest that a well-run COB program will create from $2 to $4 per member per month in additional revenue for the HMO.

Copayments require the member to pay a nominal out-of-pocket amount each time selected services are used. The rationale for such a system is that the total premium cost can be reduced somewhat by the inclusion of copayments and that copayment charges will erect a low economic barrier between the patient and the plan. Copayments provide a mechanism for rationing among members' health care services—an outcome of the pricing system; since consumers will pay something out-of-pocket (a $2 to $10 fee) every time they receive a certain service, they will not indulge unnecessarily, and members with possible hypochondria may limit their use of health services. Copayments appear to work, according to this rationale. They do increase revenues so that premium levels can be reduced and decrease utilization of physician services, and they bring the hypochondriac patient to the attention of his/her physician so that more appropriate care can be provided.

There are still some reservations concerning copayments; they may not be the most efficient or equitable way to control utilization and thus cost. This is especially true in an HMO, where prevention and early detection is such a large part of the philosophy of medical care. Copayments also discriminate against the poor; this should be considered and the use of copayments weighed against the objectives of the health plan.

DESIGN AND FORMATION

The question of what should or should not be included in a benefits package has not been fully answered. As stated previously, the HMO must meet the competition; it also must meet the requirements of any government programs whose recipients will receive its services. The HMO should have enough flexibility to allow the physician to choose from a range of treatment alternatives; the range of benefit categories should be broad enough to provide this flexibility. The major constraint in the benefits package will be the physicians themselves; can they and will they be willing to offer certain services? Physicians *must* be involved in the benefits package formulation to ensure that it is comprehensive and appropriate and to ensure their commitment to provide the services offered.

The formulation of the benefits package is an integral part of the marketing and financial planning process. Benefits should be *directly* related to the need/demand statements developed for the target populations, limited by costs and the availability of medical personnel. Moreover, benefits can be packaged in several ways. Programs offered to group members may include the individual (self only), the employee and family (self and family) or some other tiering arrangement. Some plans provide additional tiers for family membership based on the number of dependents (self and one dependent, self and two dependents, self and three dependents, and so on). Another common offering is a choice between low- and high-option programs, which differ in comprehensiveness, copayments, and deductibles. Such tiering arrangements are discussed in the next section of this chapter. By offering optional programs, the health plan may more effectively meet the needs and expectations of its members and employer purchasers.

Generally, HMOs follow three methods of package design, two of which provide programs tailored to specific groups of members.

1. Standard and supplementary sets of benefits that roughly match the requirements of the population and providers are developed from the lists in Table 11-2. The health plan then makes available to groups the standard package and the option of adding benefits from the supplementary set to develop benefit levels that meet the group's particular needs.

2. Totally custom-made packages for all groups may be developed. Thus, there may be as many benefits packages as there are groups of members.

3. The health plan may offer a standard plan only, with no custom programs or supplementary sets of benefits.

There are advantages and drawbacks in all three methods. Freedom of choice and flexibility in meeting special needs are the most important advantages of the custom package, but they create management difficulties for the HMO. Keeping track of covered/noncovered services as members arrive for care requires sophisticated computerized management information systems, for example. The standard plan offers great administrative ease, but lacks the custom approach peculiar to HMOs. All require that each benefit be "rated" to determine its financial effect on the cost of the benefits package, although the standard plan plus supplemental and custom packages may require more effort to create. Finally, the costing of benefits is a process of balancing the comprehensiveness of benefits against the use of deductibles and copayments and meeting the competition. Thus, initial packages will likely go through a metamorphosis as cost estimates are more fully developed and cash flow analyses are completed.

A clear, precise statement of benefits is required to estimate the costs of delivery, to develop marketing and advertising materials, to assist in determining staffing needs, to describe the member's financial responsibility regarding copayments, and to assist in resolving disputes regarding covered and noncovered services. Well-defined benefit statements also allow management to determine how services will be allocated among the many providers. These issues are exemplified in Table 11-3;[6] a proposed benefits package is analyzed

---

[6] For the convenience of the reader, Table 11-3 appears at the end of this chapter, following the references.

as to specific benefits and noncovered services, the medical group's and hospital's responsibilities under a capitation contract, and the member's role in copayments.

Please note that the following acronyms are defined as follows:

OP: outpatient services provided by the physician group.

IP: inpatient services provided by the hospital.

PC: the professional component of services provided by physicians in the medical group. For example, diagnostic X-ray exams are technically provided in the hospital that is responsible for the use of the equipment to provide the service, but the radiologist is a member of the medical group and thus is responsible for the professional component of the X-ray services; the physician's time is covered by the capitation to the group.

TC: the technical component of service delivery: medical devices, equipment and supplies, the facility and its upkeep, and so on. For example, physicians in the medical group are responsible for providing the medical group physician- or technician-administered inhalation therapy, while the hospital is responsible for the technical equipment and space.

Actuarial Aspects

PREMIUM DEVELOPMENT

A part of the strategic financial planning activity consists of *rate making,* the process of pricing the services that are to be sold. In the case of health plans, the price is called a premium—a fixed fee, paid in advance, that provides a plan member with all specified medical care and services. Before premiums can be calculated, rates (or charges) for each benefit unit (service) or unit of exposure must be developed. This function is a part of the total strategic planning and management processes undertaken by the HMO's management team. It is based on a deep understanding of the organization's goals and objectives, the plan's philosophy of health services delivery and finance, its underwriting rules and policies, and its basic principles of rate making. Some underwriting rules were provided in the discussion of underwriting groups earlier in this chapter. Other desirable characteristics and principles of rate making are provided below.

Characteristics and Principles of Rate Making

Six characteristics of rate making are important in establishing proper premium rates.[7] These include (1) adequacy of the rate structure, (2) competitiveness of rates, (3) equity among policyholders, (4) simplicity (ease of understanding and implementation), (5) flexibility/adaptability (degree of difficulty in making changes or adapting to new conditions), and (6) consistency.

Adequacy refers to the ability of the rates to maintain solvency and profitability; rates should adequately cover expenditures and allow for contingency reserves and profit/surplus. *Competitiveness* refers to the attractiveness of the rates as compared to other health plans; it relates to the skillfulness and resourcefulness of the HMO in establishing rates that will meet the competition and attract prospective policyholders to the HMO. *Equity* refers to the basic "fairness" of the rates—that all classes of policyholders are charged a rate that reflects the probability of loss to which the group or class is subject, constrained by law. This principle suggests that differences in rates should have a reasonable explanation. Although in principle equity is logical, in practice it may be difficult to accomplish because of the need to community rate by federally qualified plans, the need to cross-subsidize groups, the changing characteristics of the groups enrolled, and so on. *Simplicity* relates to ease of administration and understanding the rating system. As will be discussed in the next few pages, the development of rates is usually a complicated process of applying statistics, formulas, and adjustments; it is clear why the principle of simplicity may not always be followed. The fifth principle is that of *flexibility/adaptability*—the ability of the rating system to adapt to special circumstances or changing conditions. The sixth characteristic is *consistency;* a consistent method of establishing prices must be followed if policyholders and others are to have faith in the fairness, adequacy, and equity of the premium rates. This is especially important if the HMO is negotiating a Medicare risk contract with the Health Care Financing Administration and state Medicaid agencies.

Rate Making

The rate-making process follows the principles noted above. In this regard, three rating systems are available: community rating, manual rating, and experience rating. It is common today for HMOs to use all three rating systems rather than rely on one system only. Plans, for example, may be pressured by very large employers to experience rate their group, while the HMO finds it imperative to aggregate its smaller groups and use a communuity or manual rating system to arrive at its premiums. Federally qualified plans have

---

[7] Health Insurance Association of America. *Principles of Group Health Insurance*, pp. 131–133; and Charles William Wrightson, Jr., *HMO Rate Setting and Financial Strategy*, Ann Arbor, Mich., Health Administration Press Perspectives, 1990, pp. 117–120.

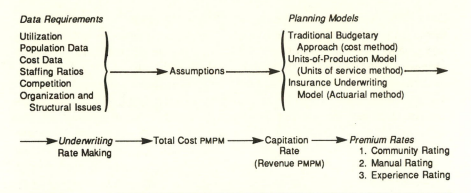

FIGURE 11-3   Capitation/premium rate setting process.

additional constraints placed on their ability to use pure manual or experience rating and thus will use modified systems that meet HCFA regulations.

Before discussing the three rating procedures, it might be useful to place the capitation/premium rate setting process in perspective. Figure 11-3 outlines the process by which HMOs establish their rates. The first step in this financial planning process is to collect data regarding the service area and its population so that planning assumptions can be realistically constructed. Estimates of need/demand for services and health insurance are made by HMO management. With planning assumptions (which are based on the demand estimates) in hand, one of the planning models is used to ultimately develop total costs PMPM. These cost estimates become the basis for establishing the capitation rate—the revenue PMPM. Premium rates are then calculated using the methodologies discussed below, for example, the use of community, manual, or experience rating.

Community rating is a system that embodies the total experience (or projected use level) of all the members in the health plan; these data are used to determine a capitation rate that is common for all groups, regardless of the utilization experience of an individual or of any one group. This rating system spreads utilization and expense costs over the total membership of the health plan, creating cross-subsidies between low- and high-risk groups. Distinctions may be made among the major risk classes (i.e., over age 65 versus under age 65, individual versus group enrollees, indigency versus solvency), but premiums are not adjusted or loaded according to the loss experience of any one enrollee or group. Each person or family who enrolls under a specific benefits package should pay exactly the same premium as every other member in the same package. Given the attitude that no windfall from lowered utilization or loss from above-average use should accrue to any group or individual, but that the surplus or deficit should be spread over the entire enrollee population, there has been a traditional attitude that there is no advantage to the HMO manager to incur the expense of projecting use data by particular classes or groups of enrollees. By carrying this operating philosophy one step farther, the manager relies on the operational aspects of capitation, that is, equal assignment of costs to each plan member. Under a purely community-rated system, no adjustments to this capitation rate would be permitted; thus, the capitation rate and premium rate would be the same. Some social welfare advocates suggest that this is desirable, because it is a good way to insure the high-risk segments of the population by averaging the costs across the entire membership. With the passage of federal welfare programs designed to cover some costs of high-risk groups (i.e., Medicare and Medicaid), however, community rating becomes less important for cost redistribution. Moreover, HMO managers have found that in the current competitive environment, the HMO must obtain use data by class or groups of members to adequately estimate the health plan's costs and to set premiums competitively.

Manual rating relies on a manual of rates containing schedules of premium rates for the benefits offered. The rate manual or book is developed over time, based on historical use experienced by broad classes of risk and characteristics of groups. The HMO manager uses this rate book to determine premium rates for the different benefit products covered by the policy. Thus, the rates reflect only the most broad and important factors that affect morbidity and health plan expenses; individual policies, thus, are not rated on the basis of detailed characteristics of the individual person as one might see in experience rating. Insurers may, however, use the manual rating system to set rates (known as tabular rates or class rates) for groups and then may adjust these rates (load or discount), based on their knowledge of the group and the HMO manager's underwriting judgment.

Most federally qualified HMOs rely on manual rates at the start and incorporate this system into their unique rating activities. This is called community rating by class, where the plan considers factors such as sex, age, industry and its size and location, and so on. But, even though these specific characteristics that affect utilization and costs might be considered, the HMO's rates must still be based on the experience of all members, not just on the experience of specific groups.

Experience rating is the third rating system used by HMOs and health care insurers. This system allows for a variation in the rates for benefit units, computed on the basis of the experience (or projected use) of the group or individual. Information on past use and expenses incurred by the HMO for each group of members is used to adjust rates for benefit units that have been developed in the actuary process or those rates that are found in rate manuals. It is a method by which premiums paid by a group policyholder are directly related to the actual utilization and expense experience of the group. Consequently, the experience-rating system modifies manual rates or rates developed in the underwriting process for broad classes of risk, usually based on a group of employees, a union, or an association.

Although Blue Cross/Blue Shield plans and HMOs were historically established on a community-rating basis, both programs now lean toward the experience-rating system used by commercial carriers. Indeed, federally qualified HMOs are now allowed to use an adjusted community-rating system in which premium rates for specific groups are based on anticipated revenues from that group. For the nonqualified plans, experience rating is accomplished through discounts or loading factors that provide adjustments to rates for major classes of risks. The basis for defending this system of rate making is that there is greater equity among policyholders: those with greater risks pay higher premiums. Moreover, competition among insurers has forced health plans to more systematically evaluate policyholders and to attempt, with reasonable premium rates, to retain groups with favorable experience. Until the passage of the HMO Amendments of 1988, this widespread policy of experience rating was placing federally qualified HMOs at a disadvantage for adverse selection; initially, qualified HMOs were restricted from using experience rating and were required to use open enrollment and community rating (except for some distinction for major risk classes). Hence, groups with poor experience and high premiums were looking toward the more liberal, qualified HMO for coverage.

CAPITATION RATE DEVELOPMENT

In the following sections, some of the approaches to capitation rate development are reviewed. Note that the first, the traditional budgetary approach, is the most common form used in the HMO field; this description expands the discussion of the budgetary model beginning on page 440 of this chapter.

Traditional Budgetary Approach

In the budgetary approach, the *planwide costs* of operation are estimated, based on the previous year's expenses and limited use of utilization rates per 1,000 members. The following steps are used:

1. Determine the level of membership to be served—a membership level that will permit the HMO to break even and create a surplus from operations. This level is equivalent to that for which the facility and program were designed, so that the greatest contribution to fixed costs can be made.

   a. Determine the size of the potential market and the expected penetration levels of each component of that market

    b. Determine the availability of resources: manpower, equipment, and capital

    c. Determine the optimal size of the facility

2. Develop a set of planning assumptions.

    a. *Utilization rates:* physician services, hospital days, laboratory tests, X-ray examinations, pharamaceuticals per member per year

    b. *Staffing ratios:* physicians, nurses, and other health personnel per fixed number of members

    c. Other assumptions

3. Convert planning assumptions to an expense budget by developing cost estimates for each of the expense areas.[8] The categories of expenses for all HMO models include:

    a. *Medical expenses:* physician and hospital services, pharmaceuticals, diagnostic services (laboratory tests and X-rays), and other medical expenses

    b. *Health plan administration:* health plan management and operation, marketing, and debt service

    c. *Medical center (clinic) operations:* salaries, building and occupancy expenses, insurance, and other center expenses

4. Convert the expense budget into a capitation rate by determining how much money is required per member to support the plan. Essentially, this is accomplished by adding the costs PMPM (minus any reinsurance recovery, COB, copayments, and interest income) to obtain a total cost PMPM. If total yearly expenses (rather than expense PMPM.) are used, then total costs PMPM are obtained by dividing total expenses by total member months.

    The capitation rate—*revenue* PMPM —is then computed; simplistically, the capitation rate is equal to the total cost PMPM.

Capitation rate development follows one of two general formulas:

1a. Annual utilization rates PMPM × unit cost ÷ 12 months = cost PMPM

1b. Annual utilization rate per 1,000 members × unit cost ÷ 12 months ÷ 1,000 = cost PMPM

  2. Total budgeted costs ÷ members ÷ 12 months = cost PMPM

---

[8] John van Steenwick, a consulting actuary, suggests that "data for about 100,000 member-years of experience (1 year's data for a 100,000-member organization; 2 years' data for a 50,000-member organization) can usually be considered a stable basis for prediction (of health plan expenses)"; Kongstvedt, *The Managed Health Care Handbook*, p. 220.

TABLE 11-4 Employer Group Capitation Rate

Quarter	Computation						Rate
	Month	×	*PMPM Cost*	+	*Month*	×	*PMPM Cost ÷ 12* =	*Rate*
1st Quarter	10	×	$126.45	+	2	×	$142.50	= $129.12
2nd Quarter	8	×	126.45	+	4	×	142.50	= 131.80
3rd Quarter	5	×	126.45	+	7	×	142.50	= 135.81
4th Quarter	3	×	126.45	+	9	×	142.50	= 138.49

Realistically, it varies by quarter of the year, because group enrollment (anniversary) dates vary. Thus, the capitation rates for each employer group will be based on the average expenses required to provide services for that group enrolled during the quarter. Using the example provided in Table 11-1, the capitation rate by quarter for an employer group is provided in Table 11-4. Note that this example is for a medical group model HMO in which an outside medical group (the plan) contracts with the HMO to deliver physician services; hence, there are no medical center operation expenses shown. These expenses are included in the physician capitation, which is $38.00 for Year 1 and $42.00 for Year 2. Thus, the health plan would use $129.12 as the rate for employer groups enrolling during the first quarter, while $135.81 would be used for groups enrolling during the third quarter. In this example, the rates would be in effect for a 12-month period from enrollment.

5. The above rates are raw capitation rates; usually these rates are adjusted, or loaded, to reflect a variety of factors, including:

    a. Start-up costs

    b. Reinsurance arrangements for initial operating losses incurred before the break-even membership is reached

    c. Relationship of the capitation to competitive packages in the market

    d. Reinsurance arrangements for special services

    e. Expected revenues from optional benefit charges and copayments

    f. Specific age, health status, social, and mobility characteristics of the enrolled population

    g. Family-loading factor, reflecting the difference between those enrollees who are covered and those who actually pay

The final capitation includes only the cost items calculated before adjusting or loading is done (i.e., before step 5). The *premium*, thus, would be the rate established by loading or discounting, as described in step 5.

Insurance Underwriting Model

The second approach to capitation rate development, the insurance underwriting model, is a continuation of the discussion of this budgeting model that

TABLE 11-5   Days of Hospital Care by Age and Sex

| Age | Expected Bed Days per 1,000 Members per Year | |
	Male	Female
0– 4	630	455
5– 9	120	80
10–14	170	170
15–19	330	340
20–24	180	460
25–29	265	660
30–34	240	530
35–39	250	410
40–44	350	360
45–49	390	425
50–54	625	590
55–59	875	600
60–64	1,380	1,010
65 +	1,595	1,492

SOURCE: Peter R. Kongstvedt. *The Managed Health Care Handbook.* Gaithersburg, Md., Aspen Publishers, 1989, p. 219. Reprinted courtesy of Aspen Publishers, Inc.

begins on page 446. This approach is built around the actuary's activities—estimates of the utilization rates of service per member or per 1,000 members. Per member per month costs or the frequency of use of each benefit line or service unit included in the benefits package are projected. Similar to the budgetary approach, the health plan analyzes the market and penetration levels, determines the optimal organizational structure and size of the facility, and then estimates its costs of operation. It is this last step that differs from the budgetary model. Instead of estimating line item costs for the health plan based on previous operations, the manager relies on the assistance of an actuary to define the costs of medical services per member. The actuary uses historical data and special studies to arrive at use rates specific to the HMO's membership. Other costs of HMO operation are then added to the medical services costs to arrive at total costs PMPM.

Services are precisely described to allow the actuary to complete as detailed an estimate as possible. This analysis begins with inpatient hospital services and other hospital-provided care, such as outpatient surgery, emergency room care, ambulance service, radiation therapy, home health, and so on. Expected bed days are estimated, based on the specific age and sex characteristics of the plan's membership. For example, Table 11-5 suggests that a population with a large over age 50 group will need substantially more days of hospital care than a population under age 50. Similarly, a health plan that enrolls predominately

TABLE 11-6 Computation of the Days of Hospital Care for an HMO

Age	Rate Male	No. of Male Members	Rate Female	No. of Female Members	Average Rate
0–4	630	60	455	65	539
5–9	120	72	80	70	101
10–14	170	110	170	90	170
15–19	330	200	340	190	335
20–24	180	280	460	300	325
25–29	265	230	660	200	449
30–34	240	460	530	480	401
35–39	250	590	410	600	331
40–44	350	400	360	450	355
45–49	390	380	425	400	408
50–54	625	300	590	390	605
55–59	875	250	600	330	718
60–64	1,380	100	1,010	120	1,178
65 +	1,595	0	1,492	0	
Total		3,432		3,685	5,915

Average rate = total of the age category averages divided by the number of age categories or 5,915 ÷ 13.

female members will experience higher hospital days than if the membership was more equally divided between males and females.

The hospital day rate to be used by the manager is based on the characteristics of projected members and their anticipated rates of services. As an example, by using the rates in Table 11-5, the average rate per 1,000 members for a fictitious membership group is provided in Table 11-6. First, the average hospital day rate for each age group is computed using the following formula: Age-specific day rate *times* the number of males in an age category, *plus* the age-specific day rate *times* the number of females in that age category, *divided* by the total number of members in that age category, *equals* the average day rate for that age category.

The average hospital day rate for our example, therefore, is 455 days per 1,000 members per year or a rate or "frequency" of .455 per member. If the average hospital day charge is $500, then the hospital cost PMPM is $18.96 ($500 × .455 ÷ 12 months) and the total yearly hospital day cost to the health plan is $1,619,117.50 ($500 × .455 ×) 7,117 members).

In some instances, HMOs have successfully negotiated contracts with more than one area hospital; as discussed in Chapter 6, these contracts range from full fee-for-service charges to prospective payments, including capitation. How are capitation rates for hospitals established by the HMO, especially if the plan is negotiating with more than one hospital as a capitated provider? The

TABLE 11-7 Computation of Capitation Rate for Hospitals

Step 1: Derive the total weighted average for each service.

Medical and Surgical Services:

Hospital	Expected Average Per Diem	Relative Utilization by HMO Members %	Weighted Average Contribution
Hospital X	$523	53	$277.19
Hospital Y	490	21	102.90
Hospital Z	580	26	150.80
		100	
Total Weighted Average For Medical/Surgical Services			$530.89

Obstetrical Services:

Hospital	Expected Average Per Diem	Relative Utilization by HMO Members %	Weighted Average Contribution
Hospital X	$760	20	$152.00
Hospital Y	840	68	571.20
Hospital Z	800	12	96.00
		100	
Total Weighted Average For Obstetrical Services			$819.20

Psychiatric Services:

Hospital	Expected Average Per Diem	Relative Utilization by HMO Members %	Weighted Average Contribution
Hospital X	$200	15	$ 30.00
Hospital Y	230	34	78.20
Hospital Z	190	51	96.90
		100	
Total Weighted Average For Psychiatric Services			$205.10

Step 2: Calculate the average per diem for all hospitalization. Assume the following utilization based on historical data or actuarial analyses:

Utilization:	%
Medical	30
Surgical	50
Obstetrical	15
Psychiatric	5

Type of Service	Average Per Diem	Relative Utilization by the HMO %	Weighted Average Contribution
Medical	$530.89	30	$159.27
Surgical	530.89	50	265.45
Obstetrical	819.20	15	122.88
Psychiatric	205.10	5	10.26
		100	
Estimated Average Per Diem			$557.86

Step 3: Compute the Capitation Rate for hospital care.

Formula: [(Bed Days/1,000/yr.) × (Combined Average Per Diem)] ÷ [Annual member months per 1,000 members].

Thus, the capitation rate for 30,000 member months per year and a projected 455 days/1,000 members is as follows:

$$[(455) \times (\$557.99)] \div 30,000 \text{ member months} = \$8.47 \text{ PMPM}$$

TABLE 11-8 Selected Rates of Service Use per 1,000 Under Age 65 Members

Service Unit	Use Rates from Several Sources (Units per 1,000)				
	Source 1	Source 2	Source 3	Source 4	
Inpatient surgery	61	–	45	38	Cases
Outpatient surgery	48	20	314	312	Procedures
Office surgery	192	58	72	76	Visits
Office visits (all)	2,480	3,300	2,682	3,095	Visits
Consultations	105	60	44	44	Visits
IP physician visits	239	315	243	182	Visits
ER physician visits	190	120	152	91	Visits
OP radiology	435	530	58	58	Procedures
OP lab and pathology	2,250	3,710	32	32	Procedures
IP lab and pathology	–	–	2,552	2,858	Procedures
Home visits	5	27	30	30	Visits
Immunizations/injections	330	–	190	190	Visits
Well-baby visits	162	–	140	140	Exams
OB delivery	18	25	26	26	Cases
OP mental health	195	200	244	190	Visits
Physical therapy	–	130	75	75	Cases
Vision/refractions	265	–	–	–	Visits
Prescription drugs	5,460	–	3,819	4,277	Scripts
Substance abuse	–	50	22	22	Visits
Extended care days	–	5	14	14	Days
Ambulance	–	10	12	12	Trips

answer to this question is provided in the following example. Assume that the health plan admits its members to three hospitals for a variety of services, including medical, surgical, obstetrical, and psychiatric care. The computations are provided in Table 11-7.

A similar approach can be used to create use rates or frequencies and costs for all other medical services included in the benefits package. Some additional examples of expected use rates and frequencies are provided in Table 11-8. These represent actual rates used by four operational HMOs in their planning process and are based on historical data for their memberships. Note the wide variation in rates among these four plans for some of the services; such variations are based on the demographics of the membership, practice patterns in the area, benefits package design, competition, members' use of outside-the-plan services, and so on. Using these and other rates, an example of the capitation rate development (total medical costs PMPM) for medical services of a fictitious HMO is provided in Table 11-9. In this example, total medical service costs per member per month are $50.33. To these costs the HMO must add the estimates of health plan administration and medical center operations. Like the bugetary model, these costs are based on estimated costs

TABLE 11-9 Development of Medical Services Costs

Service	Frequency or Rate/Member	Average Charge or Cost*	Cost PMPM†
Hospital Services:			
Inpatient days	.455	$500‡	$18.96
Outpatient surgery	.048	650	2.60
Emergency room	.190	130	2.05
Extended care	.005	160	.07
Ambulance	.010	100	.08
Subtotal			$23.76
Physician Services:			
Office visits	3.300	$ 32	$ 8.80
Consultations	.060	65	.33
IP physician visits	.239	40	.80
Office surgery	.076	650	4.12
OP mental health	.095	60	.48
Well-baby visits	.140	28	.33
Subtotal			$14.86
Other Medical Services:			
OP radiology	.435	$ 55	$ 1.99
OP lab and pathology	2.250	10	1.88
Immunizations and injections	.330	15	.41
Vision/refractions	.265	20	.44
Prescription drugs	5.465	13	5.92
Subtotal			$10.64
Outside-the-plan Services and Referrals:			
Physical therapy	.075	$ 30	$ .19
Subspecialty physician services	.050	120	.50
Substance abuse	.022	150	.28
Home health visits	.030	40	.10
Subtotal			$ 1.07
Total Medical Services Costs PMPM			$50.33

*This figure represents the amount that the HMO must pay for this service; it may be an average fee-for-service charge determined by an outside physician provider or hospital or the cost of the service computed by the HMO, based on expenses from previous periods.

†The average cost per member per month equals the frequency or rate × average cost or charge ÷ 12 months.

‡This amount represents the all-inclusive daily rate, calculated by dividing the hospital's total expenses by its total number of hospital days for the same period.

of operations; the previous year's experience usually provides the basis for these projections. Using the costs provided in the example in Table 11-9, a pro forma financial statement is provided in Table 11-10.

It is obvious that the early pro forma budgets will not balance; expenses will probably be higher than income. Management will revise its assumptions about service use, change benefits, attempt to negotiate better contracts with outside providers, add copays, increase premiums, and generally reduce operating

TABLE 11-10   Pro Forma Financial Statement for a 30,000 Member HMO

		% of Total	*PMPM*
Revenue:			
Premiums	$51,768,000	97.81	$143.80
Reinsurance recovery	324,000	0.61	.90
Coordination of benefits	216,000	0.41	.60
Copayments	540,000	1.02	1.50
Interest	0	0	0
Fees-for-service	54,000	0.10	.15
Sale of medical supplies, equipment, and prescription drugs	18,000	0.03	.05
Other	7,200	0.01	.02
Total Revenue	$52,927,200	99.99	$147.02
Expenses:			
Medical Expenses:			
Hospital services	$11,414,106	22	$ 31.70
Physician services	15,560,592	30	43.22
Other medical services	4,149,492	8	11.53
Referrals	3,630,806	7	10.08
Subtotal	$34,754,996	67	$ 96.53
Health Plan Administration:			
Management/salaries	$ 3,630,806	7	$ 10.08
Marketing	1,556,060	3	4.32
Debt service	0	0	0
Reinsurance premiums	1,037,373	2	2.88
Reserves	0	0	0
Data processing	518,686	1	1.44
Occupancy expenses	1,556,060	3	4.32
Supplies	1,556,060	3	4.32
Insurance	518,686	1	1.44
Other	0	0	0
Subtotal	$10,373,731	20	$ 28.80
Medical Center Operations:			
Salaries	$ 2,074,746	4	5.76
Occupancy expenses	2,074,746	4	5.76
Medical equipment/supplies	518,686	1	1.44
Insurance	2,074,746	4	5.76
Subtotal	$ 6,742,924	13	$ 18.72
Total Expenses	$51,871,651	100	$144.05
Net Income	$ 1,055,549	2	$ 2.94

costs. Because this process is iterative and reiterative, managers have found that computer assistance is valuable.

Other Rating Approaches

The rating method reviewed above follows the community-rating approach. Obviously, for federally qualified plans, methods other than pure community rating can be used; that is, rating by class and adjusted community rating. For nonqualified plans, adjusted community rating, experience rating, and group-specific rating methods are used. The technical aspects of these approaches are beyond this discussion. The reader is directed to Charles Wrightson's publication, *HMO Rate Setting and Financial Strategy* (see footnote 7, p. 468), for a review of the specific aspects of these other approaches.

Premium Tier Structure

After the capitation rate has been determined, the HMO can establish premium rates for each employer group. Because variations in benefits and how they are offered occur, the health plan needs to set rates by tier or contract type. In the section of this chapter on benefits package design, several premium tier structures or packaging systems (individual employee; individual plus spouse; individual, spouse, and one child; and so on) were described. Premiums are adjusted for each of these packages, using one of several available mechanisms. The simplest approach to adjusting the crude capitation rate to reflect the composition of the population and risks is described as a "straight-rate system." No loading or discounting is used in the straight-rate system; thus, the base capitation rate is multiplied by the number of individuals to be covered by the contract. An individual's premium would be multiplied by 1, individual and spouse by 2, family with one child by 3, and so on, in a step-wise expansion of the base rate. A two-step system would assign the base rate to an individual and 2 times the base rate to an individual plus family. Another method can be described as a three-step system (times 1 for an individual, times 2 for two-person families, and times 3 for families with more than two persons). Discounting, then, is accomplished by multiplying the base rate by less than 1 for each additional family member included in the family policy (i.e., the multiplier for a family with one child might be 2.75 rather than 3). Likewise, loading is accomplished by increasing the base rate by more than 1 times the base for each additional family member, as illustrated in Table 11-11.

Most plans, especially those that are federally qualified, use other methods to convert the capitation rate to a premium rate for each tier. Although the manager follows the health plan's assumption and principles for rate making, he/she must also be assured that there is a close relationship between the capitation rate (costs of operation) and the average revenue per member produced by the premium structure. The tier/premium relationships shown in Table 11-12 might be used to help assure the equivalence between costs and revenues.[9] The objective is to develop a *conversion factor* that can be used

---

[9] This discussion is based, in part, on Harry L. Sutton, Jr. and Allen J. Sorbo, *Actuarial Issues in the Fee-for-Service/Prepaid Medical Group,* Denver, Colo., Center for Research in Ambulatory Health Care Administration, 1983, pp. 52–59.

TABLE 11-11   Simple Premium Adjustment Methods

	Class of Enrollment			
	Individual	Individual + 1	Individual + 2	Family (Multiple Child)
Straight rate	1 ×	2 ×	3 ×	N ×
Two-step	1 ×	2 ×	2 ×	2 ×
Three-step	1 ×	2 ×	3 ×	3 ×
Three-step discounted	1 ×	2 ×	2.75 ×	2.75 ×
Three-step loaded	1 ×	2 ×	3.5 ×	3.5 ×

to convert the capitation rate to a single individual premium rate. Several calculations are necessary to arrive at the conversion factor, which is multiplied by the capitation rate to arrive at the single (individual) employee premium rate.

1. The average members per contract = $N1 \times 1 + N2 \times 2 + N3 \times F$. Note that this figure is the weighted average of the contract sizes.

2. The average premium per contract = $N1 \times S + N2 \times S \times R1 + N3 \times S \times R2$. Again, the average premium per contract is a weighted average of the premium rates; the single premium is an unknown at this point.

3. The capitation rate is the average premium revenue per member. Therefore, the capitation rate = the average premium per member = average premium per contract/average members per contract.

4. By substituting from formulas 1 and 2, a formula is derived in which there is only one unknown, S, the employee-only premium.

$$\text{Capitation rate} = \frac{N1 \times S + N2 \times S \times R1 + N3 \times S \times R2}{N1 \times 1 + N2 \times 2 + N3 \times F}$$

or

$$S = \text{Capitation rate} \times \frac{N1 \times 1 + N2 \times 2 + N3 \times F}{N1 \times 1 + N2 \times R1 + N3 \times R2}$$

The conversion factor, therefore, is the quotient of the formula, where $N1 \times 1 + N2 \times 2 + N3 \times F$ is the average contract size, and $N1 \times 1 + N2 \times R1 + N3 \times R2$ are the average premium units. To obtain the single employee only premium, or S, the capitation rate is multiplied by the conversion factor.

Table 11-13 shows how the premium rates for a three-tier and a two-tier product are developed using the formula for the conversion factor.

TABLE 11-12   Equivalence Rate Adjustment Method

		Class of Enrollment	
	Individual	Individual + 1	Individual + 2 or More
Distribution of contracts (% of total)	N1	N2	N3
Contract size	1	2	F
Ratio of rate	1	R1	R2
Premium rate	S	S × R1	S × R2

where: N = number of contracts
         S = single or individual employee premium
         R = ratio to the single rate
         F = family

If the group capitation rate of $129.12 from Table 11-4 (for the first quarter) is used, the single or individual employee premium is $129.12 × the conversion factor of 1.286 or $166.05.

Now, the other rates can be determined: The 2-person premium equals the single rate of $166.05 × 2 or $332.10. The family premium equals the single rate of $166.05 × 3 or $498.15.

A two-tier rate structure, assuming the same population distribution as above, can also be calculated. This process of calculating a two-tier premium rate from a three-tier rate is known as *compositing*. In the two-tier arrangement, the single-employee rate remains the same, $166.05, as in the three-tier arrangement. The family rate is derived by using the following formula:

TABLE 11-13   Conversion Factor

		Class of Enrollment	
	Individual	Individual + 1	Individual + 2 or More
Distribution of contracts (% of total)	30%	30%	40%
Contract size	1	2	4.6
Ratio to single rate	1	2	3

$$\text{Conversion factor} = \frac{.30 \times 1 + .30 \times 2 + .40 \times 4.6}{.30 \times 1 + .30 \times 2 + .40 \times 3} = 2.74 \div 2.1 \text{ or } 1.286$$

$$\frac{\text{2-person rate} \times \% \text{ of contracts} + \text{3 or more rate} \times \% \text{ of contracts}}{\% \text{ 2-person contracts} + \% \text{ 3-person contracts}}$$

Thus:

$$\text{Family rate} = \frac{\$332.10 \times .30 + \$498.15 \times .40}{.30 + .40} = \$426.99$$

Similar computations are used to develop the premium rates for each employer group if experience rating is used, or by classes of employees if the plan is federally qualified. It is obvious that the development of premium rates is somewhat technical; the previous discussion is only an introduction to this complex topic. Again, for an in-depth discussion of rate making, the reader is directed to Charles Wrightson's book, *HMO Rate Making and Financial Strategy.*

Medical Group Practice Capitation

The discussion of physician/HMO contracting in Chapter 6 suggested that the parties negotiate a reasonable capitation rate. The first step is to precisely define what medical services are to be included in the capitation and to get physician acceptance of these services (see Table 11-3 for an example of the services required of the physician's group). Both sides will then cost out these services. HMO managers will use their budgets and other studies to determine what capitation rate to offer the medical group practice. For example, Table 11-9 provides medical services costs computed by the HMO; it includes a cost for physician services along with hospital and other medical services. If it is assumed that the physicians agree to provide the services listed under Physician Services and all services under Other Medical Services except prescription drugs, then the HMO management might offer $19.58 PMPM as their physician capitation rate.

Physician Services	$14.86
Other Medical Services	10.64
Subtotal	$25.50
Less: Prescription Drugs	5.92
Total Capitation	$19.58

Conversely, the medical group will compute its estimate of costs to deliver these services. Most groups use their fee-for-service costs to estimate the costs under the capitation contract, although practice patterns of group members may change over time. For example, the physicians may hospitalize patients less and see more of them in their offices. HMO patients may demand more preventive

TABLE 11-14 Cost Development of Medical Group Practice Providing Services to 30,000 HMO Members

Cost Categories	Amount	PMPM
Physician Services:		
Average income (27 physicians @ $125,000	$3,375,000	$ 9.38
Fringe benefits @ 20% of income	675,000	1.86
Subtotal	$4,050,000	$11.24
Nonphysician Staff		
Average income (4.1 per physician @ $18,000)	$1,992,600	$ 5.54
Fringe benefits @ 15% of salary	298,890	.83
Occupancy Costs	$ 306,180	.85
Supplies	540,000	1.50
Equipment/Furniture	54,000	.15
Malpractice Insurance	202,500	.56
Debt Service	0	0
Subtotal	$3,394,170	$ 9.43
Total	$7,444,170	$20.67

services, injections, and well-baby services. Medical groups, therefore, should use a similar actuarial and budgeting approach to cost development and rate making as was used by the HMO.

Most medical groups base their estimates of costs on historical fee-for-service activity. In Table 11-14, the medical group's estimate of its costs to provide services to 30,000 members is shown. In comparison to the HMO's estimate of $19.58 PMPM, the medical group estimates it will cost them $20.67 PMPM. The plan and the medical group would reconcile the proposed capitation rates through negotiation.

Day-to-Day Financial Management

Financial management is a logical place to close a book on the planning, development, and operation of managed care systems, especially health maintenance organizations. Financial tools allow the manager to continuously evaluate the organization's progress and to recognize its level of success in meeting its objectives. This is especially true in an HMO where close fiscal management is the key to success and growth. Three financial tools are essential—the pro forma operating statements and cash flow analyses, the budget, and ratio analysis. In addition, techniques for claims liability management, claims reported but unpaid, and claims incurred but not reported are necessary for successful operation. All of these can be used to evaluate the potential level of day-to-day operation as well as success during the development and expansionary activities. Cash flow and cumulative cash flows are the most important indicators of current operations and must be positive. Budgets must be used to help set operating levels and then to periodically evaluate the actual levels attained. Financial ratios and their use in analysis enables rapid and comprehensive digestion of routine financial statements in a minimum amount of time with a maximum acquisition of useful information. Financial ratios help signal the need for new decisions about significant operational and financial issues and for reevaluation of certain areas of operation. These techniques are reviewed in the sections that follow.

CLAIMS LIABILITY MANAGEMENT—IBNR

Most discussions of HMOs deal with the prepaid nature of these systems— insurance activities and prepaid, capitated arrangements with providers. There are occasions, however, when the HMO and its physician panel incur liabilities with nonparticipating providers and others. In these situations, the HMO usually pays fees for services. Table 11-15 shows the types of services and the HMO models in which they typically occur.

Claims against the HMO or its affiliated medical group or IPA occur when nonphysician providers refer members to out-of-plan providers, or participating providers furnish services that are not under a capitation contract with the HMO. For example, a multispecialty medical group that serves HMO members under a prospective capitation contract refers a patient to a superspecialist who is not a member of the medical group. The group is responsible for the fee of the specialist—a claim that may not be received by the group for several months after services are furnished. Such claims fall into two categories. First, those that are reported to the HMO or its affiliated medical group but are unpaid; with a good management information system the HMO or group should be able to track and accurately determine and manage these claims. The second are those claims that are incurred but not reported (IBNR). These occur when members use outside services and the fee-for-service claims are not reported in a timely fashion to the HMO or medical group, or when there is a lag between service delivery and the point at which the HMO recognizes its liability in its accounting records. Specifically, IBNRs occur because HMO management fails to use notification of referrals to anticipate the cost of the service, or the notification process is faulty. Even when the notification system is operational, management may fail to obtain or analyze claims lag reports, or it uses an inappropriate technique for estimating IBNRs. Therefore, adequate management of IBNRs requires procedures and policies to govern claims generation and reporting and, secondly, techniques for tracking claims.

TABLE 11-15   Fee-for-Service Liability by Type of HMO Model

Service	HMO Model			
	Staff	Group	IPA	Network
1. Primary care physicians			X	X
2. Referrals to physician specialists	X	S	X	X
3. Hospital, long-term care, and mental health services	X	X	X	X
4. Out-of-area hospital and physician services	X	X	X	X
5. Pharmacy services	S	S	S	S
6. Ambulance	X	X	X	X
7. Home care services	X	X	X	X
8. Ancillary services	S		X	X

S = sometimes

The IBNR procedures provide a management accounting means for adjusting from a cash to an accrual basis (especially in medical group practices under a capitation contract with an HMO) and include claim forms, predefined fee schedules, required preauthorization to provide services, and so on, as the basis for managing the system.

The best method to estimate claims liabilities is to analyze the actual claims patterns from historical data; however, new and small HMOs, unfortunately, may lack such experience information. In these situations, the health plan and its capitated providers should use a combination of written and telephone notifications of referrals, hospitalizations, and out-of-plan services *prior to service delivery*. The anticipated cost of these referrals becomes the basis of the expected claims for that period. Costs are based on fee schedules, hospital per diems, published rates, previous provider claims, and so on. Then the claims lag is determined, since payment for claims incurred in one month may be received in a future month. Three time periods are important in claims lag analysis: date of service to the date of claim receipt; date of claim receipt to date paid; and date of service to date paid. The following example shows a claims lag period of 40 days.

A.	*Date of Service*	to	*Date Claim Received*		*No. of Days*
	March 1, 1990		April 2, 1990		33
B.	*Date Claim Received*	to	*Date Claim Paid*		
	April 2, 1990		April 20, 1990		19
C.	*Date of Service*	to	*Date Claim Paid*		
	March 1, 1990		April 20, 1990		52

Lag period A identified the speed with which providers submit their claims; lag period B identified the processing time; and lag period C is the sum of the two previous periods. It is period C, known as the "run-off," that affects the cash needs of the health plan and its capitated providers and is used for estimating the IBNR claims liabilities.

As historical claims data are collected, the method of determining the HMO's liabilities changes. The plan begins to identify stable patterns in lag periods. For instance, the plan will probably notice that lags are longest for out-of-area and emergency claims. The sheer volume of claims increases as membership increases, requiring sophisticated management information systems to monitor claims processing and lag periods. In addition, plans that use several capitated medical groups will probably experience wide variations in lag times among the groups.

One of the methods used in claims liability analysis is illustrated in Figure 11-4, a triangular lag table. It shows the claims received by month and the actual month payment was made, that is, the run-off for each month. The total amount of claims paid by month is shown in the third column; then, the distribution of payment for each month (by month incurred) is provided in the remaining columns. These vertical columns demonstrate the run-off or total lag factor for a given month's incurred expenses, with the percent of the month's total shown under each month of payment; see the column designated A for the lag periods for January 1990. In January, the plan paid 2 percent of the claims incurred in January; in February, the plan paid an additional 22 percent of claims incurred in January, for a cumulative total of 24 percent of all claims incurred in January, and so on. The diagonal designated B shows the consistency of the percentage paid in the month of incurral; for example, 2 percent in January, 1 percent in February, 3 percent in March, 1 percent in April, May, and June, and so on. Consistency is also evident across other time periods; for example, five months after the January incurral (June), the lag chart shows that 94 percent of the January claims were paid, 88 percent of February's claims were paid five months later (July), and so on. Unlike this example, the manager should thoroughly explore the reasons if substantial variations in the reporting and, thus, payment of claims occur. But, more importantly, HMO management should be able to project IBNR claims liability from the lag table; in the example, only 1 to 3 percent of total claims incurred during a particular month were processed and paid, approximately 20 to 27 percent were paid in the second month after they were incurred, and so on.

The final stage in IBNR management is the allocation of expected expenses each month by completing an accounting transaction. In this way the claims liability accrual is recorded in the organization's financial statements for the month. This process permits the matching of revenue and expenses by accounting period and facilitates the development of financial statements that

Distribution of Physicians Claim Payments by Month Incurred

YEAR / MONTH	CLAIMS PAYMENTS BY MONTH — TOTAL MONTHLY PAYMENT	Prior to January 1990	1990 January	1990 February	1990 March	1990 April	1990 May	1990 June	1990 July	1990 August	1990 September	1990 October	1990 November	1990 December	1991 January
1990 January	$191,100	$187,180	3,920 (2%)												
February	199,260	154,098	43,120 (24%)	2,042 (1%)											
March	199,200	97,209	54,880 (52%)	40,836 (21%)	6,275 (3%)										
April	208,213	44,696	41,160 (73%)	69,421 (55%)	50,198 (27%)	2,738 (1%)									
May	204,411	39,598	29,400 (88%)	26,543 (68%)	64,840 (58%)	42,525 (22%)	1,505 (1%)								
June	211,918	16,589	11,760 (94%)	34,711 (85%)	41,832 (78%)	54,675 (49%)	44,528 (23%)	7,823 (1%)							
July	209,806	2,147	7,840 (98%)	6,247 (88%)	25,099 (90%)	62,775 (80%)	60,720 (53%)	41,072 (25%)	3,906 (2%)						
August	207,510	3,910	2,208 (99%)	6,003 (91%)	18,824 (99%)	18,225 (89%)	58,696 (82%)	50,850 (51%)	44,924 (25%)	3,870 (2%)					
September	190,752	1,922	– (99%)	10,209 (96%)	– (99%)	12,150 (95%)	18,216 (91%)	46,939 (75%)	54,690 (53%)	42,570 (24%)	4,056 (2%)				
October	211,218	—	$1,712 (100%)	4,084 (98%)	2,092 (99%)	8,100 (99%)	16,192 (99%)	23,470 (87%)	48,830 (78%)	58,050 (54%)	44,616 (24%)	4,072 (2%)			
November	192,398	817	– (100%)	2,228 (99%)	– (100%)	– (99%)	– (99%)	13,691 (94%)	19,532 (88%)	48,375 (79%)	58,812 (53%)	44,788 (24%)	4,155 (2%)		
December	212,490	—	—	1,856 (100%)	—	1,312 (100%)	2,543 (100%)	9,779 (99%)	17,579 (97%)	17,828 (88%)	52,728 (79%)	59,038 (53%)	45,709 (24%)	4,118 (2%)	
1991 January	202,151	—*	—	– (100%)	—	– (100%)	– (100%)	1,956 (100%)	2,154 (98%)	17,002 (97%)	20,280 (89%)	50,895 (78%)	60,253 (53%)	45,302 (24%)	4,309 (2%)
Total Claims Paid to Date			$196,000	$204,180	$209,160	$202,500	$202,400	$195,580	$191,615	$187,695	$180,492	$158,793	$110,117	$49,420	$4,309

*Vertical columns demonstrate the run-off for a given month's incurred expenses, with the percent of the month's total shown under each month of payment.

†Viewing the table diagonally, the consistency of the percent paid in the month of incurral becomes evident. Consistency is also evident across other time periods (e.g., one month following incurral, etc.).

FIGURE 11-4   Lag table example: Claims received and paid.

accurately portray the organization's financial position. On the balance sheet, this activity is reflected as the "accrual claims liability." As claims are paid in future months, the organization reconciles estimated claims liability with actual paid claims. This process serves to accurately reflect claims liability over time on the financial statements.

FINANCIAL CONTROL AND EVALUATION

For HMOs in the early stages of development—from the feasibility analysis through the break-even point—many of the usual techniques of financial analysis will not adequately reflect the solvency and financial success of the plan. Concern at this stage is whether there will be sufficient assets to carry the plan through to the break-even point. Thus, the critical analysis depends on whether the sources of assets (capital, long-term debt, trade credit, gifts, and grants) are large enough to support the operation until revenues are generated from operations and then, combined with operating revenues, whether they are large enough to meet cash requirements until break-even. After break-even, the normal techniques of analysis can be used; that is, do revenues cover the expense of operation with adequate surplus or profit?

Major indicators of performance during the critical period before break-even are the ratios that follow. These ratios compare performance to preestablished normative values to determine whether the plans have developed financial programs that allow them sufficient working capital and financial strength to operate.

1. *Budget to sources of funds* (flow-of-funds analysis): If the budget is less than or equal to the sources of funds, then the plan should be adequately funded for the prebreak-even period. A ratio of 1:1 or less (i.e., 0.8:1) would indicate that the plan was satisfactory in this regard.

2. *Distribution of Expenses:*[10] A general rule-of-thumb regarding the distribution of expenses is: 35–45 percent to provide physician (medical compensation) services; 25–35 percent to provide hospital inpatient services; 12–15 percent to provide administrative services; and 10–15 percent for other medical and hospital expenses. Additional funds may be used for reserves that are required by insurance regulations, retained earnings, or dividends; these funds may be from 0–25 percent of the premium. Generally, a young plan will experience higher administrative costs than a large, mature plan—so administrative costs of 15–18 percent of premiums may be acceptable

---

[10] U.S. Department of Health and Human Services, Health Care Financing Administration, Office of Health Maintenance Organizations. *Statistical Data for Type A and B Federally Qualified HMO Population of the United States of America.* Rockville, Md., DHHS, 1985.

if enrollment is low (e.g., 2,000 to 10,000 enrollees). With enrollment over 50,000, the administrative costs should be approximately 12–14 percent of premiums. As of September 30, 1986, the Federal Government reported the following expenses for emerging Type A qualified HMOs: medical compensation averaged 40.8 percent of total expenses (down from 42.2 percent for the first quarter of 1986), hospital inpatient expenses were 29.5 percent of total expenses, other medical and hospital expenses averaged 15.3 percent of total expenses, and administrative expenses were 14.4 percent of total expenses.[11]

3. *Actual Income per Member per Month:*[12] In the first three quarters of 1986, Type A health plans averaged approximately $68.50 of income per member per month. This was up from approximately $66.00 in 1985, or an increase of approximately 4 percent per year.

4. *Actual Expenses per Member per Month:*[13] This indicator averaged $63.00 for 1985 for Type A plans, but during the first three quarters of 1986, actual expenses per member per month averaged $70.86 per member per month. A comparison with the actual income per member per month in 3 above shows a $2.36 deficit. As noted in 6 below, plans must cover their expenses to survive.

5. *Premium Income as a Percentage of Total Income:*[14] This indicator averaged around 95 percent for Type A plans before 1986, but the percentage dropped to 87.9 percent in the 3rd quarter of that year. Newly operating plans should experience a 90 percent level, while mature, well-established plans should have greater sources of nonpremium revenue; approximately 80 percent of the older plans' revenue should be from premiums.

6. *Actual Total Income as a Percentage of Actual Total Expenses:*[15] This indicator dropped during the period 1982–1985, from a high of 106 percent to approximately 95 percent for newly operational Type A plans and 103.5 percent for well-established HMOs. It should be at least 100 percent (the break-even point) or the plan will go broke—at least over the long run.

7. *Health Care Expense Ratio; Health Care Expense/Total Health Care Revenue:* Another way of viewing operations is to reverse the ratio provided

---

[11] Type A plans are federally qualified HMOs that *have not* achieved a net operating profit for three consecutive quarters nor a positive net worth, while Type B plans *have* achieved financial stability by meeting these criteria. As of April 1987, there were 281 Type A and 184 Type B plans, for a total of 465 federally qualified HMOs.

[12] U.S. Department of Health and Human Services, Health Care Financing Administration, Office of Health Maintenance Organizations, *Statistical Data for Type A and B Federally Qualified HMO Population of the United States of America.*

[13] Ibid.

[14] Ibid.

[15] Ibid.

in 6 above. This new ratio measures the portion of the total health care revenue that is paid out in the form of health care expenses. It provides a good measure of how well management is able to control health care costs; increases in the ratio imply that costs are not being controlled or premium increases are not keeping pace with medical cost increases. Obviously, the value of this ratio should not exceed 100 percent and, more logically, should be around 80 to 90 percent.

8. *Net Worth; Net Worth Plus Subordinated Liabilities Equal Intangible Assets:*[16] This test determines the amount of tangible net worth, including subordinated liabilities. The more extensive the net worth the greater the capacity to absorb any short-term negative operating results or variances; therefore, solvency is more enhanced. For 30 plans reviewed, the net worth ranged from − $1,000,000 to $4,000,000.

9. *Operating Margin; (Premium-Benefits)/Premiums:*[17] All models of HMO's have experienced an average 11.8 percent operating margin. Group models are at approximately 6.1 percent, staff models at 14.3 percent, IPA models at 12.8 percent, and network models at 9.0 percent.

10. *Return on Sales; After-tax Net Income/Premium Revenues:*[18] All plans average approximately 2.1 percent, with group models right at the average (2.1 percent), staff models at 4.5 percent, IPA models at 2.7 percent, and network models at 1.7 percent.

11. *Return on Equity; After-tax Net Income/(Reserves/Equity):*[19] The average of all plans is 29.5 percent, with group HMOs at 31.7 percent, staff HMOs at 29.5 percent, IPA HMOs at 21.4 percent, and network HMOs at 22.9 percent.

12. *Return on Total Assets; After-tax Net Income/Total Assets:*[20] All plans average 7.6 percent, with group HMOs at 6.9 percent, staff HMOs at 7.1 percent; IPA HMOs at 13.1 percent, and network HMOs at 7.5 percent.

13. *Average Collection Period (in days); Accounts Receivable/Average Daily Sales or Premiums/365:*[21] All plans average 17.9 days, with group models averaging 17.0 days, staff models averaging 16.1 days, IPA models averaging 14.8 days, and network models averaging 22.8 days.

---

[16] Illinois Department of Insurance, Solvency Surveillance Subcommittee, December 1986.

[17] U.S. Department of Health and Human Services, Health Care Financing Administration, Office of Health Maintenance Organizations. *The 1983 Investor's Guide to Health Maintenance Organizations.* Rockville, Md., DHHS, June 1983, p. 30. DHHS Publication No. (PHS) 83-50202. Note that these figures represent the median for 40 HMOs.

[18] Ibid.

[19] Ibid.

[20] Ibid.

[21] Ibid.

14. *Current Ratio (times) Current Assets/Current Liabilities:*[22] The current ratio measures short-term solvency by indicating the extent to which claims of short-term creditors are covered by assets that are expected to be converted to cash in a period roughly corresponding to the maturity of the claims. Decreases in this ratio indicate that short-term liquidity has worsened and oftentimes are an accumulation of short-term debt. For all models, it is 1.0, except for group HMOs and networks, which are at 1.1. This ratio provides an indicator of the HMO's status as a good credit risk; most users of this ratio believe that total current assets should be approximately 1.5 times as large as total current liabilities.

15. *Debt/Equity Ratio (times) Total Debt/(Reserves/Equity):*[23] This ratio measures the percentage of assets that are owed to creditors. The lower the ratio the more solvent the HMO is and the greater the cushion against creditors' losses. All models average 2.9, with group models averaging 2.7, staff models averaging 2.4, IPA models averaging 4.3, and network models averaging 4.8.

16. *Debt Service Coverage (times) (After-Tax Net Income Plus Interest Expense Plus Depreciation)/Debt Service Requirement:*[24] The average for all models is 3.0, with staff models at 3.0, group models at 3.1, IPA models at 3.6, and network models at 1.9.

17. *Profit Margin; Net Income/Total Revenue:*[25] This ratio indicates the percentage of each dollar that is ultimately realized as net income. Increases in this ratio usually indicate improved performance (more sales, more efficiency), and decreases indicate weaknesses (increased sales not producing increased net revenues, cost controls not functioning, etc). For 30 plans reviewed in December 1986 (1985 data), this ratio ranged from a −5.9 to 0.36. Seventeen plans with positive ratios had a median of 0.053, while the 13 plans with a negative ratio had a median of −1.16.

18. *Incurred but Not Reported Expenses:*[26] IBNR estimates are of vital interest; they represent an appraisal of the health plan's potential liabilities resulting from the delivery of health services that have not been reported to the health plan because hospitals and specialists frequently take lengthy periods of time to submit their bills for services for reimbursement. For a medical group under a capitation contract with an HMO, for example, IBNR expenses are generally created by referral physicians and other providers who will be

---

[22] Ibid.

[23] Ibid.

[24] Ibid.

[25] Illinois Department of Insurance, Solvency Surveillance Subcommittee.

[26] U.S. Department of Health and Human Services, Health Care Financing Administration, Office of Prepaid Health Care. Personal communication, October 15, 1986.

paid on a fee-for-service-basis but have yet to request payment for services from the capitation. From an accounting perspective, IBNR estimates provide a method for adjusting from a cash to an accrual (capitation) basis. One method to estimate IBNR is to use lag time studies, as reviewed earlier in this chapter.

19. *Cash Management:* Generally, a plan should maintain cash or other liquid assets that can be tranferred into cash in amounts equal to approximately two month's operating expenses. The health plan may find, through experience, that it will need less than the two months; some plans have been able to operate with success on a minimum of two weeks. HMOs plan their cash needs through the development of cash flow statements.

20. *Claims to Loss Ratio (Claims/Loss):* This ratio is a measure used by insurance companies to compare their actual paid claims as opposed to the premiums they have collected. Although HMOs are not insurance companies, this ratio can be applied to their operations and must have values of less than 0.85; that is, claims must be lower than total premiums collected plus administrative costs (assuming 15 percent of premiums for management).

Summary

Financial management is the administrator's method of bringing together all the components of the health plan. The tools used in financial management include budgeting and the development of pro forma financial statements; underwriting, including actuarial analysis and rate making; cash flow analysis; and ratio analysis. These allow the manager to control as well as evaluate the HMO's activities. Initial activities in the development of a good financial model are described as the financial planning process. Components of this process, which were described in Chapters 9 and 10 on HMO development and marketing, are tied together in this discussion.

Based on the goals and objectives established for the HMO, several financial planning assumptions must be developed for control of risk. These include decisions concerning staffing ratios; assumptions about the level, type, and sharing of risk; projected utilization rates; and assumptions concerning the local levels of morbidity, mortality, and disability. Estimates of the population's need and demand for medical services and additional insurance programs can be created by using ambulatory facility-focused, physician-focused, and visit-focused approaches. Underwriting rules must be developed to manage risk and govern selection concerning type of group, size of group, industry, composition of the group, location of risk, plan of insurance, cost sharing, and previous coverage and experience of the group.

Financial planning models traditionally used by HMOs include the budgetary approach and the insurance underwriting model, although the theoretical units-of-production model may also be a valuable method for considering resource allocation. In the budgetary approach, costs are developed for major expense areas based on ratios and cost assumptions. Revenues are then projected, and pro forma financial statements and a funds flow analysis are prepared. A second model, the comprehensive insurance underwriting model, is built around the insurance functions of risk taking, actuarial analysis, incentive/risk-sharing formulas, and rate making. In this model, the manager segments the populations chosen and completes estimates of penetration. After data concerning the population are collected, underwriters are asked to analyze the population to determine the risk of providing services. Once risks are calculated that, in effect, describe the types and levels of services that will be required by the enrolled population, financial analyses can be completed in the form of budgets and pro forma financial statements.

A third approach that combines some elements of the other two is the comprehensive units-of-production model, developed for the National Center for Health Services Research and Development, DHHS. This mainly theoretical model fully integrates the marketing aspects of population segmentation and penetration to develop a statement of demand; again, ratios of encounter-to-population are used to complete this first step. Plan capacity (staff, equipment, facilities, supplies) is then matched to the demand statement using consumption rates by resource. The final step is the application of a cost-per-unit of resource and a revenue-per-encounter to project a budget and a cash flow analysis. The model provides a highly sophisticated approach to demand, capacity, and financial estimation, but it also requires substantial data on which to make these estimates. Because of possible limitations in data, and the excessive time and specialized ability of managers to use this model, its usefulness may be clearly limited, although excellent results can be achieved through its use.

In general, each model develops estimates of costs that include medical services, hospitalization, and administration. These costs are compared with revenue that will be generated from several sources—premiums, fees for service, copayments, sales of drugs and supplies, government payments, loans, grants, and so on. Cash flow analysis can then be completed to determine whether the program will be financially feasible. Adjustments are normally required to bring costs and revenues into alignment. The results of these financial planning efforts are usually described as costs per member per month, and the per capita revenue is the capitation rate. The capitation or base rate is then converted to premium rates in the underwriting process by loading or discounting adjustments.

One of the major functions required in the financial planning process is risk management. Underwriting is the activity by which health plans evaluate and determine the risks of accepting populations as group members. In addition to following the underwriting rules mentioned earlier, managers control risks by designing appropriate benefits packages, using actuarial analyses and suitable rate-making methods as part of the underwriting process, sharing risks through the use of capitation payments and withholds with providers, and other management techniques. In comparison to group underwriting, the enrollment of individuals follows more restrictive requirements than for groups because of the greater chance for adverse selection and billing difficulties.

Several mechanisms, in addition to placing restrictions on accepting certain high-risk groups, may be used to control risks. These include reinsurance and limitations on certain coverage, such as catastrophic illnesses, epidemics, or disasters. Good marketing analysis and underwriting (i.e., good management) may be the most important methods for handling risks.

Benefits packages are built around a basic set and other optional benefits. Generally, the programs offered to group members are tailored to the needs of the group. Exclusions, limitations, and copayments may be included in the policy to limit or control risk and to prevent inappropriate use of services. Through the use of copayments, it is hoped that revenues from this source will help maintain low premium levels and control, to a certain extent, unnecessary utilization of physician services. Three basic models are followed in designing benefits packages—standard plus supplementary sets of benefits, a totally custom-made package, and a standard (no option) plan to all subscribers.

Pricing of the benefits packages (the premium) is traditionally the responsibility of an actuary, although many health maintenance organizations place this responsibility with the chief financial manager or the plan administrator. Rates for services to be included in the benefits package are established so that the revenue from premiums will adequately cover total costs and allow for a surplus. Rates also must be equitable, simple to understand and implement, flexible and adaptable, and consistent among groups. In this regard, three rate-making systems can be used—community, manual, and experience rating. Each system has its advantages and its drawbacks. In using any of the systems, however, certain adjustments may be applied to the intermediate (capitation) rate, with the ultimate effect of adjusting the premium rate to reflect the risk level of the subscriber group.

A review of the premium rate development as part of the traditional budgetary approach continues the discussion of the financial planning model; in this approach, the costs and revenue at the break-even enrollment level are estimated, based on fee-for-service experiences and assumptions concerning utilization of services. The total costs are then divided by the total enrollment level, then divided by 12 to reflect a monthly capitation. Loading of the capitation rate to reflect various differences in groups produces the premium. A second method, the insurance underwriting or actuarial approach, is used by many HMOs and is consistently used by commercial insurance companies. This method is built on the development of a manual of premium rates—charges for each benefit unit. Adjustments are then made, based on the experience of the group being underwritten.

The development of capitation rates for affiliated medical groups and hospitals is also a part of the financial planning process. From the HMO's perspective, group practice capitation rates are based on the estimated medical expenses generated by the financial planning model, while the hospital capitation rate proposed by the HMO may be based on the hospital's all-inclusive daily rate, or a weighted average of the expected per diem by major service for the hospital. If more than one hospital is used, then the weighted average cost for each hospital is combined to produce an average rate across all of the participating hospitals. Because negotiation plays a major role in the development of capitation contracts, both sides will propose rates they feel are appropriate for the situation. For example, the medical group may use its fee-for-service data to estimate the expenses of providing services to HMO members; this rate may be substantially different than the actuarially created rate the HMO proposes. An accommodation is attained in successful contracting.

A part of the overall financial management of the health plan is the administrator's use of pro forma operating statements, cash flow analyses, budgets, accounting-ratio analyses, and claims liability management, especially incurred but not reported claims using lag table analyses. All these financial tools help the administrator guide the plan to success.

References

Health Insurance Association of America. *Principles of Group Health Insurance I.* Chicago, Ill., HIAA, 1972.

Herbert, Michael E. *A Financial Guide for HMO Planners.* Minneapolis, Minn., InterStudy, 1974.

"IBNR: Crucial Guesswork." *GHAA News,* 28(11/12):11, 13–14, November/December 1987.

Kongstvedt, Peter R. *The Managed Health Care Handbook.* Gaithersburg, Md., Aspen Publishers, Inc., 1989, pp. 205–229.

Neal, Patricia A. *Management Information Systems, Going Prepaid Series.* Denver, Colo., Center for Research in Ambulatory Health Care Administration, 1986.

Sutton, Harry L., Jr., and Allen J. Sorbo. *Actuarial Issues in the Fee-for-Service/Prepaid Medical Group.* Denver, Colo., Center for Research in Ambulatory Health Care Administration, 1983.

U.S. Department of Health and Human Services, Health Care Financing Administration. *Claims Liability Management in Health Maintenance Organizations. Office of Health Maintenance Organizations.* Rockville, Md., DHHS, April 1981, DHHS Publication No. (PHS) 81-50165

U.S. Department of Health, Education, and Welfare, Health Services and Mental Health

Administration, Health Maintenance Organization Service. *Financial Planning Manual*. Rockville, Md., DHEW, 1972. DHEW Publication No. (HSM) 73-13007

Wrightson, Charles William, Jr. *HMO Rate Setting and Financial Strategy*. Ann Arbor, Mich., Health Administration Press Perspectives, 1990.

TABLE 11-3   Example of a Proposed Benefits Package

Benefits	Capitation	Enrollee Pays
A. Physician Services		
Office visits for preventive care, diagnosis, and treatment, including specialists' care, family planning, services for infertility, and well-baby care	Physicians	No charge
Elective examinations (not to exceed one exam per enrollee per year) in accordance with accepted medical practice; such examinations include medical history, physical exam, blood pressure testing, and necessary lab, X-ray, and diagnostic tests as indicated by the age, sex, history, and physical condition of the enrollee	Physicians	No charge
In hospital services, including daily care, surgery, and medically necessary consultations as authorized by an HMO physician	Physicians	No charge

Sterilization procedures as follows:
    Vasectomy
    Tubal Ligation
	Physicians	No charge

Although general dental services are not provided, limited oral surgical procedures will be provided in an outpatient or inpatient setting in connection with injury to the jaw bone or surrounding tissue, acute accidental trauma to sound natural teeth, gum and bone tumors and cysts, and medical conditions, provided such a condition occurred on or after the effective date of coverage, including congenital anomalies in newborn children associated with the need for oral surgery	Physicians	No charge
Anesthesia for in- and outpatients	Physicians	No charge
B. Outpatient Testing/Procedures		
Diagnostic tests and procedures: Lab tests, including but not limited to cytology examinations and venereal disease tests; X-rays; nuclear medicine procedures, including radioisotopes, sonograms, pulmonary function studies, cardiovascular studies, CT scans, EEG, EKG, and other diagnostic studies (PC and TC)	Physicians	No charge

TABLE 11-3 *(Continued)*

Nuclear medicine procedures, including radioisotopes used for the treatment of cancer, radiotherapy (PC and TC), etc.	Physicians	No charge
Annual hearing and eye exams for all eligible enrollees	Physicians	No charge
Allergy treatment and materials	Physicians	No charge or copay
Injection medication (other than in connection with allergy treatments)	Physicians	No charge or copay
Pediatric and adult immunizations in accordance with accepted medical practice	Physicians	No charge or copay
Family planning and counseling services and infertility services (limited to specifically prescribed procedures by the HMO physician)	Physicians	No charge
Appropriate outpatient supplies	Physicians	No charge
Services that can be provided through ambulatory care, including radiotherapy, dialysis, chemotherapy, outpatient surgery, and short-term rehabilitative therapy, as ordered by an HMO or authorized referral physician	Physicians	No charge
Prescribed short-term (up to 6 weeks per episode) physical therapy, inhalation therapy, and short-term speech and occupational therapy rehabilitation services on either an outpatient or inpatient basis, as determined by an HMO physician, for medical conditions as authorized; cardiac rehabilitation will be paid for up to 12 weeks	Physicians for OP Hospital for IP	No charge Nocharge

C. Hospital inpatient Services

Room (semiprivate accommodations and board; private room when medically necessary), meals, and special diets when medically necessary; use of the OR and related facilities; general nursing, special duty nurse when prescribed as medically necessary; and use of intensive care unit and services when prescribed	Hospital	No charge

TABLE 11-3 *(Continued)*

Drugs, medications, and biologicals; dressings and casts, anesthesia, and oxygen services	Hospital	No charge
Diagnostic tests and procedures: Laboratory tests, X-rays, nuclear medicine procedures, including radioisotopes, sonograms, pulmonary function studies; cardiovascular studies, CT scans, EEG, EKG, and other diagnostic studies	Physicians for PC Hospital for TC	No charge No charge
Nuclear medicine procedures including radioisotopes used for the treatment of cancer; radiotherapy	Physicians for PC Hospital for TC	No charge No charge
Chronic and acute hemodialysis and other out-of-area hospital services	Physicians for PC Hospital for TC	No charge No charge
Short-term rehabilitation when medically necessary, including inhalation therapy	Physicians for PC Hospital for TC	No charge No charge
Discharge planning and medical-social service counseling	Hospital for TC	No charge
D. Pharmacy		
Outpatient prescription drugs and medications	Physicians	Copay per prescription
E. Extended Care		
Physician services:	Physicians	No charge
100-day skilled nursing facility level of care per enrollee per calendar year when prescribed by an HHP or authorized referral physician, including semiprivate room, general nursing care, meals and special diets, all ancillary services that are available to hospital inpatients, and care and treatment by an HMO or authorized referral physician	Skilled nursing facility	No charge
F. Home Health Care		
Physician services as medically necessary: HHP physician prescribes part-time intermittent nursing services of registered nurses, public health nurses, a licensed vocational nurse, or home health aides; and service of medical social workers	Physicians	No charge

TABLE 11-3 *(Continued)*

G. Maternity Care

Maternity services will be provided for all female enrollees when such services are provided by or arranged through an HMO or authorized referral physician and include:

Complete physician care for prenatal care, delivery, and postnatal care	Physicians	No charge
Related anesthesia services	Physicians	No charge
Laboratory exams and X-ray	Physicians for OP	No charge
Inpatient hospital services	Physicians for PC	No charge
Hospital for TC	No charge	
Care and treatment of complications	Physicians for PC	No charge
Hospital for TC	No charge	
Medically necessary consultations	Physicians	No charge

H. IP and OP Mental Health

Diagnostic evaluation and individual and group therapy on an outpatient basis as may be necessary and appropriate for short-term evaluation or crisis intervention mental health services up to 30 outpatient visits per enrollee	Physicians	$30 charge per individual session (maximum of 15 individual visits per year) $10 per group per calendar year
Up to 30 days per enrollee each calendar year for inpatient services for the treatment of nervous and mental conditions, alcoholism, and drug addiction, including professional services and as authorized by an HMO physician	Physicians for PC mental health facility for TC	No charge No charge

I. Emergency Care

Emergency care obtained from hospitals or emergency rooms by care plan providers within HMO service area for life-threatening emergencies or illness requiring immediate medical treatment; if treatment is not received under the direction of an HMO physician then plan must be notified within 72 hours	Physicians	No charge

TABLE 11-3   *(Continued)*

Out-of-area emergency care is covered in full provided a life-threatening condition exists; the plan must be notified within 72 hours that such treatment has occurred	Physicians	No charge
J. Urgent Care		
Urgent medical care is defined as any unexpected injury or illness that is not life threatening but requires prompt medical attention; if a condition requiring urgent care develops while in the service area, treatment should be obtained at the HMO facility; HMO physicians are on call 24 hours each day	Physicians	No charge
Should a condition requiring urgent care develop outside the HMO service area, the enrollee should proceed to the nearest interplan hospital, and HMO must be notified within 72 hours; the treatment must be a covered service and is subject to approval by HMO	Physicians	No charge
K. Ambulance Service		
Ambulance services are provided when there is a life-threatening illness or accident; if not ordered by an HMO physician or an authorized referred physician, the plan must be notified within 72 hours	Physicians	No charge
L. Health Education		
Health education services for specific conditions, such as diabetic counseling, post-coronary counseling, and nutritional counseling	Physicians	No charge
Education in appropriate use of HMO and information regarding personal health behavior and care	Physicians	No charge
M. Alcoholism and Drug Abuse		
Medically necessary diagnostic and medical treatment for alcoholism and abuse of drugs, including detoxification for alcoholism or drug abuse on either an outpatient	Physicians for OP Physicians for IP, PC Others for IP, TC	No charge No charge No charge

TABLE 11-3 *(Continued)*

or inpatient basis, is covered when ordered
or approved by an HMO physician; see
mental health benefits section for details

N. NonCovered Services

1. Abortions
2. The cost of blood, blood plasma, or blood products such as Rh factor, immuno-globulins, and Rh immune globulins (may be covered)
3. Contraceptive devices, including IUDs and diaphragms
4. Cosmetic surgery and/or treatment, except reconstructive surgery to correct a congenital disease or anomaly that has resulted in a functional defect, or when performed to correct a condition resulting from accidental injury or incidental surgery if such accident or surgery occurred on or after the effective date of the member's coverage; removal of moles will be a coverable service
5. Custodial, domicillary, and convalescent care
6. Dental services, except for emergency dental services that are required to treat injuries caused by an accident that occurred while covered under this certificate (the initial visit only); examples of noncovered exclusions are treatment and surgical repair of temporal mandibular joint dysfunction or impacted wisdom teeth, facial pain syndromes that are the result of malocclusions and dental conditions
7. Durable medical equipment such as crutches, wheelchairs, and hospital beds
8. Emergency procedures, including experimental transplants and implants
9. Eyeglasses, contact lenses or the fitting of contact lenses, hearing aids or the fitting of hearing aids, and dentures
10. Homemaker services
11. All medical services terminate upon termination of coverage under the certificate, including hospitalization and skilled nursing facility services
12. Nutritional food supplements and parental nutritional products (nonprescription)
13. Orthopedic devices such as knee braces and clavicle collars (better definition needed)
14. Personal convenience items, such as telephone and television, that are billed by a hospital or skilled nursing facility
15. Physical examinations and/or hospitalizations that are required by public or private agencies, and the completion of administrative requirements
16. Prescriptions not written by an HMO or authorized referral physician, or received at other than at the HMO or contract pharmacy
17. Psychiatric conditions such as chronic, organic, or not subject to significant improvement through short-term treatment
18. Replacement of external prosthetic devices
19. Reversal of voluntary, surgically induced sterility
20. Any services or supplies for which coverage is available through federal, state, or local government agencies, worker's compensation, or Social Security (excluding Medicaid)
21. Services that are not medically necessary, as defined in the benefits package
22. Services that are not provided and/or authorized by HMO physicians
23. Service-connected disabilities covered by the VA, if provided in a VA facility
24. Services or supplies received prior to the effective date of coverage or after the cancellation date of coverage
25. Counseling services (needs to be clarified)

TABLE 11-3 *(Continued)*

26. Rehabilitative therapy, except as otherwise defined
27. Nonsurface transportation
28. In vitro fertilization
29. Artificial insemination, homologous or donor
30. Any services or prescriptions and/or therapy issued while a member but filled or used after loss of coverage or disenrollment (the member will be responsible for the standard charge)

GLOSSARY

AAPCC (adjusted average per capita cost): Medicare's managed care payment system. Payment is set at 95 percent of the amount estimated by the Health Care Financing Administration that similar care would have cost in a fee-for-service setting.

AAPPO (American Association of Preferred Provider Organizations): A trade group located in Chicago, Illinois.

Access: An individual's ability to obtain medical services on a timely and financially acceptable basis. Ease of access is determined by such other factors as location of health care facilities, transportation, and hours of operation.

Actuarial Study: The calculation of risks and premiums and other statistical studies used in insurance underwriting.

Administrative Loading (or **Retention,** as in insurance): The amount added to the prospective actuarial cost of the health care services (pure premium) for expenses of administration, marketing, and profit.

Adverse Selection: Some population parameter, such as age (e.g., a larger number of persons age 65 or older in proportion to younger persons), that increases the potential for higher utilization than budgeted and increases costs above those covered by the capitation rate.

Algorithm: *See* **Protocol.**

Alternative Delivery System (ADS): A method of providing health care benefits that departs from traditional indemnity methods. An HMO, for example, can be said to be an alternative delivery system.

Ambulatory Care/Services: (*See also* **Outpatient Care**) Care given a person who does not stay overnight in a medical care facility or hospital.

AMCRA (American Managed Care and Review Association): A Washington, D.C. trade group of preferred provider organizations.

ASO (administration services only): Services provided by third-party administrators (TPAs) or insurers to self-insured employers.

Assignment (also **Authorization to Pay Benefits**): A statement, usually included on a claim form, that permits the insured to authorize the insurance company or health plan to pay benefits directly to the provider of the services.

505

Attrition Rate: Disenrollment expressed as a percentage of total membership. An HMO with 50,000 members experiencing a two-percent monthly attrition rate would need to gain 1,000 members per month to retain its 50,000-member level.

Authorization to Pay Benefits: *See* **Assignment.**

Bargaining Representative: A representative designated for collective bargaining under the National Labor Relations Act.

Basic Health Services: The health care services required of qualified HMOs, including but not limited to hospitalization, physicians' services, X-ray and laboratory services, and preventive health services.

Beneficiary (*also* **Participant**): (*See also* **Eligible Individual; Enrollee; Member**) Any person, either a subscriber or a dependent, eligible for service under a health plan contract.

Benefits: Specific areas of plan coverage or services provided, such as outpatient visits and hospitalization, that make up the range of medical services marketed by an HMO to its subscribers.

Benefits Package: Specific services provided or assured by the HMO to enrollees.

Blue Cross: A hospital insurance plan that provides benefits covering specified hospital-related services and pays member hospitals directly for services rendered.

Blue Laws: Medical and hospital service corporation laws that were originally enacted to regulate Blue Cross and Blue Shield plans. Under certain conditions, they may be used to describe the corporate form for an HMO or, in some states, may provide a mandatory form of incorporation. They generally were considered to limit the flexibility of the managed care organization structure; in most states, blue laws have been amended or modified to allow HMOs to operate.

Blue Shield: A medical service insurance plan that provides benefits covering specific physician-related services and pays either the patient or physician.

Break-even Point: The HMO membership level at which total revenues and total costs are equal, producing neither a net gain nor loss from operations.

Capitation/Capitation Fee/Capitation Payment (*also* **per Capita**): The amount of money required per person by a health care vendor (or health insurance organization) to provide (insure) covered services to a person for a specific time (usually per month).

Carrier: An insurer; an underwriter of risk. A voluntary association, corporation, partnership, or other nongovernmental organization that is engaged in providing, paying for, or reimbursing all or part of the cost of health services under group insurance policies or contracts, medical or hospital services agreements, membership or subscription contracts, or similar group arrangements, in consideration of premiums or other periodic charges payable to the carrier.

Case Unit Cost: An average cost for the treatment of illness, usually derived by completing an actuarial study and utilizing underwriting rules.

Cash Indemnity Benefits: Amounts paid to the insured after he/she has received and filed a claim for a service. Such benefits may be received directly or may be assigned to the provider of service (e.g., the doctor) by the insured.

Certificate Holder: *See* **Subscriber.**

Clinic (*also* **Health Center**): A facility for the provision of preventive, diagnostic, and treatment services to ambulatory patients, where patient care is under the professional supervision of persons licensed to practice medicine.

Closed-panel HMO: Viewed from the consumer's perspective, a closed-panel HMO limits the number of physicians from whom a member of a plan may obtain health care services. In general, this definition applies to prepaid group practice plans/group model HMOs.

Closed-panel Practice (*also* **Open-panel Practice**): The group practice of medicine where admission to the medical group is controlled by the group membership. Medical group practices are closed-panel practices whereas IPAs, which are open to all members of the medical society, are open-panel practices.

Coinsurance: A policy provision under which the insured pays or shares part of the medical bill, usually according to a fixed percentage. Major medical expense policies usually provide for coinsurance and deductibles.

Collective Bargaining Agreement: An agreement between an employer and the bargaining representative of its employees.

Community-rated Premium: (*See also* **Experience-rated Premium**) The practice by some health plans whereby net rates or premiums for plan subscribers are reasonably uniform and not dependent on individual claim experience or the experience of any one group.

Community Rating: The rating system by which a plan or an indemnity carrier takes the total experience of the subscribers or members within a given geographic area or "community" and uses these data to determine a capitation rate that is common for all groups regardless of the individual claims experience of any one group.

Communitywide Plans: Plans in which the membership is open to qualified groups or individuals in the community, rather than limited to members of specified unions or employees of specific industries.

Competitive Medical Plan (CMP): Any organization that meets specific eligibility criteria for Medicare risk contracting but is not necessarily an HMO. CMPs must be "at-risk" and provide physicians' services primarily through employees of the organization or through contracts with individual physicians or groups of physicians. The CMP enters into an agreement with HCFA to provide specific services to Medicare beneficiaries for a predetermined and prepaid capitation sum based on HCFA's adjusted average per capita cost (AAPCC) for the counties served by the CMP.

Completion Method: A method of determining outstanding claims liability, whereby the claims already paid are divided by a factor indicating the percentage of estimated claims paid to date.

Composite Rate: A uniform premium applicable to all eligibles in a subscriber group regardless of the number of claimed dependents. This rate is commonplace among labor unions and large employer groups and usually does not require any contribution by the union member or employee.

Composite Rating: A method of developing a rate structure in which the capitation rates for single and single/spouse member units include some of the medical care costs developed for a family unit. Composite rating also makes possible the development of rates for families of more than four people.

Compositing: A term used for combining a multiple-tiered rate structure into a tier structure with fewer tiers; for example, combining a rating system using two-person contracts and three-or-more-person contracts into a premium structure that includes all families of two or more persons.

Comprehensive Benefits: Included under one policy, in addition to the basic benefits, some or all of the following services outside the hospital: diagnostic services, preventive services, treatment in doctor's office or patient's home, and so on. Sometimes used synonymously with "Major Medical Expense Benefits."

Comprehensive Care: Provision of a broad spectrum of health services, including physician services and hospitalization, that are required to prevent, diagnose, and treat physical and mental illnesses to maintain health.

Contract Group: (*See also* **Enrolled Group**) A specific group of persons who are to be provided a particular program of benefits (e.g., a union local, an employer group of employees and dependents, federal employees).

Contract Type: Classification of employees into categories, usually based on enrolled dependent status. Typical would be a single employee, an employee with one dependent, or an employee with two or more dependents.

Contributory: A term used to describe a group insurance plan under which the insured (subscriber) shares in the cost of the plan with the policyholder.

Conversion Factor: An arithmetic number that is multiplied by the HMO capitation rate to produce a rate for single employees.

Conversion Privilege: The provision that allows a member enrolled through a group to convert, regardless of age or physical condition, to a direct-pay program at the time of retirement or other separation from the group.

Coordination of Benefits (COB): A typical insurance provision whereby responsibility for primary payment for medical services is allocated between carriers when a person is covered by more than one employer-sponsored health benefits program. This coordination avoids the possibility that a person will be reimbursed twice for the same medical services.

Copayment: A payment by the insured of a fee per day or per service specified within a contractual agreement and in addition to an insurance premium.

Cost Centers: Functional areas that generate the basic costs incurred in providing the plan's range of benefits.

Coverage: In general, the services or benefits that are provided, arranged, or paid for through a health insurance plan (a package of specified benefits); or the people eligible for care under such a plan.

Customary, Prevailing, and Reasonable Charges (CPR): The traditional basis of fee-for-service rates.

Deductibles: Amounts required to be paid by the insured under a health insurance contract before benefits become payable (similar to waiting periods of cash sickness insurance). Intended as a deterrent to overuse. In some health plans, deductibles are the difference between the cost for services and fixed benefits by the carrier.

Dependents: Generally the spouse and children, as defined in a contract, of a person or subscriber covered by a health plan. Under some contracts, coverage may include parents and others.

Direct Payment Subscribers (*also* **Individual Coverage**): Persons enrolled in a health plan who make individual premium payments directly to the plan rather than through a group. Rates of payment are generally higher, and benefits may not be as extensive as for a subscriber enrolled and paying as a member of a group.

Direct Service Benefits: *See* **Service Benefits**.

Direct Service Plan: *See* **Group Health Plan**.

Dual Choice (*also* **Multiple Choice**): An option offered to individuals in a group; the choice between two or more health plans (several different arrangements for prepaying medical care). In most situations, employees might be offered the option of enrolling in an indemnity insurance plan, a Blue Cross/Blue Shield program, and a health maintenance organization.

Economies of Scale: Occur when the cost of producing a good or service decreases as the number of goods or services produced increases.

Efficiency: A technical term indicating that the combination of inputs used to produce a good or service provides the maximum feasible outputs. When inefficiency exists, the output produced from a given set of inputs is below the maximum obtainable.

Eligible Individual (*also* **Participant**): (*See also* **Beneficiary; Enrollee; Member**) An employee who meets the terms and conditions established by an employer, or its designee, to participate in an existing health benefits plan.

Emergency Care Benefits: Benefits for care received from nonplan doctors and nonplan facilities in the event of accident or emergency illness, whether in or out of the plan's service area.

Enrolled Group: (*See also* **Contract Group**) A group of persons with the same employer, or with membership in common in an organization, who are enrolled in a health plan. Usually there are stipulations regarding the minimum size of the group and the minimum percentage of the group who must enroll before the coverage is available.

Enrollee (*also* **Participant**): (*See also* **Beneficiary; Eligible Individual; Member**) Any person eligible for services, either as a subscriber or a dependent, in accordance with a contract.

Enrollment: The process by which an individual becomes a subscriber for him/herself and/or his/her dependents for coverage in a health plan. This may be done either through an actual signing up of the individual or by virtue of his/her collective bargaining agreement on the employer's conditions of employment. The result, therefore, is that the health plan is aware of its entire population of beneficiary eligibles. As a usual practice, it is incumbent on the individual to notify the health plan of any changes in family status that affect the enrollment of dependents.

Enrollment Period: A period of at least 10 calendar days each year during which each eligible employee will be given the opportunity to select from among the alternative health benefits plans.

Exclusive Provider Organization (EPO): A managed care plan that requires members to use a PPO-like provider network exclusively. Care outside the network is the responsibility of the EPO member.

Expense Ratio: Ratio of HMO total expenses to earned premiums.

Experience-rated Premium: (*See also* **Community-rated Premium**) A premium that is based on the anticipated claims experience of, or utilization of services by, a contract group according to its age, sex constitution, and any other attributes expected to affect its health services utilization, and that is subject to periodic adjustment in line with actual claims or utilization experience.

Experience Rating: A rating system by which a plan determines the capitation rate by the experience of the individual group enrolled. Each group will have a different capitation rate based on utilization. This system tends to increase the premiums required of small groups with high utilization.

Federal Employees Health Benefits Program (FEHBP): Also referred to as **Federal**

Employees Plan or **FEP**. The health plans made available to federal employees as part of their employment benefits.

Fee for Service: With respect to the physician or other supplier of service, this refers to the payment of specific amounts for specific services rendered on a service unit basis—as opposed to retainer, salary, or other contract arrangements. In relation to the patient, it refers to the payment of specific amounts for specific services received on a service unit basis, as opposed to the advance payment of an insurance premium or membership fee for coverage under a plan that provides the services or payment to the supplier.

Fee Schedule: A listing of accepted fees or established allowances for specified medical procedures. As used in health plans, it usually represents the maximum amounts the program will pay for the specified procedures.

Fixed Costs: Costs that do not change or vary with fluctuations in enrollment or in utilization of services.

Foundation/Foundation for Medical Care: (*See also* **Individual Practice Association; Prepaid Individual Practice**) An association of physicians that organizes and develops a management and fiscal structure and sets a fee schedule for individual physicians who join the foundation. Foundations usually market the plan to subscribers, provide peer review, arrange claims payments, and set rates for subscribers.

Geographic Capitation: A proposed system of prospective capitation payments by the Health Care Financing Administration, DHHS, to a major health insuring and services organization, usually by region or county, which, in turn, would contract on a risk basis with other providers (physicians, hospitals, skilled nursing facilities, etc.) for the delivery of services.

Group Health Association of America, Inc. (GHAA): A Washington, D.C. trade group for health maintenance organizations.

Group Health Plan (*also* **Direct Service Plan; Health Plan; Plan; Prepaid Health Plan**): (*See also* **Group Practice Prepayment Plan**) A plan that provides health services to persons covered by a prepayment program through a group of physicians usually working in a group clinic or health center.

Group Model HMO: An HMO in which a medical group practice contracts with an HMO to provide health services.

Group Practice (*also* **Medical Group Practice**): (*See also* **Medical Group; Solo Practice**) The definition that was adopted by the American Medical Association and most commonly used is "Group medical practice is the application of medical services by a number of physicians working in systematic association with the joint use of equipment and technical personnel and with centralized administration and financial organization."

Group Practice Prepayment Plan: (*See also* **Group Health Plan**) A group model HMO.

HBO: *See* **Health Benefit Organization.**

HCFA: *See* **Health Care Financing Administration.**

Health and Welfare Fund: *See* **Welfare Fund.**

Health Benefit Organization (HBO): HBOs are Health Care Financing Administration-contracted entities that are required to provide a package of benefits that essentially matches Medicare's benefits without exceeding current program cost-sharing levels. Under the Private Health Plan Option, these are the organizations that might be contracting with HCFA; under the voucher proposals, beneficiaries could present vouchers worth 95 percent of the adjusted average beneficiary costs in an area to the HBO in return for services.

Health Benefits Contract: A legally enforceable agreement between an employer, or its designee, and a carrier to provide or make payment for health benefits or services to eligible employees.

Health Benefits Plan: Any plan that provides or makes payments for basic and supplemental health services and is offered to eligible employees and/or their dependents by or on behalf of an employer.

Health Care Financing Administration (HCFA): A part of the U.S. Department of Health and Human Services. In addition to its many other functions, HCFA is the contracting agency for HMOs that seek direct contract/provider status for provision of the Medicare benefits package.

Health Center: *See* Clinic.

Health Insurance Association of America (HIAA): A Washington D.C. trade group for health insurers.

Health Insuring Organization (HIO): Usually an organization that contracts with a state or federal agency to assure the delivery of services to beneficiaries of a state or federal program such as Medicaid or Medicare. The HIO will contract with health services organizations, either on a discounted fee-for-service or a capitated basis, for the provision of hospital and physician services.

Health Maintenance Organization (HMO): A term specifically defined in the Health Maintenance Organization Act of 1970 (P.L. 93-222) and its amendments, an HMO is any legal organization, either for-profit or nonprofit, that accepts responsibility for the provision and delivery of a predetermined set of comprehensive health maintenance and treatment services to a voluntarily enrolled group in a geographic area for a prenegotiated and fixed periodic capitation (prepaid) payment.

Health Maintenance Organization Service (HMOS) of the U.S. Department of Health, Education and Welfare (DHEW): This service was also titled the Office of Health Maintenance Organizations (OHMO); its functions are now under the Office of Prepaid Health Care in the Health Care Financing Administration, U.S. Department of Health and Human Services. These are the federal DHHS agencies responsible for managed care activities.

Health Plan: *See* Group Health Plan.

Health Services Organization (HSO): Usually a regional medical center, hospital, or medical group practice that delivers medical services. A generic term that describes organizations that deliver medical or mental health services.

HIAA: *See* Health Insurance Association of America.

HMO: *See* Health Maintenance Organization.

HMOS: *See* Health Maintenance Organization Service.

Hospital Affiliation: Hospitals with which the plan contracts to provide the hospital benefits of the plan.

Hybrid HMO: Known as "second generation" managed care systems, these organizations are extremely sophisticated in their organizational structures and product offerings. They tend to blur the differences among individual practice association model HMOs, PPOs, and managed care fee-for-service indemnity health plans; thus, hybrid HMOs offer "open option" or "open ended" products that modify the total "lock-in" of the traditional HMO enrollee to allow enrollees to use nonsystem providers but require a copayment, deductible, and the like. These offerings are also known as "triple" or "multiple" option products. The objective of such products is to allow the hybrid HMO to more effectively compete with PPOs and traditional insurance programs.

IHCC: *See* **Medical Staff/Hospital Venture Organization.**

Incentives: As related to health services delivery, this term refers to economic incentives for hospitals by means of third-party reimbursement formulas to motivate efficiency in management; or economic incentives for physicians who encourage decreased hospital utilization, promote judicious use of all resources, and increase delivery of preventive health services.

Indemnify: To compensate for damages, loss sustained, or expense incurred; to recompense for hardship.

Indemnity: Protection or security against damages or loss. Benefits are in the form of cash payments rather than medical services.

Indemnity Carrier: Usually an insurance company or insurance group that provides marketing, management, and claims payment review and agrees to assume risk for its subscribers at some predetermined level.

Indemnity Health Insurance: *See* **Indemnity Plan.**

Indemnity Plan (*also* **Indemnity Health Insurance**): (*See also* **Service Plan**) A plan that reimburses physicians for services performed or beneficiaries for health services expenses incurred. Such plans are contrasted with group health plans, HMOs, and PPOs, which provide service benefits through group medical practice and/or IPA.

Individual Coverage: *See* **Direct Payment Subscribers.**

Inpatient Care: Care given a registered bed patient in a hospital, nursing home, or other medical or psychiatric institution.

Individual (or Independent) Practice Association (IPA): (*See also* **Foundation/Foundation for Medical Care; Prepaid Individual Practice**) A legal entity established by individual physicians who own stock in the organization. The IPA acts as an economic bargaining unit for the member physicians. It is a medical management organization engaged in arranging for the coordinated delivery of all or part of health care services to members enrolled in an HMO. The IPA enters into a service arrangement with physicians who are generally practicing on an individual basis rather than a group or salaried basis.

Integrated Health Care Corporation (IHCC) *see* **Medical Staff/Hospital Venture Organization.**

IPA: *See* **Individual Practice Association.**

Lag Factor: A general term indicating a percentage of claims incurred in a given accounting period but received, processed, and paid in specified months following the close of the accounting period.

Loading: (*See also* **Risk Load**) Used, in conjunction with discounting, to adjust rates for individuals and groups. Loading is an integral part of experience rating but is not used in community rating. A factor multiplied into the rate to offset some adverse parameter in the group to which the HMO is delivering care, the risk load provides more money in reserves to offset expected deficits.

Loss Ratio: The ratio of HMO actual incurred expenses to total premiums; the relationship between money paid out for services and the amount collected in premiums.

Managed Care Organization (MCO): A generic term that describes organizations that manage and control medical service. It includes HMOs, PPOs, CMPs, managed indemnity insurance programs, and managed BC/BS programs.

Managed Health Care Association: An informal group of 77 major employers with an interest in managed care benefits, located in Morristown, N.J.

Manual Rates: A commercial insurer's standard rate tables that are included in its rate manual or underwriter's manual and used to develop premium rates.

Market Share/Market Penetration: That portion of the local health service population served by the health plan, usually a percentage of the total potential or targeted members.

MCO: *See* **Managed Care Organization.**

Medical Group (*also* **Medical Group Practice**): A group of physicians organized to provide medical services to members of a group health plan under a specified contract. A medical group in prepaid health plans includes a broad range of medical specialties having the capability to meet most needs in providing medical diagnosis and treatment, including primary and specialty care (with the ability to purchase services beyond its capabilities on a fee-for-service basis). The group operates under common employment, or with common financial interest, under a capitation arrangement or some system for payment other than fee for service; has available group offices and facilities, equipment, and the services of paramedical personnel and nonmedical assistance; and has responsibility for the care of a defined group of enrolled members.

Medical Group Practice: *See* **Group Practice; Medical Group.**

Medically Insured Group (MIG): A program that is part of the Federal Government's effort to offer multiple options to Medicare eligible retirees under its PHPO concept.

Medical Staff/Hospital Venture Organization (MES/H or IHCC) (*also* **Integrated Health Care Corporation**): An organization developed by the medical staff and hospital that establishes a structure to provide various health care delivery services such as utilization review, reimbursement analysis, hospital and medical group management services, and the like. The MES/H may become a PPO with insurance carriers, unions, employers, HMOs, and others.

Member (*also* **Participant**): (*See also* **Beneficiary; Eligible Individual; Enrollee; Subscriber**) An individual enrolled for health services or benefits under a contract with a health plan.

MES/H: *See* **Medical Staff/Hospital Venture Organization.**

MIG: *See* **Medically Insured Group.**

Multiple Choice: *See* **Dual Choice.**

National Committee for Quality Assurance (NCQA): A Washington, D.C. group that develops HMO accreditation standards.

National Physician PPO: Panels of participating physicians, established by county Medicare carriers, who provide services to Medicare recipients and receive higher fee updates than nonparticipating physicians, but who are subject to strict utilization review.

Network: An arrangement of several delivery points (i.e., medical group practices) affiliated with a managed care organization; an arrangement of HMOs (either autonomous and separate legal entities, or subsidiaries of a larger corporation) using one common insuring mechanism such as Blue Cross/Blue Shield; a broker organization (health plan) that arranges with physician groups, carriers, payer agencies, consumer groups, and others for services to be provided to enrollees.

Net Working Capital: *See* **Working Capital.**

Network Model HMO: An HMO contracts with two or more independent group practices and/or other delivery sites to provide health services.

Noncontributory Arrangement: An arrangement under which the employer, union, or other third party pays the full premium.

Nonprofit or **Not-for-profit Plan:** A term applied to a prepaid health plan under which no part of the net earnings accrues, or may lawfully accrue, to the benefit of any private shareholder or individual. An organization that has received 501-C-3 or 501-C-4 designation by the Internal Revenue Service.

Office Visit: A formal face-to-face contact between the physician and the patient in a health center, office, or hospital outpatient department.

Open Enrollment: A period during which members in a dual/multiple choice health benefits program have the opportunity to select the alternative health plan being offered them. Most frequently, open enrollment periods are negotiated and held for one month every one or two years.

Open-panel Practice: *See* **Closed-panel Practice.**

Out-of-area Benefits: Those benefits that the plan supplies to its members when they are outside the geographical limits or service area of the HMO. These benefits usually include emergency care benefits and stipulate that within-the-area services for emergency care will be provided until the member can be returned to the plan area for medical management of the case.

Outpatient Care: (*See also* **Ambulatory Care/Services**) Services provided at an HSO to a person who is not bedridden and does not require overnight hospitalization.

Participant: *See* **Beneficiary; Eligible Individual; Enrollee; Member.**

Peer Review Organization (PRO): Designated by HCFA to monitor physicians who provide care to Medicare recipients.

Penetration: The percentage of business that a managed care plan is able to capture in a particular member group or in the market area as a whole. For example, signing 10 enrollees out of 100 eligible members yields a 10-percent penetration.

Per Capita: *See* **Capitation/Capitation Fee/Capitation Payment.**

PHPO: *See* **Private Health Plan Option.**

Physician Services: Services involving a face-to-face contact with a physician.

Plan: *See* **Group Health Plan.**

Plan Administration: The management unit having responsibility to manage and control the health plan—includes accounting, billing, personnel, marketing, legal services, purchasing, possible underwriting, management information, facilities maintenance, and servicing of accounts. This group normally contracts for medical services and hospital care.

Plan Sponsorship: The group that organizes the plan, finances its facilities, and/or makes up its governing board.

Policyholder: Under a group purchase plan, the policyholder is the employer, labor union, or trustee to whom a group contract is issued and in whose name a policy is written. In a plan contracting directly with the individual or family, the policyholder is the individual to whom the contract is issued.

PPA: *See* **Preferred Provider Organization.**

PPO: *See* **Preferred Provider Organization.**

Preexisting Condition: A physical condition of a member that existed prior to the issuance of his/her policy or enrollment in a plan, which may or may not limit the contract on coverage or benefits.

Preferred Provider Organization (PPO and PPA): A limited grouping (panel) of providers (doctors and/or hospitals) who agree to provide health care to subscribers for a negotiated, usually discounted, fee and who agree to utilization review. The arrangement, created among the providers and others (employers, unions, commercial insurers, HMOs, etc.), is called the PPA or preferred provider arrangement.

Premium: A prospectively determined rate that a member pays for specific health services. Generally, a comprehensive prepaid health plan will have a premium rate established for single members and for families.

Prepaid Group Practice: Prepaid group practice plans involve multispecialty associations of physicians and other health professionals who contract to provide a wide range of preventive, diagnostic, and treatment services on a continuing basis for enrolled participants.

Prepaid Health Plan: *See* **Group Health Plan.**

Prepaid Individual Practice: (*See also* **Foundation/Foundation for Medical Care; Individual Practice Association**) Plans that use the services of individual solo physicians in their private offices. Most of these plans are included under the category of IPA model HMOs.

Prepayment: A method of providing, in advance, for the cost of predetermined benefits for a population group through regular periodic payments in the form of premiums, dues, or contributions, including those contributions that are made to a health and welfare fund by employers on behalf of their employees and payments to HMOs and CMPs made by federal agencies for Medicare eligibles.

Primary Care: Professional and related services administered by an internist, family practitioner, obstetrician/gynecologist, or pediatrician in an ambulatory setting, with referral to specialists as necessary.

Private Health Plan Option (PHPO): An HCFA proposal to broaden the number of available alternatives to standard Medicare coverage by developing contracts between HCFA/SSA and HMOs, CMPs, employers, commercial insurers, unions, combinations of employers and their unions, or others responsible for the medical expenses of health care to groups of Medicare-eligible retirees. PHPO is the administration's euphemism for capitation and its effort to privatize Medicare.

PRO: *See* **Peer Review Organization.**

Protocol (*also* **Algorithm**): A decision tree that describes a course of treatment or established practice patterns.

Provider: A person or organization providing health services.

Quality Assurance: A formal set of activities to measure the quality of services provided; these may also include corrective measures.

RAPs: DRGs for radiologists, anesthesiologists, and pathologists used by HCFA to reimburse these specialists for care to Medicare recipients.

Rate Structure: A classification of dependency options and related premiums applicable to a given member group. Most groups use one of the following rate structures in their health benefits programs: (1) a composite rate or one-tier rate, (2) a two-tier rate, (3) a three-tier rate, or (4) a four-tier rate.

RBRVS: *See* **Resource Based Relative Value Scale.**

Reciprocity: The right of a member of a health plan, temporarily away from home, to receive necessary medical care from a health plan in the area where he/she is a visitor.

Reinsurance: The dividing of risk through transfer of a portion of the risk of one carrier insurance company or other third party to another organization, company, or group. Reinsurance also may be used by carriers to lessen the risks of catastrophic losses to health insurance plans.

Relative Value System (Studies) (RVSs): (*See also* **Resource Based Relative Value Scale**) A method of valuing medical services, especially physician services. Based on the California relative value studies of the 1960s through the 1980s, the Federal Government will change to an RBRVS physician payment system in early 1992, an RVS payment system for physician services to Medicare recipients.

Reserves: A fiscal method of withholding a certain percentage of premiums to provide a fund for committed but undelivered health care and such uncertainties as higher hospital utilization levels than expected, overutilization of referrals, accidental catastrophies, and the like.

Resource Based Relative Value Scale (RBRVS): (*See also* **Relative Value System**) On January 1, 1992, Medicare payments will be based on a resource-based relative value scale, replacing the customary and prevailing charge mechanism for fee-for-service providers participating in the Medicare program. The objective is that physician fees should reflect the relative value of work performed, their practice expense, and malpractice insurance costs.

Risk: Any chance of loss, or the possibility that revenues of the health plan will not be sufficient to cover expenditures incurred in the delivery of contractual services.

Risk Control Insurance: *See* **Stop Loss.**

Risk Load: (*See also* **Loading**) A factor that is multiplied into the rate to offset some adverse parameter in the group.

Risk-sharing: A provision of most HMOs where at least part of the provider's income is directly linked to the financial performance of the plan. If the plan's costs exceed its budget, the providers are responsible for covering at least part of the deficit.

RVSs: *See* **Relative Value System (Studies).**

Self-administered Plan: A plan administered by the employer or welfare fund without recourse to an intermedicate insurance carrier. Some benefits may be insured or subcontracted while others are self-insured.

Self-insured: An employer-managed and -controlled health plan that offers a benefits package to its employees and dependents and pays providers for services from funds set aside for such purposes. Some employers may contract with PPOs for services and may use third-party administrators (TPAs) or administrative services only (ASOs) organizations for day-to-day operation of the plan.

Service Area: The geographic area covered by the plan within which it provides direct service benefits.

Service Benefits (*also* **Direct Service Benefits**): Benefits provided by the plan itself.

Service Charges: Any extra charges specified in the contract for certain services not fully covered through the premium.

Service Plan: (*See also* **Indemnity Plan**) A plan that provides benefits in the form of medical care and services for a stated premium.

Skilled Nursing Facility (SNF): A nursing or convalescent home offering skilled nursing care and rehabilitation services.

Solo Practice: (*See also* **Group Practice**) Individual practice of medicine by a physician who does not practice in a group or does not share personnel, facilities, or equipment with three or more physicians.

Staff-model HMO: Health services delivered through a physician group that is controlled by the HMO unit.

Stop Loss (*also* **Risk Control Insurance**; often incorrectly referred to as **Reinsurance**): Insuring with a third party against a risk that the plan cannot financially and totally manage. For example, a comprehensive prepaid health plan can self-insure hospitalization costs or it can insure hospitalization costs with one or more insurance carriers.

Straight Rating: A single rate multiplied by the total number of people in a family to give the family rate.

Subrogation: Seeking, by legal or administrative means, reimbursement from others responsible for certain categories of medical expenses such as worker's compensation, third-party negligence liability, or no-fault auto medical coverage.

Subscriber (*also* **Certificate Holder**): (*See also* **Member**) The person in whose name an individual or family certificate is issued. Other family members are "dependents." Note that the subscriber can, but need not, be the policyholder.

Third-party Administrator (TPA): Manages claims payment without assuming insurance risk.

Third-party Payment: The payment for health care when the beneficiary is not making payment, in whole or in part, on his/her own behalf.

Token Payment: A partial payment or copayment made for a service or supply item. For example, some comprehensive prepaid health plans charge $10 for each office visit. Sometimes also known as "nominal" or "hesitation" payments.

TPA: *See* **Third-party Administrator**.

Transferability: The right of a member of a group health plan who changes his/her place of residency to receive medical services in a group health plan in his/her new place of residency, with benefits and obligations as defined under prior agreement between the plans.

Underwriting: The process by which an insurer determines whether or not and on what basis it will accept an application for insurance.

Union-sponsored Plan: A program of health benefits developed by a union. The union may operate the program directly or may contract for benefits. Funds to finance the benefits are usually paid from a welfare fund that receives its income from employer contributions, employer and union member contributions, or union members alone.

Utilization: The extent to which a given group uses specific services in a specified period of time. Usually expressed as the number of services used per year per 100 or per 1,000 persons eligible for the services; utilization rates may be expressed in other types of ratios, that is, per eligible person covered.

Voluntarily Enrolled Group: An enrolled group of persons, each of whom has exercised an option to join the program.

Welfare Fund (*also* **Health and Welfare Fund**): A fund into which employer and/or employee contributions for health care are placed and that is administered by a board, usually with equal representation from labor and management. When the welfare fund provides health benefits, it either pays directly, purchases insurance, or provides service benefits.

Working Capital (*also* **Net Working Capital**): Refers to an institution's investment in short-term assets—cash, short-term securities, accounts receivable, and inventories. *Gross* working capital is defined as an institution's total current assets. *Net* working capital is defined as current assets minus current liabilities. If the term "working capital" is used without further qualification, it generally refers to net working capital.

INDEX